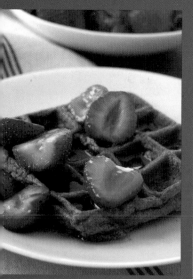
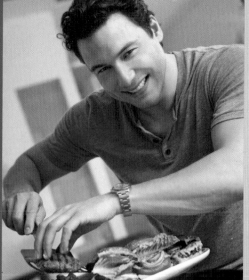
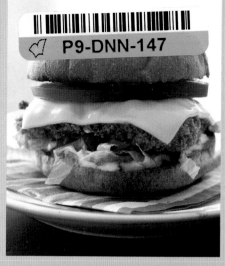

P9-DNN-147

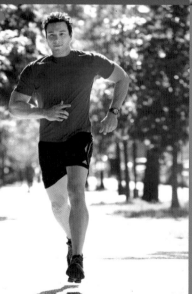
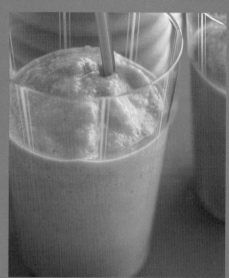
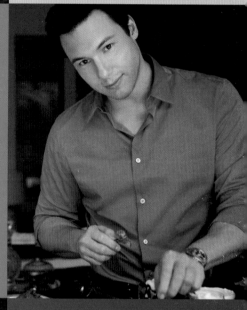

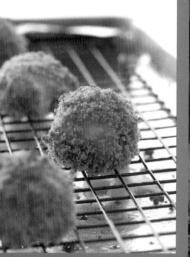
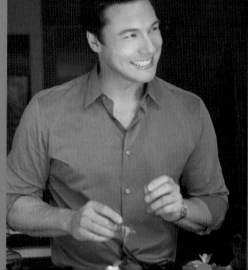
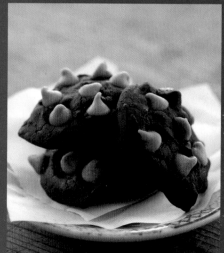

Also by
# Rocco DiSpirito

· · · · · · · · · · · · · · · · · · · · · · · · · · · · · · · · · · · · · · · · · · · · · · · · · · · · · · · · · · · · · · ·

**FLAVOR**

**ROCCO'S ITALIAN-AMERICAN**

**ROCCO'S 5 MINUTE FLAVOR:**
Fabulous Meals with 5 Ingredients in 5 Minutes

**ROCCO'S REAL LIFE RECIPES:**
Fast Flavor for Every Day

**ROCCO GETS REAL:**
Cook at Home, Every Day

**NOW EAT THIS!:**
150 of America's Favorite Comfort Foods,
All Under 350 Calories

# NOW EAT THIS! DIET

## ROCCO DISPIRITO

foreword by
Mehmet C. Oz, MD

GRAND CENTRAL
Life & Style

NEW YORK · BOSTON

Neither this diet nor any other diet program should be followed without first consulting a health care professional. If you have any special conditions requiring attention, you should consult with your health care professional regularly regarding possible modification of the program contained in this book.

Copyright © 2011 by Flavorworks, Inc.
All rights reserved. Except as permitted under the U.S. Copyright Act of 1976, no part of this publication may be reproduced, distributed, or transmitted in any form or by any means, or stored in a database or retrieval system, without the prior written permission of the publisher.

Food photography and photo on page 3 by Kritsada
All other photography by Jonathan Pushnik

Grand Central Life & Style
Hachette Book Group
237 Park Avenue
New York, NY 10017

www.HachetteBookGroup.com

Grand Central Life & Style is an imprint of Grand Central Publishing.

The Grand Central Life & Style name and logo are trademarks of Hachette Book Group, Inc.

The publisher is not responsible for websites (or their content) that are not owned by the publisher.

Book design by HSU+ASSOCIATES

Printed in the United States of America

First Edition: March 2011
10 9 8 7 6 5

Library of Congress Cataloging-in-Publication Data

DiSpirito, Rocco.
  Now eat this! diet / by Rocco DiSpirito. — 1st ed.
    p. cm.
  Includes index.
  ISBN 978-0-446-58449-4
  1. Reducing diets—Recipes.  I. Title.
  RM222.2.D5785 2011
  641.5'635—dc22
                                        2010048158

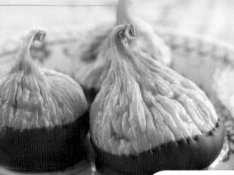

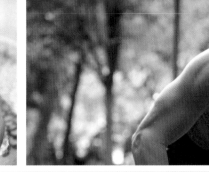

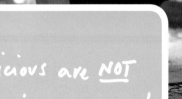

*Healthy & delicious are NOT mutually exclusive anymore!*

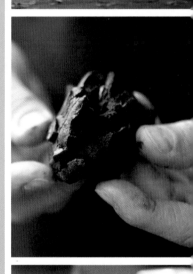

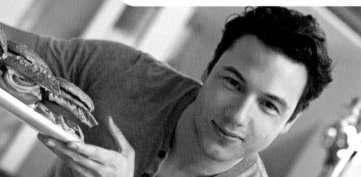

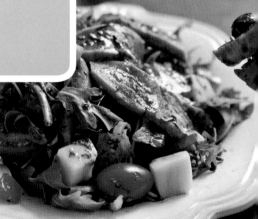

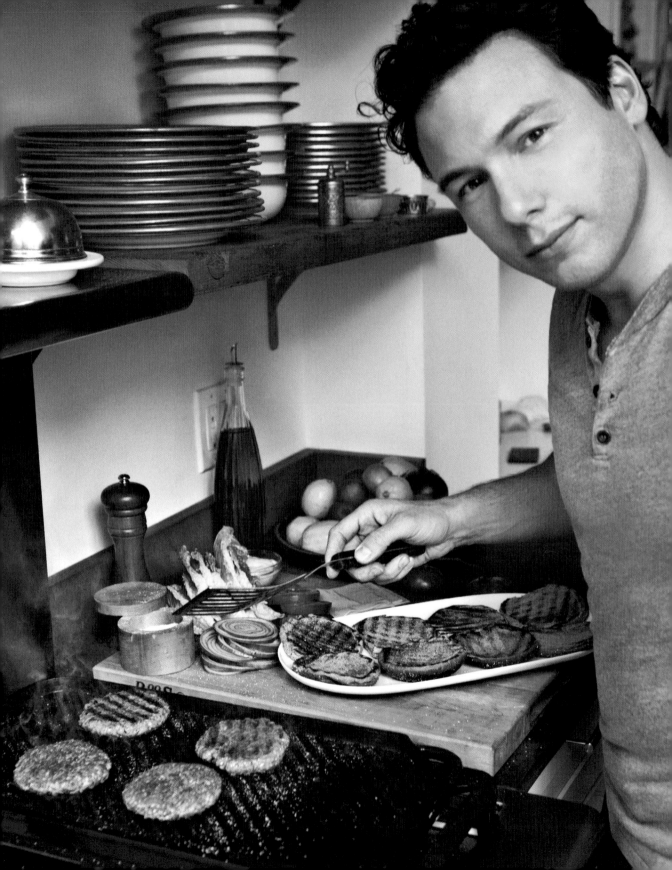

# Dedication

It nearly brings me to tears when I think about how we are given a life full of possibilities and with the choices we make we slowly and methodically strip them away. Most of us wake up every day and make a series of decisions and often don't even know what informs them. And for at least 67% of us, those choices can be devastating to our health, to the health of our families, and to our health care system.

The information I'm sharing on these pages will help you make better health and nutritional choices. It is information that has helped me achieve my best weight and get to the finish line of many grueling triathlons, lowered my cholesterol and my blood pressure, and generally made me a healthier, happier, and more productive person.

This book is dedicated to all of those who are committed to maximizing their lives and to passing on their passion for great health to others. I know you're in that group, or you wouldn't be holding this book in your hands. I know it's not easy to make changes, but even the smallest change is heroic, and I applaud your courage and determination. A healthy, balanced life, full of energy and possibilities, is yours for the taking.

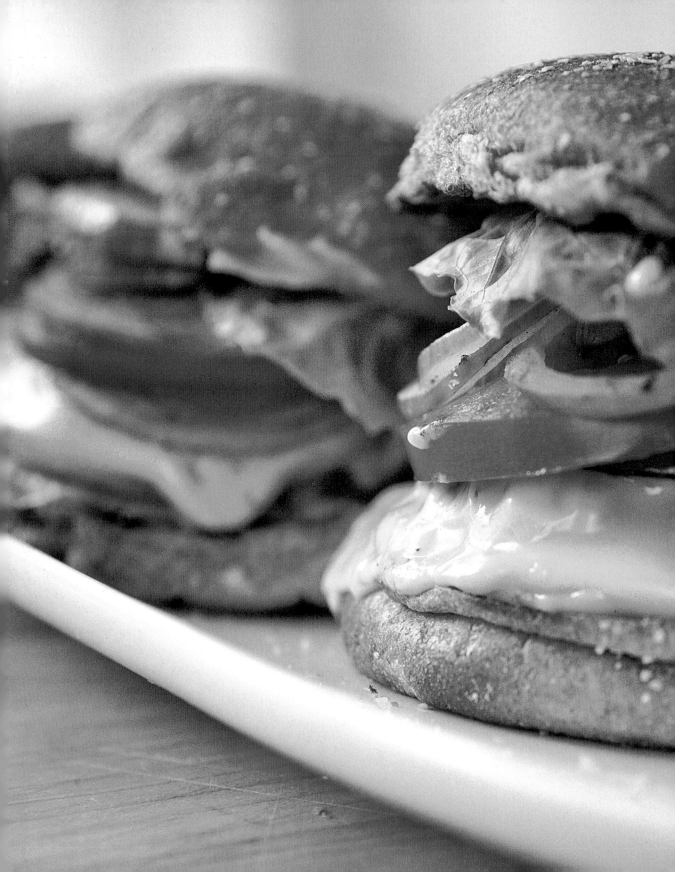

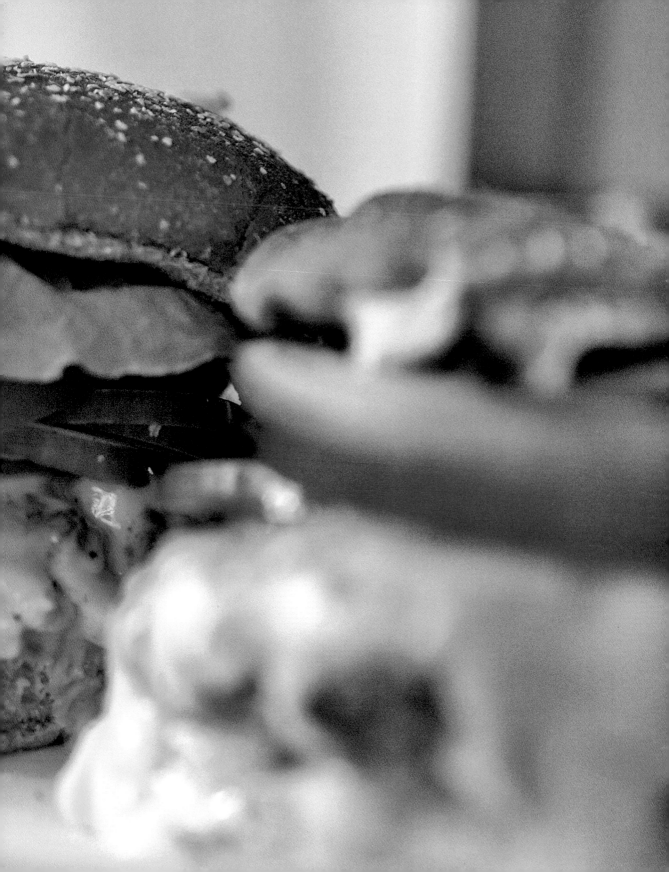

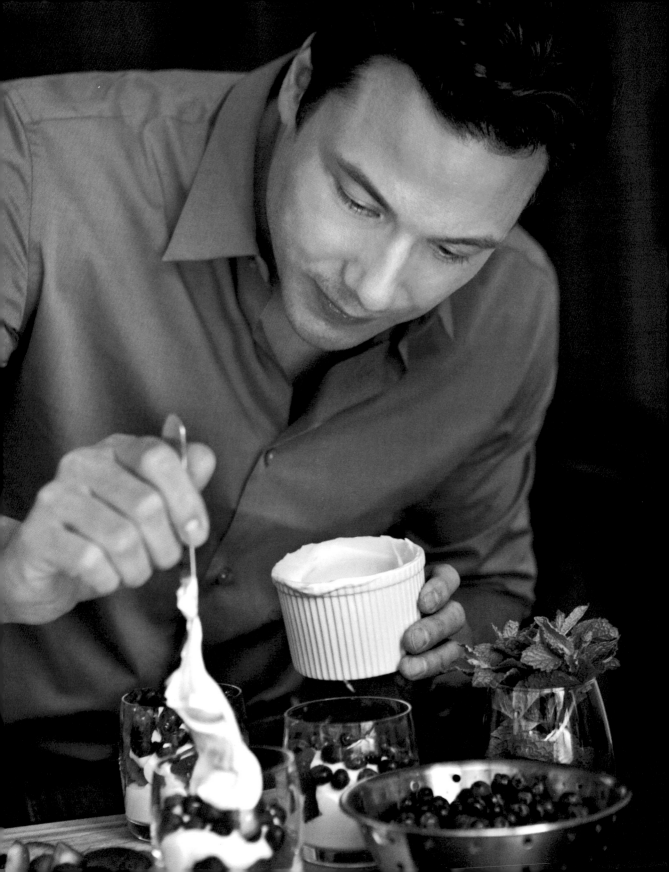

# Contents

· · · · · · · · · · · · · · · · · · · · · · · · · · · · · · · · · · · · · · · · · · · · · · · · · · · · · · · · · · · · · · · · · · · · ·

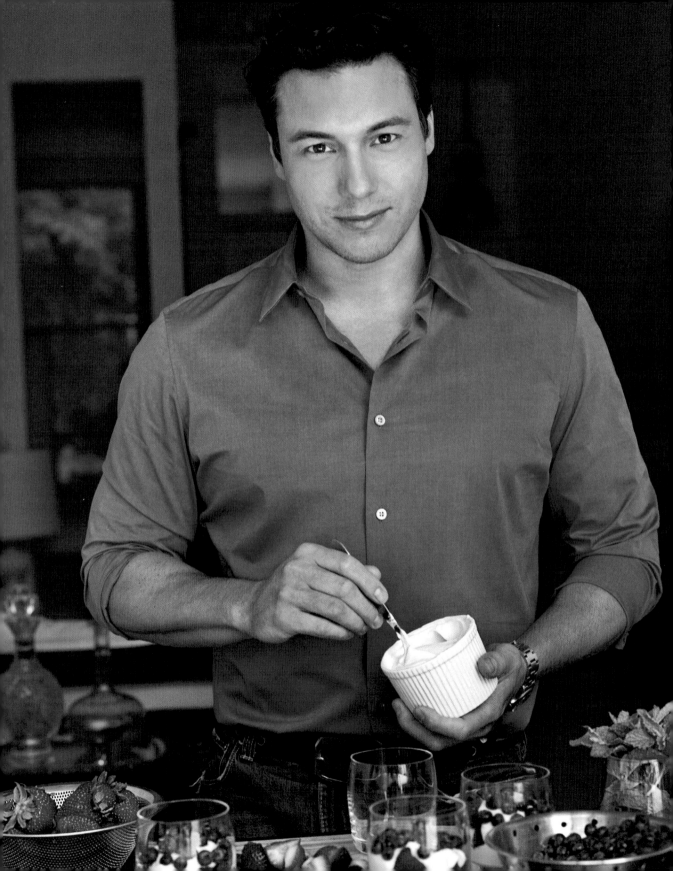

# Acknowledgments

· · · · · · · · · · · · · · · · · · · · · · · · · · · · · · · · · · · · · · · · · · · · · · · · · ·

With tremendous gratitude to all those whose contribution to this work merits more than a casual inclusion in a long list of names. You always take my calls, generously share your ideas, listen to mine, and work exceptionally hard to help make everything I do better than I imagined. You know who you are, and I really couldn't do it without you.

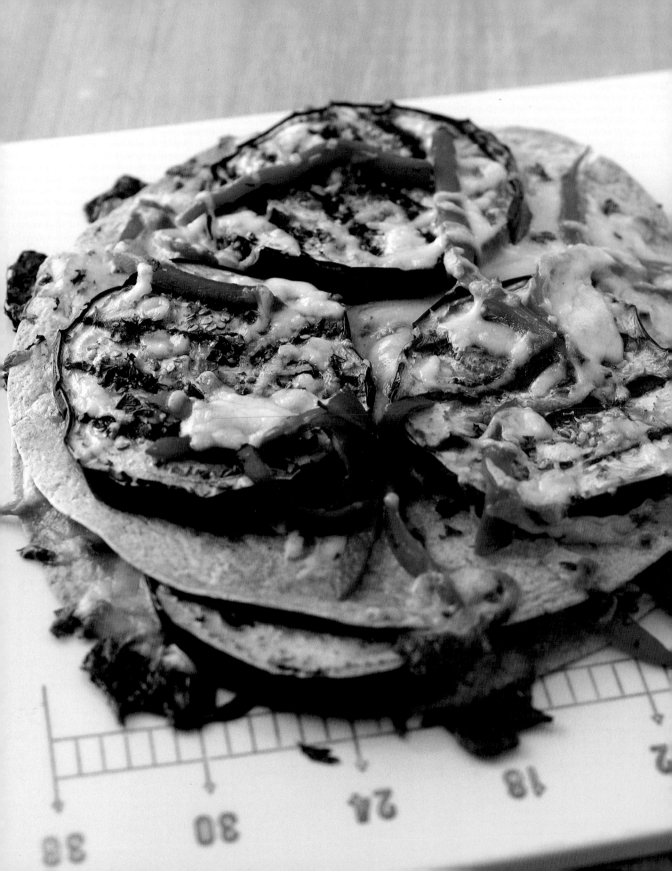

# Foreword
## Mehmet C. Oz, MD

Doctors enter and exit the lives of our patients, changing them, we hope for the better. Often the favor is returned and a patient or family comes along to change us for the better by what they teach us. I met Rocco the way most doctors meet people: Someone was sick and needed my help. It was November 2005, right after Thanksgiving. His charming mother, Nicolina, had suffered a massive heart attack on her way to a doctor's appointment. She practically died in Rocco's arms. She was rushed into surgery, and thankfully, her life was saved.

As is sometimes the case, Nicolina would ultimately need a pacemaker, a heart-valve replacement, and a stent to keep one of her arteries propped open. A friend of Rocco's suggested that he get in touch with me to perform these procedures. Of course I agreed. I sat down with Rocco and his mom and talked as best I could in plain, everyday language about what the surgery and recovery would entail.

Heart surgery, like all surgeries, is serious business. When you treat and care for people undergoing surgery, you get to know them and their families at an intensely personal level. You prepare them emotionally and physically for the operation and encourage them through the rougher parts of recovery. You become very close with the families as you study what is best for them. Through the experience, I discovered that Rocco and I had many shared interests—health, cooking, living a balanced life. Rocco had the same mission I had: to fundamentally change how we treat ourselves—mind, body, and soul. We became fast friends.

And then I discovered his amazing talent for cooking healthy food and asked Rocco to get involved with HealthCorps, a charity I founded. Its mission is to empower teens in underserved populations to make simple lifestyle changes to enhance their health and well-being and take the message to friends, families, and neighbors. Rocco prepared and donated dinners for HealthCorps events and gave talks on healthy cooking at several of my symposiums. I invited Rocco to be on my television show as a regular guest, and he's a hit whenever he appears to create some of his fabulous, healthy dishes.

If you don't know already, Rocco can take the most fattening, heart-unhealthy recipes and turn them into miraculous nutrient-packed, delectable, mouthwatering meals. He cuts the calories, the trans fats, the saturated fats, the simple carbs, the sugar—all the bad stuff—without cutting the flavor.

This kind of cooking is just what America needs right now, and Rocco delivers.

You can use this book every day of your life to take care of the most precious thing that you ever inherited: your body. When you take care of your body, your body will take care of you.

For losing weight, not much of what most of us have tried will work. Whether no-carb, low-carb, low-fat, no-fat, cabbage soup, or whatever else your diet ploy is, please know it will not work over the long term.

Repeat after me: will—not—work for the years of healthy living you crave.

Let that sink in. Take a moment. Mourn all that money you've spent on various diet books and shakes and memberships.

Rocco's book *Now Eat This! Diet* offers a strategy that *will* work because you get to eat healthy, delicious, natural foods—your favorite foods, in fact—in satisfying proportions that allow steady, progressive weight loss.

So forget the usual boring list of diet foods. Get ready to serve up fettuccine, cookies, crème brûlée, waffles—all the stuff you thought was bad for you.

Start eating the meals in this book, and you'll feel so much better, physically, mentally, emotionally—and for a lifetime. We doctors can medicate you to cover up the poor food choices you make, but that's just like painting over cracks in a foundation. We can put mechanical devices in, but those are poor imitations of what you were born with. Only you can change what you put in your mouth, and you are best able to achieve this goal if you crave the foods that are good for you. Let this book be your nudge to starting better nutritional habits.

By this time next week, I expect this beautiful book of yours to be covered with muffin crumbs, barbecue sauce drippings, spaghetti sauce, and other remnants of the great dishes you've prepared.

Oh, and by the way, do I use this book, as well as Rocco's other cookbooks? You bet I do. My whole family does. Our favorites: Pita Chips with Charred Eggplant Dip and Crunchy Tomato Bread, to name just a couple. Embrace this book, start cooking, reboot your taste buds, lose weight, and feel alive once more. Now, if you'll excuse me, I have some No-Boil Mushroom Lasagna in the oven . . .

# NOW EAT THIS! DIET

NOW
EAT
THIS!
DIET

# Introduction

I'm really sick and tired of hearing that losing weight means eating less, giving up sweets, and exercising your ass off. How much denial can we endure? All of this diet food and low-fat cooking is choking the life out of our psyches, our taste buds, and our bodies. How did we even get to this point?

For the most part, diet food is boring and painfully bland because the health and medical community has overemphasized the discipline of dieting and underemphasized the flavor of food. And, unfortunately, unlike chefs, most of these experts lack the skills to create delicious, filling, satisfying food that is also low in calories and fat. Making food taste good is what chefs do for a living. And the "experts" expect us to suck it up and eat platefuls of cottage cheese and grapefruit, even if we absolutely hate those foods! The fact that we as consumers have been so underserved in this regard annoys me, especially since obesity and obesity-related diseases are killing us.

So let's take a permanent sabbatical from boring diets, calorie-burning pills, infomercial fat-zapping products, and cabbage soup.

Let's try something different: a diet that feels good and tastes good. One that lets you eat all the delicious foods you love and doesn't require any inner struggle or self-denial. One that takes off ugly pounds as easily as you gained them and still lets you eat all your favorite foods.

Wouldn't you just love that?

Well, guess what—it's here, and you're holding it in your hands: the Now Eat This! Diet. It is an entirely new and different way to lose weight: one that will satisfy your hunger and your taste buds and help you get to your best possible weight. It fixes the number

one problem with diets today: food that's unappetizing and tastes bad. It's time for *healthy* and *culinary* to stop being mutually exclusive.

I guarantee you'll love this new way of dieting. How does French toast sound for breakfast? Or pizza for lunch? How about a juicy steak for dinner? I could go on and on with a long list of delicious foods you get to eat and still lose weight. The point is, you do not have to eat like a bird or subsist on tasteless crap to be healthy and lose weight.

I can sum it up like this: You know all that stuff you avoided on your last diet? Now you can eat it.

Yes, now you can eat those foods and more—all your favorite foods, all those wonderful comfort foods you love. Now you can eat them six times a day—and lose weight without sacrifice, struggle, or willpower.

The Now Eat This! Diet is happiness ever after, so start buying smaller sizes immediately. I can say this with confidence because you will now lose weight— up to 2 to 3 pounds a week, depending on how much weight you need to lose and how many calories you consume per day right now.

Week by week, you'll experience an awesome transformation in the way you look and feel, whether you need to lose 5 pounds or 30 pounds or more. This is a plan you can live with for life.

You're asking yourself, "Is this really possible?" Yes, it is. This new way of eating feels good and tastes good every step of the way. You'll love the food. You'll love the way you feel about yourself. And you'll love the results.

I know you might be wondering what a chef could possibly know about diets and weight loss. True, most diet books are written by doctors, dietitians, and health experts, and I have consulted with a number of medical and nutritional authorities on this book. I hate to blow my own horn, but I'll do it just loud enough to register a pleasant, memorable note: I've accomplished what most health experts have not and cannot: I've reinvented "diet food" so that it's no longer boring or tasteless. Too often, in the glut of diet plans available, the doctor, dietitian, or other experts tend to deemphasize taste, eye appeal, the use of flavor-enhancing ingredients, and the originality of flavor combinations. Some of my dishes actually taste *better* than their fattening original counterparts. When I modify my recipes, health is always in the back of my mind, but my first priority is always flavor. This is the critical difference between this diet and most other diets you've tried.

I also know a thing or two about losing weight. A few years ago, I looked like I had spent a year sitting on the couch with cheesecake and a remote. I love to eat, and because of my Italian origins and years of working as a chef, I ate a lot of very good food. My body, without consulting me, started converting truffle risotto, homemade pasta, braised short ribs of beef, foie gras, and gianduja into rolls of fat. My doctor went from routinely saying "Nothing's wrong" to saying "I think we have a problem." So I said, "That's the end of that." I shed my weight—almost 30 pounds, and most of it was fat. How did I do it? By doing everything I'm asking you to do in this book.

My Italian instincts tell me that you need to love what you eat and enjoy preparing it, sharing it, and talking about it to the fullest. So I wanted to take the foods we all love—no matter how bad they might be for us—and make them healthy and flavorful, something that

I really wanted to eat. I figured out how to turn America's favorite comfort foods into delicious meals and a weight-loss plan that makes pounds melt away.

I didn't do it by using a lot of fake ingredients, either. Those always felt like a bad choice to me. They have scary multisyllabic names that make you feel like you need a degree in chemistry to understand them. (I've often wondered if you could make weapons of mass destruction with some of this stuff.) No, I used the freshest, healthiest, and most natural ingredients I could find: whole wheat pastas . . . natural sweeteners like agave nectar . . . healthy, great-tasting cheeses . . . fresh fruits . . . and more.

It's just not healthy to be overweight. It's misery. It compromises your life span and lifestyle. That's no secret. I know one thing for sure: When I'm in my proper range of weight, I have more energy, I think better, I am more productive, funnier, nicer, and I just generally feel great.

I know that the best way to shed pounds is by eating for flavor and pleasure, treating yourself well, and savoring the foods you love. Who wouldn't enjoy losing weight like that?

On the Now Eat This! Diet, you won't even know you're dieting. How could you, when you're eating oatmeal raisin cookies, mushroom lasagna, and blueberry pancakes?

Do I hear a collective "Yippee"?

Great. To hell with boring diets. Now, let's eat and lose weight. Your most difficult decision will be which recipes to try first!

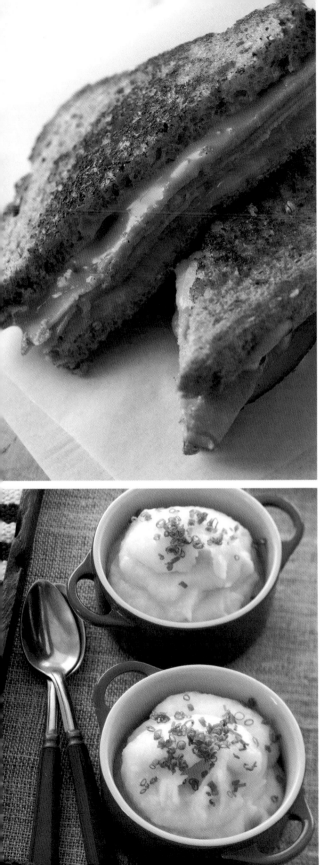

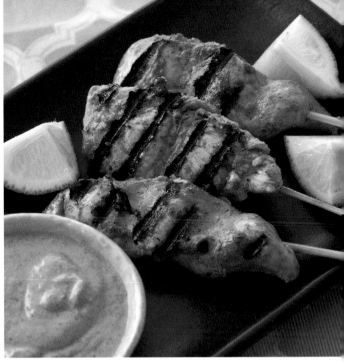

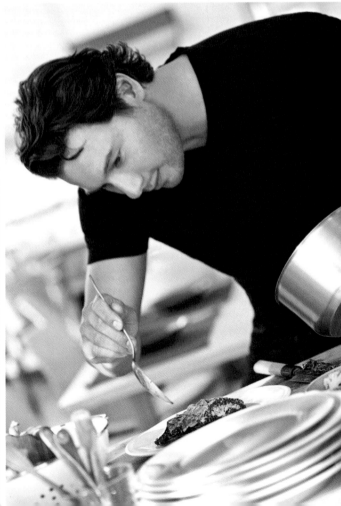

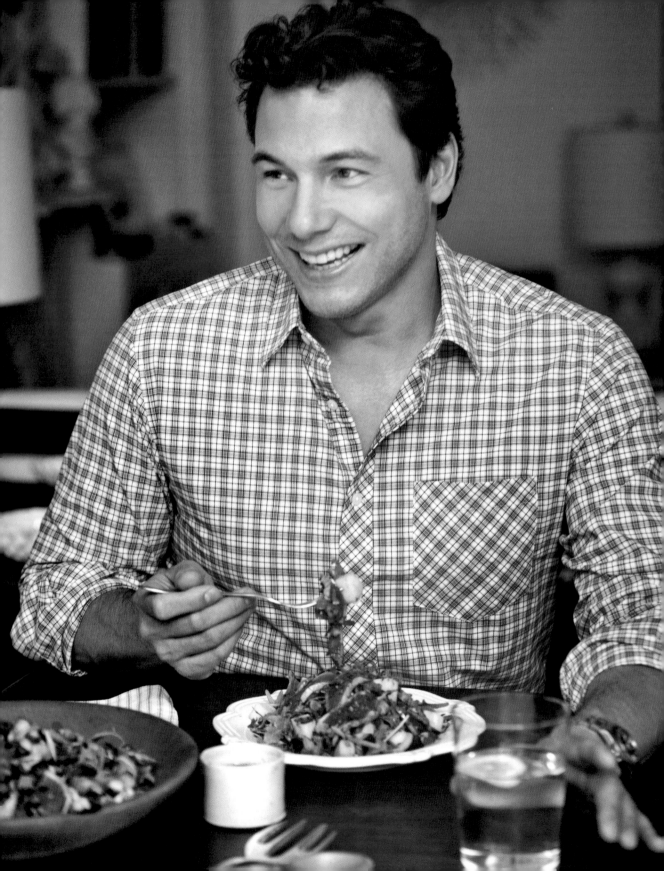

# PART ONE

# Now You Can Really Lose Weight

So let's eat what you love, and lose weight.

If a cheeseburger makes you happy, go right ahead and eat it. Or cookies, or quesadillas—plate them up.

On this plan, you can have it all. For instance:

*Potatoes and sweets.* If you love these things—and who doesn't?—don't deny yourself. Help yourself to mashed potatoes, oatmeal raisin cookies, chocolate mousse, and more.

*Have pasta!* You'll be happy to learn that you can finally eat linguine and not be hunted down by carb cops trying to catch you in the act of eating pasta and bread. We Italians love and eat pasta from the minute we're born until the day we die. We usually live long lives, too. So if you've been avoiding pasta because you heard it was fattening, well, I'll introduce you to some noodles you can eat to your heart's content.

*Juicy beef.* Most people believe they have to give beef and other meat the boot if they want to

lose weight or prevent a heart attack. Well, that's bullshit. Certain cuts of meat can be as low in fat and as heart-healthy as chicken—and taste incredible.

*No-no sandwiches.* On what diet have you ever sunk your teeth into a BLT or a grilled cheese? On this diet, now you can eat all your favorite sandwiches, and the calories won't count against you.

*Do you love junk food?* What do you do when your family insists on fattening meals and snacks? Whip up my healthier, de-junked versions of jalapeño poppers, chicken tenders, potato skins, or mac and cheese. No one will know the difference.

*Craving chocolate?* If chocolate has your number, go for it. Now you can eat chocolaty foods like chocolate milk shakes, chocolate crème brûlée, and the others you tried—unsuccessfully—to resist in the past. On this diet, you can stop fighting food cravings and enjoy your favorite foods again.

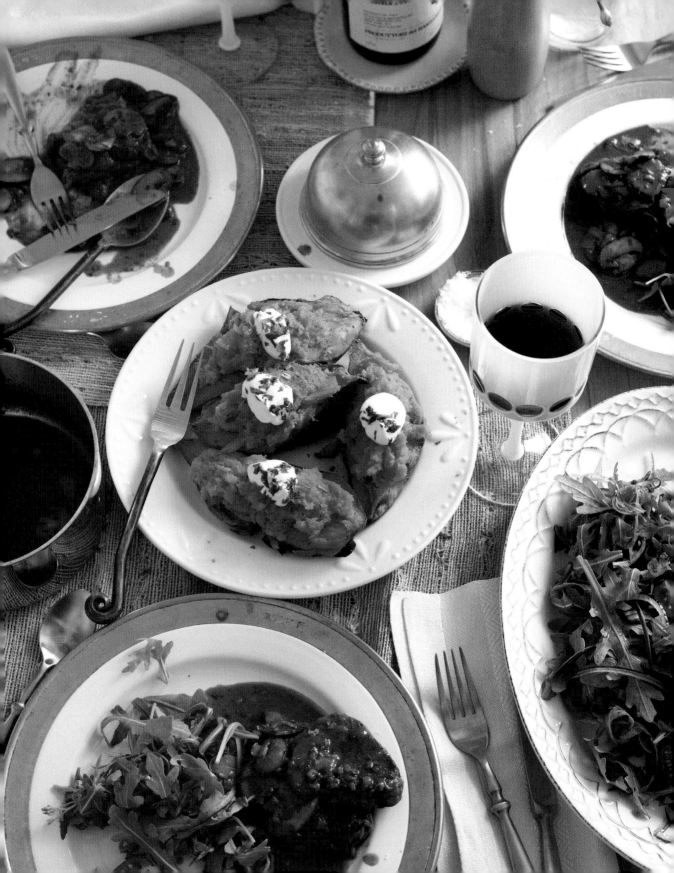

chapter

# 1

☺

# The Now Eat This! Diet

Thanks to this plan, the foods you love—and that you may have thought of as diet breakers—can be eaten in good conscience and good health. How is all this possible?

In my previous book, *Now Eat This!*, I transformed everyone's favorite comfort foods into deliciously healthy versions, all with few bad carbs, few bad fats, less sugar, and maximum flavor. This book goes a step further. It contains eighty all-new healthy recipes—say hello to everything from Italian dishes to stir-fry to classic comfort foods like tuna casserole, BBQ pork, and fudgy fruit and nut bars—but it shows you how to put those recipes into a program that is based on three simple principles:

- Watch Your Calories.
- Learn to Cook.
- Exercise.

I'll briefly summarize each one for you.

## Watch Your Calories

The Now Eat This! Diet is based on controlling your calories. Yes, the calorie is back. Well, technically the calorie never left (it's not as if it's been vacationing in the Bahamas), but it sure has gotten short shrift lately in our fat-free, low-carb, high-protein world.

To put it in simple terms, calories are the energy in food. Most of the calories you take in every day are used to get you through life, meaning your body requires a certain number of calories to perform duties you take for granted, like breathing, maintaining a steady heartbeat, and keeping the blood pumping through your body. Everything that automatically goes on in your body without your even thinking about it requires energy.

Another name for this, which you may have heard before, is *resting metabolic rate*. If you did nothing for a whole day and just sat still, your body would burn between 1,200 and 1,700 calories. Everyone burns calories at a different rate. So, without getting technical, if your body burns 1,200 calories just from the mechanics of living, and you eat 2,000 calories in a day, then your body is going to store that additional 800 calories as fat if you do nothing to expend those extra calories through exercise or additional daily tasks, like getting up off that couch.

The only way to lose weight is to cut or burn calories.

Some diet gurus sell a lot of books by making it seem otherwise and overselling the gimmicks instead of focusing on the basics. But while a given diet plan may tell you to count the carbs or the fat, your body is still counting calories. It doesn't matter if they are carb calories or fat calories or protein calories—your body sheds pounds when you reduce them.

Here's the math of weight loss: 1 pound of fat = 3,500 calories. So, if you can engineer a deficit of 500 calories a day, you should theoretically lose a pound a week. The easiest way to reduce your normal calories by 500 per day is through diet and exercise. You can cut 250 calories from your diet and burn the other 250 with extra exercise, for instance. Or, on more energetic days, you could exercise off 350 calories and eat 150 fewer calories. Weight loss just won't happen without calorie control.

Some diets promise unrealistic weight loss, like 8 to 10 pounds a week. But all you're losing on those fad diets is water and muscle. Your weight bounces right back the moment you go off the diet.

This diet is carefully calibrated to provide between 1,200 and 1,400 calories a day for women and between 1,400 and 1,600 calories a day for men and is based on what doctors and dietitians recommend for safe, effective weight loss. Translation: You'll eat enough every day—and up to six times a day! You never want to take your calories too low (below 1,000 per day), or you'll reduce your metabolic rate and your weight loss might slow down. Eating the right amount of calories daily will get you to your best possible weight.

But don't worry. I'm going to show you a simple way to watch your calories that doesn't involve using a calculator or doing any head-scratching math.

## Learn to Cook

Here's what hardly anyone realizes: One of the keys to successful weight control and good health is to cook at home more often and eat out less. Wait—don't close this book!

Hear me out: The decline of home cooking worldwide is an underlying cause of obesity. That's the conclusion of several research studies done in the past few years. Adults, teens, and kids who eat out a lot are more likely to consume lots of fat, sodium, and soft drinks and lower amounts of nutrient-dense foods, such as vegetables.

I'd like to see us eat together more often as families—at home. Eating together is almost a lost art in America, with breakfast on the run, prepared lunches at school or work, and few sit-down dinners on a regular basis. Some intriguing news: A few years ago, Australian researchers found that teenagers who regularly eat with their families are less likely to be overweight.

This made me think of my childhood and how I was raised. Our family always ate together, and we lingered over our meals for hours, nurturing each other with love, laughter, and lasagna. I remember all the wonderful smells that wafted out of the kitchen, where my mother and grandmother cooked for hours, feeding anyone who would sit at their table. I was always allowed to help out, and that, too, made me feel that I was part of something magical. My grandmother, who is probably cooking up pots of marinara sauce in heaven, is no doubt shaking her head in dismay and praying for the lost souls who don't understand the importance of enjoying great food and breaking bread with family and friends.

The bottom line: You can't eat out all the time and expect to be thin and healthy. You must cook more often for yourself, and everyone can cook *something*. By the way, if you've made a peanut butter and jelly sandwich or heated up soup, you know how to cook. Cooking more often at home is absolutely necessary if you want to get in great shape, inside and out.

Don't worry about time, either. I'll show you how to get a meal on the table in less time than it takes for a pizza to arrive. I am always looking for ways to save time and simplify cooking, so I use a lot of shortcuts, simple ingredients, and labor-saving techniques, and you'll learn about them in this book. Few recipes in this book take longer than 30 minutes to prepare.

While we can't control every aspect of our lives, we have the ability to control the fuel we put into our bodies. So cook for yourself (and your family)! By cooking at home, you're in charge: of the ingredients, the calories, the sodium, the sugar, the fat, the portion size—everything that's important to your weight and health.

Most things are better when we make them at home, just because they are usually more fresh and healthy. So skip driving to your favorite restaurant every night of the week, waiting around for a table, and paying top dollar for food that's making you fat. Don't avoid the kitchen because you think you can't cook. (You can!) Stop using your countertops as a space for today's mail. Stock your home with quality ingredients and foods. Shop to select the food you will really use each week, rather than a collection of stuff you may never touch. I'll give you ingredient lists that will make shopping a cinch. Have basic equipment on hand, like a good heavy, large cutting board, two sharp knives, measuring cups and spoons, a few large spoons and spatulas, a blender, three pans, a sheet tray, and a 9 x 13-inch baking dish. Most recipes can be made using basic utensils.

Instead of watching others cook, join in the fun, and amaze yourself and your family with how delicious healthy cooking can be. I hear from people all the time who have made the decision to cook at home more often. Here's what they're saying:

*I made sweet potato gnocchi tonight. Add that to the list of delish recipes from Rocco!* — Twitter

*I made the replacement for the mashed potatoes tonight and another thumbs up. Thanks.* — Twitter

*I made your Indian Curry with Shrimp a few nights ago and got a lot of praise 4 it ... It was delish!!* — Twitter

Get used to reading recipes, measuring ingredients, and at the very least, boiling or microwaving a few things. Don't worry about looking like a total culinary failure. I've made plenty of mistakes; I've burned rice, overcooked meat, and underbaked bread. Before long, you'll start enjoying yourself. I promise! Everyone is doing it!

## Exercise

I'll tell you a weight-loss secret—sort of a "duh" secret because it's obvious, although some of us don't act as if it's true: You've got to exercise. A lot of people think weight gain comes from eating too much. That's only half the problem. Successful weight loss requires exercise. You don't need to join a gym or exercise for hours; just get more active in every phase of your life. Of course, a regular program of walking, jogging, or cycling will increase the effect, but even mowing the lawn, walking your dog, or climbing stairs can help. It is also helpful to lift weights and increase muscle tone because muscles burn calories.

I've got an easy way to look at exercise: Translate calories into exercise. I've written an entire chapter devoted to this. Knowing the amount of time you need to engage in certain activities to burn off the calories is a great way to speed up your weight loss.

## How I Developed This Plan

As I wrote in the introduction, I, too, struggle with weight. Five years ago I was 30 pounds heavier, with an unhealthy 20 percent body fat. The weight gain bothered me, but I always told myself, "I'll take care of it." I rationalized that at six foot one and 216 pounds, I wasn't really that heavy. Yet deep down I knew that if I didn't start watching my weight, it could really get out of control.

What I did not realize was that there were health problems percolating under the extra flab. One day I went in to see my doctor for the results of my annual routine screening tests. I was shocked by what he told me. My cholesterol and blood pressure tests registered several times what is considered healthy. The scene began to take on the otherworldliness of a short film about heart disease, I couldn't believe he was talking to me. Basically, if I didn't turn this around fast, my answer to that ubiquitous question "Where do you want to be 10 years from now?" could have been: "Not in a cemetery or hospital."

The last thing I ever expected was to be a candidate for heart problems that young. I was down and discouraged, but I knew I had to do something, anything. Realizing my own mortality slammed me into gear.

I had to make some changes—not easy for a guy who grew up eating meatballs, sausage, homemade bread, and pastas like manicotti, lasagna, and ravioli at will, and in any quantity. My mother was always cooking or offering us something to eat. But it never seemed silly to me; that gesture was the most warm, maternal thing I could imagine. It was her absolute expression of love and one of her supreme ways of fulfilling her life's destiny, which, as she saw it, was to nurture her family and take care of other people.

I started making changes incrementally. The first to go was sugar. Sugar was a big deal but easy to eliminate. Little by little, I reduced sugar and limited my alcohol intake. I stopped guzzling soft drinks. I ate high-protein foods, vegetables, and good carbs and eliminated starchy, oily, and junk food completely. No more eating Chinese takeout five times a week and pounding out two to three orders of creaky chicken a day. I don't think my local Chinese restaurant ever recovered financially from the sudden loss of my business. I started eating something healthy at regular intervals. This increased my metabolism, helping me to lose weight. Within six months, I started feeling stronger and more energetic. The difference I felt in my system was incredible.

Feeling driven to do more, I began cooking at home more often, although I wasn't sure I had time. (Yes, even chefs fall prey to that too-busy-to-cook nonsense.) But I knew that if I cooked at home I could better control my nutrition and eat healthier food. Home cooking proved to be much more difficult than cooking in restaurants: I didn't have an army of prep cooks, the big muscular stove, and the endless stream of clean cookware, and I found I had to do the shopping, the prep work, and the cleaning myself. It was a pretty rude awakening.

One of my biggest challenges was finding a way to fit my passion for food and cooking into my healthier lifestyle. After hours of trial and error, I found I could modify my favorite foods and make them low in fat, yet delicious. One of the first dishes to undergo a makeover was my favorite food, lobster bisque. After about twenty-five tries, I nailed it, amazed that it tasted even better than the original but had one-fifth the calories. It more than satisfied the deep lobster-bisque-loving corners of my soul. You'll find this delicious recipe in my previous book, *Now Eat This!*

The more I cooked like this, the more the pounds began coming off, and when I started exercising (usually cardio), they seemed to melt away. I didn't feel deprived. This way of eating is part of my healthier lifestyle now.

## Killing Ourselves with Bad Food

My experience in shedding pounds got me interested in why so many of us are fat. In my case, I knew it was a combination of bad habits, working around rich food, lack of exercise, and indifference to the quality, caloric content, and nutritional value of the foods I ate. But why is it so easy to fall into this kind of harmful eating trap and so difficult to escape from it?

In my experience as a chef, it seemed that nobody was really interested in eating healthy, because *healthy* meant tasteless and bland. So as a society, I think we gravitated to a diet that's arguably designed to make us fat: more processed foods; fewer fruits, vegetables, and whole grains;

and loads of added sugar, salt, fat, and preservatives—a calorie-maximized prescription for poor health.

That way of eating is a radical departure from the diet of our grandparents and great-grandparents, who ate mostly freshly grown plants and grains and fresh meat and fish—which they cooked and prepared themselves. The way my grandmother lived on Long Island was just like the way she lived in Italy. She had rabbits, chickens, and every kind of vegetable and fruit you can think of: fig trees, apple trees, cherry trees, lettuce, tomatoes, everything. Everywhere you looked, something was growing. There was no running to the grocery store. Practically everything she needed was homegrown and home raised. She made unbelievable dinners, almost everything fresh from her garden. In the winter she used ingredients she preserved from her summer garden.

We just don't eat enough fresh, wholesome food anymore, and it's killing us. One of the most credible sources on our nation's health is the Centers for Disease Control (CDC). The CDC says that, since 1990, annual deaths due to overeating and lack of exercise climbed 33 percent to four hundred thousand (almost as many deaths as caused by tobacco).

So basically we're eating ourselves into early graves. The CDC has warned time and again that today's children may have shorter life spans than their parents do. Further, public officials at the CDC cite all the usual reasons for Americans getting fatter, like sedentary jobs and lives, but they also underline the following: too much fast food and too little cooking at home!

Part of the benefit of growing all of that food was the physical activity of tending the garden. Now, I'm not suggesting you start a garden to lose weight, although it's not a bad idea! But commercial food makers, including restaurants, put boatloads of sugar, salt, and fat in food. I know this firsthand, since I'm a chef and have worked in and owned several restaurants. I'll let you in on something: As chefs, we used to love to figure out how much fat we could put in a dish to make food taste good. Per square inch, the density of fat is usually five or six times what a home cook would use. Example: For a dinner party of ten people, I might use 8 pounds of whole butter in a multi-course meal. Yes, you read that right: *8 pounds.* Not all that fat ends up in the food (although that was certainly my goal), but more than half of it will. And the fat I'd use is the full-flavor, heart-clogging, saturated-to-the-max type; I'd even use goose fat.

So much of our culture revolves around irresponsibly prepared food. By that I mean food that's high in artery-clogging fats, added sugar, and calories, and low in fiber, vitamins, and minerals—any food that's prepared without much regard to health. This kind of food is advertised on television, on billboards, and in publications. It's in restaurants and grocery stores, and even our own families prepare it, whether they realize it or not. It's even in "healthy" foods. Take fat-free foods, for example. I'm sure food makers had good intentions in creating them, but many of these foods have nearly as many calories as, or even more calories than, their full-fat counterparts. The label *fat-free* creates a kind of delusion that encourages us to eat more food that's often high in calories, such as processed starches and foods loaded with sweeteners, including artificial ones.

## FAST-FOOD CALORIES

Meals eaten in fast-food restaurants contain an absolutely unbelievable number of calories. To put these numbers in perspective, realize that the average person needs to eat around 2,000 calories a day—so if you had a combo meal for lunch or dinner, you've spent a whopping portion of that budget! I can't tell you how ridiculous these calorie counts are.

| FAST-FOOD CATEGORY | CALORIES |
|---|---|
| HAMBURGER | 857 |
| SUB SANDWICH | 734 |
| FRIED CHICKEN | 931 |
| PIZZA | 766 |
| TACO | 900 |
| COMBO MEALS (SANDWICH, FRIES, DRINK) | 1200 |
| FRIES | 334 |
| SALAD WITH DRESSING | 450 |
| NUGGETS | 365 |

*Source:* T. Dumanovsky, C. A. Nonas, C. Y. Huang, L. D. Silver, and M. T. Bassett, "What people buy from fast-food restaurants: Caloric content and menu item selection, New York City 2007," Obesity 17 (2009): 1369–1374.

Irresponsibly prepared food is absolute garbage and will kill you faster than you realize. If you are in your thirties, forties, or fifties and are eating poorly most of the time, in ten years, you're going to have serious problems that you aren't going to be able to fix. We absolutely must stop the madness and the obesity and the increase in life-shortening diseases. Americans are raising the most unhealthy generation of children in our history because we feed this junk to our kids!

My solution is to return to the healthy, wholesome foods you enjoy and to get creative with them. The point of this book is to get you to be in control of what you put in your body—so that you can lose weight and stay fit and healthy.

## BARGAIN OR NO BARGAIN?

When you supersize a meal at a fast-food joint, you're paying 67 cents more, on average. But that's not all. There are hidden financial costs. You're spending more on health care and gasoline, according to researchers at the University of Wisconsin–Madison. They calculated that for a single instance of paying 67 cents to make a fast-food meal larger, the total daily cost for increased energy needs, gasoline,* and medical care would be between $4.06 and $7.72 for men and between $3.10 and $4.53 for women, depending on body type. The more you overeat, the greater your financial cost.

So let's say you eat at a fast-food restaurant ten times a month and supersize your meal each time. Here's what that might cost you in *extra* money per year.

| MEN | $487–$926 |
|---|---|
| WOMEN | $372–$544 |

* An increase in weight in a vehicle decreases its gasoline efficiency. If you gain a lot of weight, you might find yourself buying more gas.

Source: R. N. Close and D. A. Schoeller, "The financial reality of overeating." *Journal of the American College of Nutrition* 25 (2006): 203–209.

# The Biggest Losers and Me

I saw what a profound impact healthy foods and healthy cooking could make on people's lives in 2008 when I got a call from the producers of NBC's hit show *The Biggest Loser*. The producers wanted me to cook and to teach the contestants how to prepare healthy versions of their favorite foods—foods like chicken Alfredo, pizza, fried chicken, chocolate chip mint ice cream, and other "downfall dishes" that got them in trouble in the first place.

I had been doing the very same thing for myself. Now I had the opportunity to do it on a grander scale. I was excited. The show had some specific cooking guidelines, too: no sugar, no salt, no white flour, barely any fat, nothing artificial. Only organic fruits and vegetables, except those with high sugar content—grapes, mangoes, pineapples, beets, and potatoes. Protein was allowed, but it had to be superlean and organic. I couldn't wait to rise to the challenge to see if I could match the flavor profiles I expected from myself. After all, I'm known as the flavor guy. People expect me to make *anything* taste good.

All of my experience told me that I had to think and cook in a completely different way than ever before. I dug deep down in my culinary bag of tricks. I remembered that in cooking, if you know the basics, you can work around just about any obstacle. People's health and lives were hanging in the balance. I had to take it seriously.

I went into my "lab"—my kitchen—and started experimenting. Dish by dish, I figured out even more ways to replace the fat and sugar in foods without sacrificing their intrinsic flavors. Replacing the fat was the biggest challenge. Fat does two things. It gives a rich mouthfeel, and it carries flavor. I began to experiment with alternative ingredients like vegetable puree, onion puree, garlic puree, evaporated milk, cornstarch, chicken stock, and nonfat yogurt to provide the same thickness and creaminess that we associate with foods like cream and butter. It worked.

For example, one of the *Biggest Loser* contestants I was working with loved fried chicken. True fried chicken weighs in at about 700 calories a serving, so drastic reductions in fat were required. I didn't want to make just the same-old, same-old oven-fried chicken you see in all the low-fat cookbooks. My standards are higher than the average diet-food standards, and I knew people were counting on me to deliver above-average results.

I did some homework and spoke to nutritionists, doctors, and even a renowned food scientist. After experimenting a lot, I concluded and confirmed that the amount of fat absorbed in frying is a function of time, not a function of the quantity of fat. I realized that if I fried chicken for a very short amount of time—a method called flash frying—it would absorb very little fat but still achieve a crispy coating. By flash frying, I was able to eliminate 20 grams of fat and 500 calories from traditional fried chicken, and it tastes as good as, if not better than, the original.

Next out of my bag of tricks: sugar replacement. Here's where I get gray hairs: trying to make something taste naturally sweet but leaving out all the calories. To ease back on the sugar in recipes, I experimented with agave nectar, extracted from the plant that's used to make tequila. Although it has more calories than sugar—about 20 calories per teaspoon—agave nectar is sweeter, so I could use less of it.

For desserts like brownies, cookies, and bars, I began experimenting with ingredients outside the traditional sphere of flour. I found that beans and legumes make excellent structural replacements for flour in desserts like cookies, brownies, and bars. In fact, Japanese cooks use red beans all the time in their desserts. So, by using various types of beans, I was able to get rid of the flour, and then I used natural sweeteners like agave nectar or stevia for sweetening. In the Red Velvet Chocolate Squares recipe on page 263, I used beet, rather than flour, as the base. It was an extraordinary discovery for me.

The results of my experiments were miraculous. I found I could modify people's favorite foods and make them low in fat, bad carbs, sugar, and calories, yet mouthwatering and delicious. I could take every comfort food ever known and transform it into a dish that would promote health, not damage it.

In the world of weight loss, I discovered that "diet food" has the potential to be really wonderful. And the impact it had on the *Biggest Loser* contestants stirred me deeply as a chef. One contestant, Mark Kruger, confided that he used to eat a tub of mint chocolate chip ice cream every night. He loved it. When he ate my revised version, he teared up with gratitude. He thought he'd never be able to enjoy his favorite ice cream again. I gave him the ice cream machine so he could keep on making it.

I knew the food I made for the contestants was good, but with every dish I made, their oohs and aahs and heartfelt thanks confirmed it. It was then that I realized that this type of cooking can make an impact. It can really change people's lives and life expectancy for good.

Cooking is about nurturing and entertaining people with an experience, an atmosphere, and big flavors, and for many years I enjoyed the gratification of just cooking for kicks. But here I saw that when you cook to entertain and to help people achieve their health goals and possibly extend their lives, the gratification is profound.

And so I've become passionate about this new way of cooking and eating. Earlier in my career I was a French-trained chef intrigued by Southeast Asian foods. I got a kick out of mixing old-school techniques with ingredients from around the world—the newer or more unusual the ingredients, the better—to see how their flavors would coalesce.

Both my journey toward better health and the *Biggest Loser* experience opened my eyes to good food that is good for you. Afterward, I began incorporating the concepts of healthy cooking and eating into my work. I now write cookbooks on healthy cooking, and I talk about healthful eating on television shows all the time. I'm dedicated to bringing flavorful, healthful food to more people around the country.

This plan was born from all these experiences. It takes healthy cooking to a whole new level and shows you how to put nutritious, delicious recipes into an actual plan that you can live with and love.

Now, let's get started.

## TAKE OFF POUNDS, ADD YEARS TO YOUR LIFE

The average life expectancy for men and women in the United States is 77.9 years, according to the Centers for Disease Control (CDC). Being overweight, however, can take years off your life. Based on *actuarial* tables used by insurance companies, you can roughly calculate how much your weight might cost you in years. For example:

- If you are overweight by 50 pounds, subtract 13 years from your average life expectancy if you are a man, and 8 years if you are a woman.

- If you are overweight by 30 to 50 pounds, subtract 4 years from your average life expectancy.

- If you are overweight by 10 to 30 pounds, subtract 2 years from your average life expectancy.

*Adapted from:* K. R. Fontaine, et. al., "Years of life lost due to obesity," *Journal of the American Medical Association* 289 (2003): 187–193.

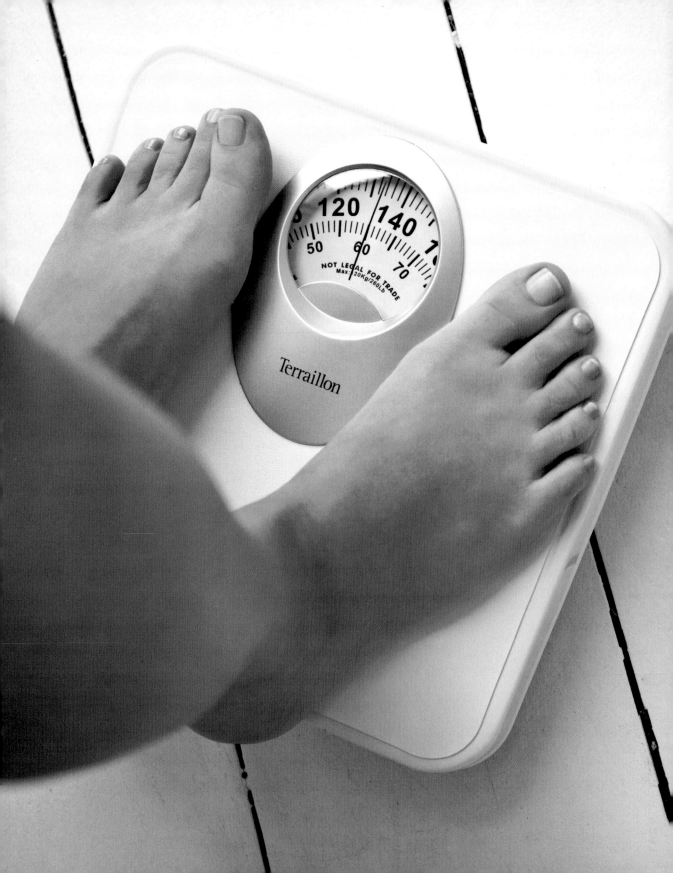

# chapter

# 2

## Eat More and Weigh Less

I t's the biggest little secret in the weight-loss world. The lucky people who know about it are losing extra pounds every week without depriving themselves. And they're not eating less food. They're eating *more* food.

You'll be eating six times a day on this diet—a pattern of eating that can help burn calories more efficiently because your metabolism gets revved up after every meal. The menus I provide are calorie controlled, and when you control calories, you burn fat and calories and lose weight.

I like variety in my menus—so that's what you'll enjoy on this diet. When your meals are monotonous—the same, day after day—you're practically guaranteed unwelcome, powerful cravings. After filling up on the healthy meals in this book, there's no way you'll feel like overindulging in junk food and blowing your results.

## Two Plans, Lots of Food

The Now Eat This! Diet is divided into two plans. The first is called the Now Eat This! 14-Day Fast-Track Plan. On it, you'll eat around 1,200 calories a day if you're a woman and 1,400 calories a day if you're a man. These daily calorie counts trigger faster weight loss and give you the incentive to keep going.

The second plan is called the Now Eat This! Lifestyle Plan. On it, you get to bump up your calorie count. You'll aim for around 1,400 calories a day if you're a woman and 1,600 calories a day if you're a man. These calorie counts are based on what most doctors and dietitians advise for safe weight loss and to ensure that you obtain all necessary vitamins and minerals.

## Calories Count, but You Don't Have to Count Them

I won't be asking you to actually count calories, just to be aware of them. Why not count? It's practically impossible to do; even a group of nutritionists in one study misjudged how many calories were on a plate by almost half! Instead, get smart about the portions in front of you—and let common sense be your guide. Plus, I'm going to show you how to get the right amount of calories easily and without too much trouble. Here's how:

I've created 18 breakfasts, which include 4 all-purpose, enjoy-anytime smoothies; 15 lunches; 16 dinners; 15 snacks; and 16 desserts for you, and I've assigned a color to each recipe. Each color corresponds to the calorie count of the recipe. My color codes work like this:

| BLUE | 350 to 450 | CALORIES |
|---|---|---|
| YELLOW | 250 to 350 | CALORIES |
| GREEN | 150 to 250 | CALORIES |
| ORANGE | 75 to 150 | CALORIES |
| PURPLE | UNDER 75 | CALORIES |

The color coding makes meal planning fun and easy. Let's suppose you're eating 1,400 calories a day. Here's how you'd put together your meals for one day:

For a 200-calorie breakfast, select one of my **GREEN** breakfasts, such as Scrambled Eggs with Smoked Salmon on Toast.

For a 300-calorie lunch, select one of my **YELLOW** lunches, say, my Individual Crispy "Loaded" Pizza.

For a 400-calorie dinner, select one my **BLUE** dinners, like No-Boil Mushroom Lasagna.

Have a 200-calorie dessert after lunch or dinner; select one of my **GREEN** desserts, such as Silken Chocolate Mousse.

At this point, you've spent around 1,100 calories. That leaves you 300 calories to spread out over three snacks. For example:

Include fresh fruit as one or more of your snacks. A medium pear, for example, would be an **ORANGE** snack.

Make up a batch of my Decadent Lemon Bars, Red Velvet Chocolate Squares, Oatmeal Raisin Cookies, or

Fudgy Fruit and Nut Bars to have on hand for another ORANGE snack.

For your third snack, grab something quick and easy like a 6-ounce carton of yogurt. It's an ORANGE snack, too.

So here's how your daily menu might look, using my color-coded recipes:

### BREAKFAST

Scrambled Eggs with Smoked Salmon on Toast (214 calories)

### LUNCH

Individual Crispy "Loaded" Pizza (316 calories)

### DINNER

No-Boil Mushroom Lasagna (388 calories)

Silken Chocolate Mousse (161 calories)

### SNACKS

Medium pear (96 calories)

Red Velvet Chocolate Square (106 calories)

6-ounce carton of yogurt (100 calories)

Using my color codes, you can quickly add up your calories and see that this delicious day of eating weighs in at nearly 1,400 calories. In the two chapters that follow, I'll make this even easier for you by doing your menu planning for you, so you can eat three satisfying meals, enjoy up to three or even four snacks, eat every two hours if you wish, and come out with the right amount of calories each day for weight loss.

## How Fast Will I Lose Weight?

That's a tough question to answer. The rate at which people burn calories may be as distinctive as their fingerprints, and it does rather depend on your starting average daily caloric intake and starting weight. Big eaters and very overweight people will lose weight more quickly than someone with only a small amount to lose. But research shows, on average, that with a diet in this caloric range, you could shed about 1 to 2 pounds per week, maybe more if you exercise.

If you want to get a rough idea of how much you might lose, at least initially, here's what to do:

First, record everything that passes your lips in an average day—most people eat more than they think. In fact, I would do it for three days and then average it out. Use a website like www.calorieking.com or www.fitday.com to figure out your daily calories. That's your baseline.

Second, keep a tally of your daily exercise. You will be surprised at how much you actually move around. Find a website like www.nutristrategy.com that gives you a calorie count for daily activities.

Once you've done those two steps, you can figure out how fast you might lose weight. Estimates vary a lot, but most people eat around 2,500 to 3,500 calories a day. I even encountered a study by the UN Food and Agriculture Organization that claims that the per capita daily consumption in America is 3,790 calories! So you see, the more calories you eat before this diet, the more weight you'll lose when you cut them down to my recommendations. Let's say you're a woman and you eat 2,500 calories a day. On my 14 Day Fast-Track Plan, you'll eat around 1,200 calories a day, so you'll be decreasing your calories by 1,300 a day (1,200 down from your usual 2,500). That means you could lose about 2½ pounds a week, initially (1,300 x 7 = 9,100 ÷ 3,500 = 2.6 pounds). Add in some exercise every day, like taking a brisk walk for 60 minutes, which burns about 300 calories, and you'll burn off an extra pound a week for a total of 3½ pounds.

Now let's say you're a man who eats a staggering 3,790 calories per day. On my 14 Day Fast-Track Plan, you'll eat around 1,400 calories a day, so you'll be decreasing your calories by 2,390 a day (1,400 down from your usual 3,790). That means you could lose nearly 5 pounds a week, initially (2,390 x 7 = 16,730 ÷ 3,500 = 4.78 pounds). Your success ultimately depends on how consistently you follow the diet and how long and how often you exercise.

## Now Eat All This

When deciding how to spend your calories, experts agree that your body performs best when you include all of the macronutrients—protein, carbohydrates, and fats—in your diet. The American Dietetic Association recommends a diet that contains 30 percent calories from fat, 55 percent from carbs, and 15 percent from protein.

The Now Eat This! Diet weighs in very close to this recommendation. It features five nutritious food groups: protein foods, whole grains, vegetables, fruits, and healthy fats. Proportionately, the diet is higher in protein (around 20 to 30 percent of total daily calories), moderate in carbohydrates (50 to 55 percent of total calories), and moderate in fat (around 25 percent of total calories). This nutritional breakdown is also compatible with an active lifestyle.

Generally, the Now Eat This! Diet breaks down like this:

## PERCENTAGE OF CALORIES

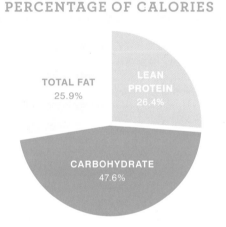

TOTAL FAT
25.9%

LEAN PROTEIN
26.4%

CARBOHYDRATE
47.6%

## Lean Proteins for a Lean Body

The research on weight loss says that protein is essential for healthy weight loss, so this plan is generous in lean proteins. Examples include beef, fish, shellfish, turkey, chicken, whey protein, beans, tofu, and yogurt.

Protein builds shapely muscle, curbs your appetite, and helps your body shed fat more quickly. It's a must if you exercise, because without it, your workouts are wasted. You need the amino acids in protein to repair and build your muscles and help your body recover properly. Protein, combined with strength training, is what makes your muscles firm. There's little that protein doesn't do, except maybe jog around the block for you.

I've included a lot of great seafood recipes using tuna, salmon, shrimp, and other gifts from the sea. They are loaded with omega-3 fatty acids (only if not farm raised). The fat consumed from fish isn't readily stored. That's because it's prioritized for important physiological processes (like promoting heart and joint health and funneling carbs into muscles for energy).

Many of my recipes use Greek yogurt, which is high in protein and rich in calcium. Plus, it's low in calories and fat.

I use vegetarian proteins in many of my recipes, too. Beans are a good example. They're packed with fiber, which increases the feeling of fullness and prolongs emptying of the stomach, making us feel fuller, longer. In all of my protein-rich recipes, you'll find many easy, creative variations on chicken, turkey, fish, meat, beans, and other healthy proteins.

## Good-for-You Carbohydrates

Please stop hating carbs. My Italian grandmother's prescription for any problem was some pasta with a little marinara sauce. She would have found a way to sentence all the carb haters to hard time and have them eat pasta three times a day for extra punishment. The simple fact of the matter is that carbohydrates are a necessary part of any diet; they provide us with the fuel our bodies need to get through the day.

Not all carbohydrates are bad for you. All you need to do is make sure you eat the good ones and in the right amounts: wheat, barley, rye, brown rice, oats, 100 percent whole-grain bread and pastas, and other whole grains; fresh fruits; vegetables; and beans and legumes. Good carbs like these are absorbed more slowly than processed carbs. Brown rice, for instance, takes longer to digest than white rice, and that's exactly what you want. Slower-digesting foods keep the body's chemistry consistent throughout the day, preventing sluggishness and cravings for more food. These foods are especially high in disease-fighting antioxidants and fiber.

As for bad carbs, get rid of anything white immediately, before even reading the next page: white rice, white flour, and white sugar. That's what I did, and it was one of the best nutritional decisions I ever made because it helped me lose weight and feel more energetic.

These foods are highly refined and stripped of their

nutritional value. Plus, they're quickly digested, causing blood sugar to spike soon after they're eaten (so you feel hungry again, tend to eat more, and consequently put on weight).

You won't miss this stuff, either. Why? Because I've transformed them into identical-but-healthy twins by using smarter carbs like whole grains. Now you can eat carbs like Strawberry Malted Belgian Waffles, Garlic Mashed Potatoes, Banana Walnut Muffins, and a lot more.

## Where's the Fat?

The Now Eat This! Diet was designed to be moderate in fat, particularly good fats such as olive oil and avocados. Fat simply makes meals more satisfying, so you're not as likely to get hungry between meals.

Reducing the fat slightly in recipes does help reduce their calories. Some simple things you will learn from me include:

- Using egg whites or egg substitutes instead of whole eggs

- Using evaporated skim milk, yogurt, or silken tofu instead of cream to make rich, creamy desserts like my Silken Chocolate Mousse

- Substituting plain low-fat or nonfat yogurt for sour cream in Mexican dishes

- Sautéing vegetables in a pan coated with nonstick vegetable spray, not oil

- Trying lime juice on salads and other foods instead of vinaigrettes, as in my Flash-Fried Chicken "*Carnitas*"

## Good Sugar, Bad Sugar

I don't need to tell you that sugar is bad for you. But I'm going to anyway. Sugar is *really bad for you*. In fact, it's the worst thing you can eat if you want to lose weight. When you eat a lot of sugar, your body cannot tap into its fat cells for energy, and very little fat is burned. We are eating *far* too much sugar. Hey, don't just take my word for it.

According to the USDA, we are eating more than twelve times the amount of sugar our great-grandparents consumed. That's roughly equivalent to 154 pounds of sugar per person per year. Now, imagine filling up your car

or bathtub or bedroom with 154 of those 1-pound boxes of sugar you buy at the grocery store. Really get an image of it. Okay, maybe you don't eat as much as everyone else. Cut it in half. That's still a huge pile, don't you think?

The body can't use that much sugar, so it stores it as fat for later. If you ease back on your sugar intake, your body has a chance to ignite its fat-burning response. When I eliminated sugar from my diet, I noticed that the weight was dropping off. I was losing about 10 pounds a month.

That said, you do get to eat dessert on this plan. The desserts I've created are low in calories, fat, and sugar, but of course high in flavor. They incorporate a little bit of what I call "good sugars"—more natural sweeteners that have some nutrients and are better for you than added sugars found in many processed, packaged foods, which I consider "bad sugars."

## Volume-Rich Foods

I use a lot of "volume-rich foods" in my recipes—foods that have a high fiber or high water content but don't carry many calories: fruits, vegetables, and broth-based soups. Their weight comes from water, so they're great foods to eat when you're trying to fill yourself up without consuming a lot of calories. Enjoy them as snacks or as filling side dishes.

Examples include my Blueberry Vanilla Smoothie (page 107), Ginger Peach Lassie (page 105), Strawberry Protein Punch Smoothie (page 103), White Bean and Kale Soup (page 152), Spinach and Bacon Salad (page 151), Boston Blue Chicken and Apple Salad (page 160), Garlic Mashed Potatoes made with cauliflower (page 221), and Apple Cinnamon Cranberry Cobbler (page 280).

Researchers believe that water in food empties from the stomach more slowly than water you drink, making you feel full longer. Water also increases food's volume or weight, which signals that you're full even though you're eating fewer calories. In general, too, the more water a food contains, the lower the calories (as with fruits and vegetables), while foods with less water are more dense and contain more calories—think fats and concentrated sugary foods. Foods that naturally contain a lot of water also are bulky and take longer to chew, making you feel full with fewer calories.

Eating watery fruits like watermelon and grapefruit or fresh watery vegetables is also a good way to hydrate your body. Water makes you feel better and helps your skin to look younger and clearer.

All fruits and vegetables are volume rich, but the table below shows those with the highest water content, and thus the most "fill power."

## How Much Food Do I Eat Now? My 3-2-1 Matrix

Often, many people don't know how much protein, carbs, and vegetables they need to eat at a meal. I recommend following what I call the "3-2-1 matrix." To keep this as simple as possible, visualize a round, regular-size dinner plate (9- to 10-inch diameter) and divide the plate into six compartments. Fill one compartment with a lean protein; fill two compartments with a good carb such as brown rice, sweet potatoes, or other starch. Vegetables earn the biggest space, so fill the rest of the plate—three compartments—with high-volume vegetables such as broccoli, green beans, or a salad. You can use the 3-2-1 matrix for breakfast, too. Fill one compartment

with cooked eggs, two compartments with two slices of 100 percent whole-grain toast, and the rest with chopped fresh fruit. This is how I came up with my menus, and if you use this approach for most meals, you will get the nutrients you need and keep calories in check without having to obsess over them.

## General Guidelines While Following the Now Eat This! Diet

I know every dieter has come across this advice at least a thousands times before, so I'll be as brief as possible:

1. Watch your portions. Each recipe is portion controlled for you, so you don't have to worry about measuring things out. The portion size of these recipes can also teach key lessons, like what a single portion of chicken or rice really should look like. And I think you'll be pleasantly surprised at how large some of the portions are. But if you can't quite picture what a moderate serving is, you have a built-in

| VEGETABLES | CALORIES PER CUP | FRUITS | CALORIES PER SERVING |
|---|---|---|---|
| BROCCOLI, COOKED | 50 | APPLE, 1 MEDIUM | 90 |
| CABBAGE, COOKED | 30 | BERRIES, 1 CUP | 50 |
| CARROTS, COOKED | 70 | CANTALOUPE, ½ SMALL | 125 |
| CAULIFLOWER, COOKED | 30 | CHERRIES, 8 FRUITS | 40 |
| CUCUMBERS, RAW, SLICED | 10 | CRANBERRIES, 1 CUP | 40 |
| EGGPLANT, COOKED | 35 | GRAPEFRUIT, ½ MEDIUM | 50 |
| KALE, COOKED | 40 | LEMON, 1 FRUIT | 20 |
| LETTUCE, RAW | 10 | LIME, 1 FRUIT | 20 |
| ONION | 64 | ORANGE, 1 MEDIUM | 70 |
| RED BELL PEPPERS, RAW | 24 | PEACH, 1 MEDIUM | 50 |
| SPINACH, RAW | 20 | PLUM, 1 MEDIUM | 45 |
| SQUASH, SUMMER, COOKED | 36 | WATERMELON, 1 THICK SLICE | 50 |
| TOMATO | 35 | | |
| WATERCRESS, RAW | 8 | | |
| ZUCCHINI, COOKED | 26 | | |

*Source:* USDA Nutrient Data Laboratory, http://grande.nal.usda.gov/NDL/index.html.

food gauge: the palm of your hand. No matter what you eat, it should almost always be able to fit inside the palm of your hand (not including your fingers). Whether it's rice, oatmeal, vegetables, a sweet potato, a piece of fruit, or a serving of protein, the palm of your hand is considered a medium-size (or moderate) portion.

② Drink lots of water. In fact, drink it all day, so that you get in at least ten 8-ounce glasses a day. When I started training for triathlons, I noticed that the athletes I worked with *always* had a bottle of water with them: one in their hand and another one ready to drink. Water will help you feel full. It boosts your immunity so you get sick less often. Plus, it helps keep your metabolism charged up. Water will not bloat you, either. When you don't drink enough, your body starts to feel like it's stranded in the desert, and it holds on to whatever moisture is on hand. The result: You may begin to bloat and retain water. So drink up, and drink until you pee clear. The color of your urine is a good indication of your level of hydration. The clearer your pee, the better.

If you hate water, try a water-based beverage with flavor: iced tea, or water with lemon juice, cucumber, a little agave nectar, vanilla or almond extract, or a few drops of coconut milk.

Or cut your water with a healthy, unsweetened juice. Examples include 100 percent pomegranate juice, Concord grape juice, prune juice, cranberry juice, or fortified orange juice. Avoid store-bought juice "drinks," also called "cocktails" or "punches"; they may contain as little as 5 percent juice and a lot of added sugar. Check the label to see what you're getting. Your juice of choice should be 100 percent fruit juice, made without added sugar.

The key is to drink water like an elephant at a watering hole in sub-Saharan Africa. The more water you drink, the less soda, sugar-ridden juices, and alcohol you'll desire.

Drinking water is fundamental—no arguing! After two weeks of your new water-drinking habit, you'll love it. Trust me on this. And with every sip and every trip to the bathroom, you'll get thinner and healthier, and you may even go a year before catching a cold again.

③ Eat multiple meals. This charges up your metabolism. I've been eating five or six small meals every day now for many years, and it helped change my weight. On the Now Eat This! Diet, you get to eat up to six times a day, within your designated calorie ranges.

④ Don't skip breakfast. People who skip breakfast will find themselves snacking on junk food all day long. In fact, studies show that people who eat breakfast are less likely to overeat during the day. On this diet, you have so many great breakfast choices, from quick-fix smoothies to pancakes to frittatas—dishes you won't want to miss.

⑤ Eat most of your calories the first half of your day— from breakfast through lunch. That way, you're more likely to burn them up. We're supposed to fuel the day, not the night.

There you have it: my overview of the Now Eat This! Diet. Let's get started with the 14-Day Fast-Track Plan to kick-start your weight loss.

*eat more and weigh less*

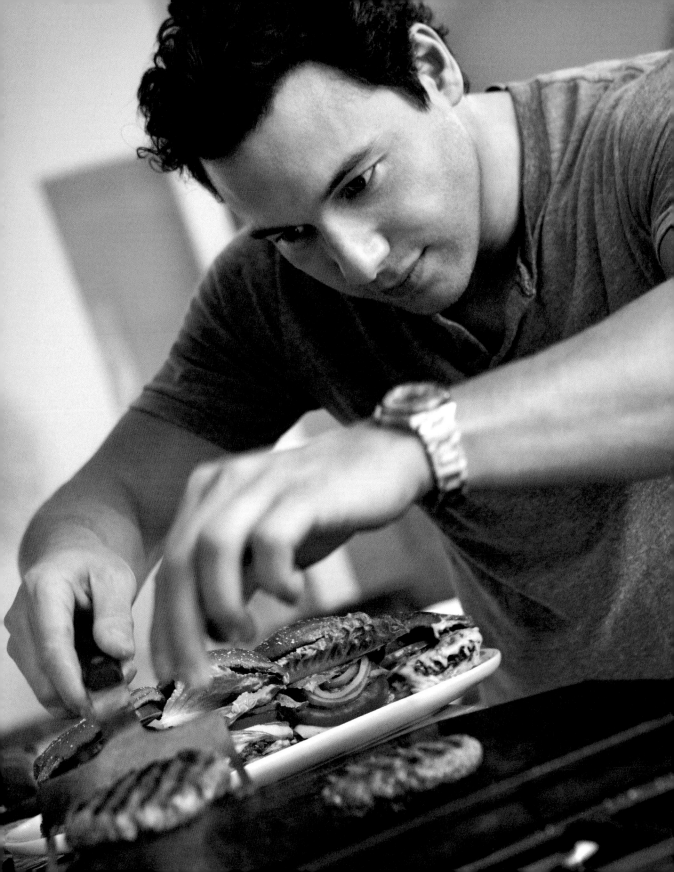

chapter

# 3

☺

# The Now Eat This! 14-Day Fast-Track Plan

Most people I know would like to lose weight at blinding speed. If you're among them, I have come up with the Now Eat This! 14-Day Fast-Track Plan. This plan suggests cutting calories to 1,200 a day if you're a woman and 1,400 calories a day if you're a man to produce early rapid weight loss. Starting off with two weeks of major calorie cutting will actually help you segue into the more moderate Now Eat This! Lifestyle Plan.

There's nothing wrong with losing weight a little faster at the start. Yes, it's the reverse of the usual advice that slow and steady wins the weight-loss race, but recent research suggests otherwise. A study done in 2010 at the University of Melbourne showed that people on a rapid weight-loss regimen designed to trim 3 pounds a week stuck to the diet better and had greater weight loss than did people on a gradual-loss regimen designed to produce a 1-pound loss a week. The bottom line is that once you see the results, you'll want to keep going. So following the Fast-Track Plan is a delicious way to kick-start your weight loss and keep your morale high as you continue losing more weight on the Lifestyle Plan.

Please note: You'll stay on the Fast-Track Plan for 14 days.

## Planning 1,200-Calorie Fast-Track Meals (Women)

Let's see what 1,200 calories a day actually looks and feels like.

- Green Tea Watermelon Super Punch (page 109)
- Pepper, Onion, and Goat Cheese Frittata (page 111)
- Scrambled Eggs with Smoked Salmon on Toast (page 113)
- Sweet Potato and Blue Corn Egg Casserole (page 115)
- Creamy Stuffed Crepes with Orange Butter Syrup (page 117)
- Banana Walnut Muffin (page 278) with 2 scrambled egg whites
- Blueberry Cream Muffin (page 271) with 6 ounces of Greek yogurt

### GENERIC BREAKFAST SUGGESTIONS

- 2 scrambled egg whites, 1 piece of whole wheat toast, and ½ grapefruit
- 1 cup of cut-up fresh fruit with 6 ounces of Greek yogurt
- ½ cup of high-fiber cereal (such as All-Bran) with ½ cup of soy milk and a sliced fresh peach (Look for unsweetened cereal with at least 5 grams of fiber per serving.)
- 1 piece of whole-grain toast, 1 tablespoon of reduced-fat cream cheese, 2 ounces of lox, and 1 medium orange
- 6 ounces of Greek yogurt mixed with ½ cup of high-fiber cereal and 1 cup of blueberries

## GREEN BREAKFASTS
### (150 TO 250 CALORIES)

Each morning, choose one of these breakfasts. Have a different breakfast every day, or stick to a few breakfasts you love. Smoothies are great for breakfast, too; anyone can make them in a matter of minutes. In one glass, you get all the nutrition you need for the morning. What could be simpler? Or make up a batch of muffins ahead of time and pair them with scrambled egg whites or some yogurt for a quick, complete breakfast. Other breakfast options are 200-calorie generic breakfasts that will fit your calorie budget on this plan.

## YELLOW LUNCHES
### (250 to 350 Calories)

Each day, choose one of these lunches. Have a different lunch every day, or stick to a few you love. Use my lunch recipes to help you plan. I've included other lunches that will fit your calorie budget on this plan.

- Red Beet, Goat Cheese, and Walnut Salad (page 145) with a Red Velvet Chocolate Square (page 263) for dessert
- Mediterranean Tuna, Bread, and Cheese Salad (page 157)

- Beef and Orzo Soup (page 159)
- Boston Blue Chicken and Apple Salad (page 160)
- Yellow Curry Shrimp and Green Pea Soup (page 162)
- Faux-Fried Filet o' Fish Sandwich (page 164)
- Individual Crispy "Loaded" Pizza (page 166)
- Chicken and Mushroom Quesadilla (page 171)
- Grilled Cheese and Ham (page 173)
- Rich Beef and Noodle Pho with Lime and Bean Sprouts (page 147) with 5 whole wheat crackers and 1 cup of mixed chopped fruit

### GENERIC LUNCH SUGGESTIONS

- Brown-bag turkey sandwich: 2 slices of light whole wheat bread, 2 ounces of turkey breast, 1 teaspoon of light mayonnaise, tomato slices, lettuce or baby spinach leaves, and 1 teaspoon of mustard
- Vegetarian sandwich: 2 slices of whole wheat bread, ¼ of an avocado, mashed, a 1-ounce slice of Swiss or Jarlsberg cheese, alfalfa sprouts, and tomato slices
- Vegetable salad: 2–3 cups of mixed salad greens with tomatoes, mushrooms, onions, beets, ½ cup of chickpeas, and 1 tablespoon of light Italian dressing, and 1 piece of fruit, such as an orange, an apple, or a pear, or 1 cup of berries
- Pita sandwich: 2 ounces of turkey breast, 1 whole wheat pita pocket, ½ cup of sprouts (alfalfa or broccoli), ¼ cup of chopped tomato, and 2 teaspoons of mustard

## BLUE DINNERS
**(350 to 450 Calories)**

Flip to the dinner entrée section beginning on page 177 and choose a dinner that appeals to you. Have a different one every day, or to save time through the week, cook in bulk and enjoy leftovers. The protein in each dish is complemented with one or two vegetables for a complete, healthy meal. When there's caloric room, add a dessert to your dinner.

- Crispy-on-the-Top Tuna and Green Pea Casserole (page 203)

- Grilled Salmon with Curried Cauliflower (page 205)
- Fettuccine Alfredo with Shrimp (page 207)
- Chicken Pesto Pasta (page 208)
- No-Boil Mushroom Lasagna (page 211)
- BBQ Pork Chops (page 212)
- Mac and Cheese with Ham and Broccoli (page 215)
- Sautéed Steak with Mushrooms (page 195) with a Coconut Cream Mango Pop (page 267) for dessert
- Turkey Dinner with All the Trimmings (page 191) with a Red Velvet Chocolate Square (page 263) for dessert
- Chicken Amandine with Green Beans and Lemon Butter (page 196) with a Decadent Lemon Bar (page 259) for dessert
- Ginger Sweet Chicken and Broccoli Stir-Fry (page 186) with a Fudgy Fruit and Nut Bar (page 265) for dessert
- Roast Beef with Brussels Sprouts and Balsamic Jus (page 179) with Silken Chocolate Mousse (page 276) for dessert

## SNACKS

With breakfast, lunch, and dinner on this plan, you've used around 900 calories so far. That leaves you a full 300 calories for snacks. Try to incorporate two to three snacks in your meal planning each day. The snacks I recommend are made with natural ingredients, nothing overly processed. Other healthy snacks include fresh fruits, raw veggies, vegetable juices, Greek yogurt, protein bars, and nuts. Here are some ideas:

## SNACKS
**(75 to 150 Calories)**

### NOW EAT THIS! SNACKS
Decadent Lemon Bars (page 259)
Red Velvet Chocolate Squares (page 263)
Oatmeal Raisin Cookies (page 261)

### FRUIT AND DRIED FRUIT
Apple, 1 medium
Banana, 1 medium
Cantaloupe, ½ small

Guava, 1 cup diced
Mango, 1 cup diced
Pear, 1 medium
Pineapple, 1 cup diced
Raisins, 1-ounce package

## NUTS
Almonds, dry roasted, 20
Brazil nuts, 6
Cashews, dry roasted, 16
Mixed nuts, dry roasted, 15
Peanuts, dry roasted, 25

## OTHER SNACKS
Carrot juice, 1 cup
V8 V-Fusion, 1 cup
6 ounces of yogurt (plain, nonfat, or sugar-free, fruit flavored)

# SNACKS
**(under 75 Calories)**

## NOW EAT THIS! SNACKS
PBJ Cookies (page 254)
Double Chocolate Chip Cookies (page 256)

## FRUIT
Apricots, 2 medium
Apricots, dried, 8 halves
Berries, 1 cup
Cherries, 8
Figs, dried, 3
Grapefruit, ½
Grapes, 1 cup
Kiwi, 1 medium
Nectarine, 1 medium
Orange, 1 medium
Papaya, 1 cup diced
Peach, 1 medium
Tangerine, 1 medium
Watermelon, 1 thick slice

## OTHER SNACK CHOICES
Baby carrots, 8
Fresh, cut-up veggies, unlimited amounts
Vegetable juice, 1 cup

# Sample 1,200-Calorie Menu

Here's what a typical menu might look like if you mix and match your meals from the color-coded lists.

| BREAKFAST | CALORIES |
|---|---|
| GREEN TEA WATERMELON SUPER PUNCH (PAGE 109) | 176 |
| **LUNCH** | **CALORIES** |
| BROWN-BAG TURKEY SANDWICH | 300 |
| **DINNER** | **CALORIES** |
| MAC AND CHEESE WITH HAM AND BROCCOLI (PAGE 215) | 399 |
| **SNACKS (3 DAILY)** | **CALORIES** |
| OATMEAL RAISIN COOKIE (PAGE 261) | 84 |
| PEAR, 1 MEDIUM | 96 |
| APPLE, 1 MEDIUM | 90 |
| TOTAL | 1,145 CALORIES |

# Your Daily Menu Planner

It may help you to plan your meals using the following worksheet. Using the meal lists, simply fill in what you will eat each day. Planning your meals can help you stay on track.

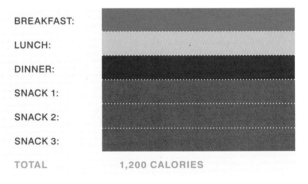

| | |
|---|---|
| BREAKFAST: | |
| LUNCH: | |
| DINNER: | |
| SNACK 1: | |
| SNACK 2: | |
| SNACK 3: | |
| TOTAL | 1,200 CALORIES |

# Planning 1,400-Calorie Fast-Track Menus (Men)

Let's go through the same planning process for a 1,400-calorie diet for a man on the Fast-Track Plan.

## YELLOW BREAKFASTS
### (250 to 350 Calories)

Each morning, choose one of these breakfasts to net you around 250 to 350 calories. Have a different breakfast every day, or stick to a few breakfasts you love. Smoothies are quick to make, especially if you don't have a lot of time in the morning. My smoothie recipes begin on page 103. Enjoy some whole wheat toast or one of my muffins with your smoothie, and you've got a filling breakfast that's quick and easy to make. I've included several generic breakfast options, too, that will fit your calorie budget on this plan.

- Strawberry Protein Punch Smoothie (page 103) with 2 slices of whole wheat toast and 1 tablespoon of all-fruit jam
- Green Tea Watermelon Super Punch (page 109) and a Banana Walnut Muffin (page 278)
- Ginger Peach Lassie (page 105) and a Blueberry Cream Muffin (page 271)
- Blueberry Vanilla Smoothie (page 107) with 2 slices of whole wheat toast and 1 tablespoon of all-fruit jam
- Pizza Egg Bake (page 121)
- Apple and Cranberry Granola Cereal (page 123)
- Sunrise Sandwich (page 126)
- Cherry Red Oatmeal (page 129)
- Blue on Blueberry Silver Dollar Pancakes (page 130)
- French Toast à L'Orange (page 133)
- Rocky Road Oatmeal (page 134)
- South of the Border Scramble with Chorizo and Salsa (page 137)
- Blueberry Graham Cheesecake Oatmeal (page 138)

## GENERIC BREAKFAST SUGGESTIONS

- 1 cup of high-fiber cereal (such as All-Bran) with ½ cup of soy milk and a sliced fresh peach (Look for unsweetened cereal with at least 5 grams of fiber per serving.)
- 1 toasted whole wheat English muffin, 6 ounces of Greek yogurt, and 1 sliced fresh pear
- 1 cereal bar, 6 ounces of Greek yogurt, and 1 cup of fresh berries
- 2 slices of whole-grain toast, 2 tablespoons of reduced-fat cream cheese, 2 ounces of lox, and 1 medium orange
- 6 ounces of Greek yogurt mixed with 1 cup of high-fiber cereal and 1 cup of blueberries

## YELLOW LUNCHES
### (250 to 350 Calories)

Each day, choose one of these lunches in the 250 to 350 calorie range. Have a different lunch every day, or stick to a few you love. Use my lunch recipes to help you plan. I've included other generic lunches that will fit your calorie budget on this plan.

- Mediterranean Tuna, Bread, and Cheese Salad (page 157)
- Beef and Orzo Soup (page 159)
- Boston Blue Chicken and Apple Salad (page 160)
- Yellow Curry Shrimp and Green Pea Soup (page 162)
- Faux-Fried Filet o' Fish Sandwich (page 164)
- Individual Crispy "Loaded" Pizza (page 166)
- Chicken and Mushroom Quesadilla (page 171)
- Grilled Cheese and Ham (page 173)
- Red Beet, Goat Cheese, and Walnut Salad (page 145) with a Red Velvet Chocolate Square (page 263) for dessert
- Rich Beef and Noodle Pho with Lime and Bean Sprouts (page 147) with 5 whole wheat crackers and 1 cup of mixed chopped fruit

## GENERIC LUNCH SUGGESTIONS

- Brown-bag turkey sandwich: 2 slices of light whole wheat bread, 2 ounces of turkey breast, 1 teaspoon of light mayonnaise, tomato slices, lettuce or baby spinach leaves, and 1 teaspoon of mustard

- Vegetarian sandwich: 2 slices of whole wheat bread, ¼ of an avocado, mashed, a 1-ounce slice of Swiss or Jarlsberg cheese, alfalfa sprouts, and tomato slices

- Vegetable salad: 2–3 cups of mixed salad greens with tomatoes, mushrooms, onions, beets, ½ cup of chickpeas, and 1 tablespoon of light Italian dressing, and 1 piece of fruit, such as an orange, an apple, or a pear, or 1 cup of berries

- Pita sandwich: 2 ounces of turkey breast, 1 whole wheat pita pocket, ½ cup of sprouts (alfalfa or broccoli), ¼ cup of chopped tomato, and 2 teaspoons of mustard

- Chicken Amandine with Green Beans and Lemon Butter (page 196) with an Oatmeal Raisin Cookie (page 261) for dessert

- Ginger Sweet Chicken and Broccoli Stir-Fry (page 186) with a Fudgy Fruit and Nut Bar (page 265) for dessert

- Lemon Pepper Shrimp (page 185) with a Coconut Cream Mango Pop (page 267) for dessert

- Roast Beef with Brussels Sprouts and Balsamic Jus (page 179) with Silken Chocolate Mousse (page 276) for dessert

## SNACKS

With breakfast, lunch, and dinner on this plan, you've used around 1,000 calories so far. That leaves you a full 400 calories for snacks. Try to incorporate three snacks in your meal planning each day. Here are some ideas:

## BLUE DINNERS
**(350 to 450 Calories)**

Here are dinner suggestions that weigh in at 350 to 450 calories. Have a different one every day, or to save time through the week, cook in bulk and enjoy leftovers. When there's caloric room, add a dessert to your dinner.

- Crispy-on-the-Top Tuna and Green Pea Casserole (page 203)

- Grilled Salmon with Curried Cauliflower (page 205)

- Fettuccine Alfredo with Shrimp (page 207)

- Chicken Pesto Pasta (page 208)

- No-Boil Mushroom Lasagna (page 211)

- BBQ Pork Chops (page 212)

- Mac and Cheese with Ham and Broccoli (page 215)

- Sautéed Steak with Mushrooms (page 195) with a Decadent Lemon Bar (page 259) for dessert

- Spicy-Sweet Linguine alla Vodka (page 189) with a Red Velvet Chocolate Square (page 263) for dessert

- Turkey Dinner with All the Trimmings (page 191) with an Oatmeal Raisin Cookie (page 261) for dessert

## SNACKS
**(150 to 250 Calories)**

NOW EAT THIS! SNACKS
Curried Chicken Skewers (page 230)
Pita Chips with Charred Eggplant Dip (page 233)
South of the Border Loaded Potato Skins (page 234)
Tuna Croquettes with Dill Relish (page 236)
Banana Walnut Muffins (page 278)
Crunchy Tomato Bread (page 238)
"Fried" Cheese Balls (page 241)
Mama's Mini Meatball Bites (page 242)
Eggplant and Roasted Red Pepper Torta (page 244)
Hogs Undercover (page 246)
Chicken Tenders with Ranch Dressing (page 248)
Shrimp and Cheddar Tostada with Salsa Verde (page 250)
Green Tea Watermelon Super Punch (page 109)

NUTS
Macadamia nuts, 7
Pecans, 20
Pistachios, shelled, 45

OTHER SNACKS
Any protein bar between 150 and 250 calories

## SNACKS
### (75 to 150 Calories)

NOW EAT THIS! SMOOTHIES
Strawberry Protein Punch Smoothie (page 103)
Ginger Peach Lassie (page 105)
Blueberry Vanilla Smoothie (page 107)

NOW EAT THIS! SNACKS
Decadent Lemon Bars (page 259)
Oatmeal Raisin Cookies (page 261)
Red Velvet Chocolate Squares (page 263)
Fudgy Fruit and Nut Bars (page 265)
Coconut Cream Mango Pops (page 267)
Chocolate Malted Milk Shake (page 269)
Blueberry Cream Muffins (page 271)
Any Berry Parfait (page 273)

FRUIT AND DRIED FRUIT
Apple, 1 medium
Banana, 1 medium
Guava, 1 cup diced
Mango, 1 cup diced
Pear, 1 medium
Pineapple, 1 cup diced
Raisins, 1-ounce package

NUTS
Almonds, dry roasted, 20
Brazil nuts, 6
Cashews, dry roasted, 16
Mixed nuts, dry roasted, 15
Peanuts, dry roasted, 25

OTHER SNACKS
Carrot juice, 1 cup
V8 V-Fusion, 1 cup
6 ounces of nonfat Greek yogurt such as 0% Fage
Total

## SNACKS
### (under 75 Calories)

NOW EAT THIS! SNACKS
PBJ Cookies (page 254)
Double Chocolate Chip Cookies (page 256)

FRUITS
Apricots, 2 medium
Apricots, dried, 8 halves
Berries, 1 cup
Cherries, 8
Figs, dried, 3
Grapefruit, ½
Grapes, 1 cup
Kiwi, 1 medium
Nectarine, 1 medium
Orange, 1 medium
Papaya, 1 cup diced
Peach, 1 medium
Tangerine, 1 medium
Watermelon, 1 thick slice

OTHER SNACK CHOICES
Baby carrots, 8
Fresh, cut-up veggies, unlimited amounts
Vegetable juice, 1 cup

# Sample 1,400-Calorie Menu

Here's what a typical menu might look like if you mix and match your meals from the color-coded lists.

| BREAKFAST | CALORIES |
|---|---|
| SUNRISE SANDWICH (PAGE 126) | 279 |
| LUNCH | CALORIES |
| INDIVIDUAL CRISPY "LOADED" PIZZA (PAGE 166) | 316 |
| DINNER | CALORIES |
| BBQ PORK CHOPS (PAGE 212) | 398 |
| SNACKS (3 DAILY) | CALORIES |
| "FRIED" CHEESE BALLS (PAGE 241) | 177 |
| STRAWBERRY PROTEIN PUNCH SMOOTHIE (PAGE 103) | 107 |
| GRAPES, 1 MEDIUM BUNCH | 125 |
| TOTAL | 1,402 CALORIES |

# Your Daily Menu Planner

Plan your meals using the following worksheet. Using the meal lists, simply fill in what you will eat each day. Planning your meals can help you stay on track.

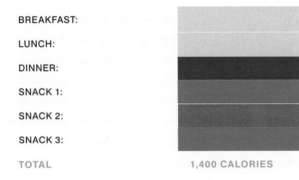

| | |
|---|---|
| BREAKFAST: | |
| LUNCH: | |
| DINNER: | |
| SNACK 1: | |
| SNACK 2: | |
| SNACK 3: | |
| TOTAL | 1,400 CALORIES |

If you follow these guidelines—mixing and matching your meals according to your color codes, it's easy to figure out what to eat each day. It's simple and fuss-free—you don't have to count calories. Just choose meals you enjoy and start losing weight.

## 14 Days of Sample Menus

Here's a day-by-day plan if you like to follow preset menus. It guides you as to what to eat each day. It's fuss-free—you don't have to count calories or buy complicated ingredients. Shopping lists are included on pages 35–40. Remember, you can substitute one dinner or lunch for another dinner or lunch. These are all simple, great-tasting meals your whole family can enjoy, too.

### DAY 1

| BREAKFAST | CALORIES |
|---|---|
| SCRAMBLED EGGS WITH SMOKED SALMON ON TOAST (PAGE 113) | 214 |
| GRAPEFRUIT, ½ MEDIUM | 50 |
| **LUNCH** | **CALORIES** |
| YES, A CHEESEBURGER! (PAGE 175) | 368 |
| **DINNER** | **CALORIES** |
| ROAST BEEF WITH BRUSSELS SPROUTS AND BALSAMIC JUS (PAGE 179) | 246 |

| | |
|---|---|
| TOSSED MIXED GREENS SALAD WITH REDUCED-FAT SALAD DRESSING | 50 |
| **SNACKS (3 DAILY)** | **CALORIES** |
| DOUBLE CHOCOLATE CHIP COOKIE (PAGE 256) | 74 |
| APPLE, 1 MEDIUM | 90 |
| RED VELVET CHOCOLATE SQUARE (PAGE 263) | 106 |
| **TOTAL/WOMEN** | **1,198 CALORIES** |
| MEN: ADD MY GREEN TEA WATERMELON SUPER PUNCH (PAGE 109) TO ANY OF THESE 3 SNACKS | 176 |
| **TOTAL/MEN** | **1,374 CALORIES** |

### DAY 2

| BREAKFAST | CALORIES |
|---|---|
| APPLE AND CRANBERRY GRANOLA CEREAL (PAGE 123) | 253 |
| **LUNCH** | **CALORIES** |
| BACON LETTUCE TOMATO ROLL (PAGE 155) | 245 |
| DOUBLE CHOCOLATE CHIP COOKIE (PAGE 256) | 74 |
| **DINNER** | **CALORIES** |
| ROASTED PORK TENDERLOIN WITH BUTTERNUT SQUASH MASH AND TARRAGON GRAVY (PAGE 199) | 343 |
| **SNACKS (3 DAILY)** | **CALORIES** |
| COCONUT CREAM MANGO POP (PAGE 267) | 115 |
| PEAR, 1 MEDIUM | 96 |
| CHOCOLATE MALTED MILK SHAKE (PAGE 269) | 126 |
| **TOTAL/WOMEN** | **1,252 CALORIES** |

| | |
|---|---|
| MEN: ENJOY A PROTEIN BAR WITH ANY OF THESE 3 SNACKS | 200 |
| **TOTAL/MEN** | **1,452 CALORIES** |

## DAY 3

| BREAKFAST | CALORIES |
|---|---|
| PEPPER, ONION, AND GOAT CHEESE FRITTATA (PAGE 111) | 182 |

| LUNCH | CALORIES |
|---|---|
| GRILLED CHEESE AND HAM (PAGE 173) | 337 |
| RICH BEEF AND NOODLE PHO WITH LIME AND BEAN SPROUTS (PAGE 147) | 172 |

| DINNER | CALORIES |
|---|---|
| GRILLED SALMON WITH CURRIED CAULIFLOWER (PAGE 205) | 367 |

| SNACKS (3 DAILY) | CALORIES |
|---|---|
| DOUBLE CHOCOLATE CHIP COOKIE (PAGE 256) | 74 |
| PLUM, 1 MEDIUM | 45 |
| STRAWBERRY PROTEIN PUNCH SMOOTHIE (PAGE 103) | 107 |
| **TOTAL/WOMEN** | **1,284 CALORIES** |
| MEN: ENJOY ONE OF MY COCONUT CREAM MANGO POPS (PAGE 267) WITH ANY OF THESE 3 SNACKS | 115 |
| **TOTAL/MEN** | **1,399 CALORIES** |

## DAY 4

| BREAKFAST | CALORIES |
|---|---|
| ROCKY ROAD OATMEAL (PAGE 134) | 327 |

| LUNCH | CALORIES |
|---|---|
| MEDITERRANEAN TUNA, BREAD, AND CHEESE SALAD (PAGE 157) | 278 |

| DINNER | CALORIES |
|---|---|
| MAC AND CHEESE WITH HAM AND BROCCOLI (PAGE 215) | 399 |

| SNACKS (3 DAILY) | CALORIES |
|---|---|
| COCONUT CREAM MANGO POP (PAGE 267) | 115 |
| TANGERINE, 1 MEDIUM | 47 |
| PBJ COOKIE (PAGE 254) | 55 |
| **TOTAL/WOMEN** | **1,221 CALORIES** |
| MEN: ENJOY CURRIED CHICKEN SKEWERS (PAGE 230) WITH ANY OF THESE 3 SNACKS | 159 |
| **TOTAL/MENS** | **1,380 CALORIES** |

## DAY 5

| BREAKFAST | CALORIES |
|---|---|
| SOUTH OF THE BORDER SCRAMBLE WITH CHORIZO AND SALSA (PAGE 137) | 328 |

| LUNCH | CALORIES |
|---|---|
| YELLOW CURRY SHRIMP AND GREEN PEA SOUP (PAGE 162) | 302 |

| DINNER | CALORIES |
|---|---|
| CHICKEN PESTO PASTA (PAGE 208) | 385 |

| SNACKS (3 DAILY) | CALORIES |
|---|---|
| TANGERINE, 1 MEDIUM | 47 |
| BLUEBERRY CREAM MUFFIN (PAGE 271) | 145 |
| 6 OUNCES NONFAT GREEK YOGURT | 90 |
| **TOTAL/WOMEN** | **1,297 CALORIES** |
| MEN: ENJOY MY BLUEBERRY VANILLA SMOOTHIE (PAGE 107) WITH ANY OF THESE 3 SNACKS | 134 |
| **TOTAL/MEN** | **1,431 CALORIES** |

## DAY 6

| BREAKFAST | CALORIES |
|---|---|
| BLUEBERRY GRAHAM CHEESECAKE OATMEAL (PAGE 138) | 339 |

| LUNCH | CALORIES |
|---|---|
| WHITE BEAN AND KALE SOUP WITH ROSEMARY AND PARMIGIANO-REGGIANO (PAGE 152) | 234 |
| FUDGY FRUIT AND NUT BAR (PAGE 265) | 110 |

| DINNER | CALORIES |
|---|---|
| NO-BOIL MUSHROOM LASAGNA (PAGE 211) | 388 |

| SNACKS (3 DAILY) | CALORIES |
|---|---|
| STRAWBERRIES, 1 CUP SLICED | 50 |
| CHOCOLATE MALTED MILK SHAKE (PAGE 269) | 126 |
| BABY CARROTS, 8 | 28 |
| TOTAL/WOMEN | 1,275 CALORIES |
| MEN: ENJOY A PROTEIN BAR WITH ANY OF THESE 3 SNACKS | 200 |
| TOTAL/MEN | 1,475 CALORIES |

## DAY 7

| BREAKFAST | CALORIES |
|---|---|
| CREAMY STUFFED CREPES WITH ORANGE BUTTER SYRUP (PAGE 117) | 239 |

| LUNCH | CALORIES |
|---|---|
| NO-BOIL MUSHROOM LASAGNA (LEFTOVERS) (PAGE 211) | 388 |

| DINNER | CALORIES |
|---|---|
| TURKEY DINNER WITH ALL THE TRIMMINGS (PAGE 191) | 323 |
| FUDGY FRUIT AND NUT BAR (PAGE 265) | 110 |

| SNACKS (3 DAILY) | CALORIES |
|---|---|
| STRAWBERRY PROTEIN PUNCH SMOOTHIE (PAGE 103) | 107 |
| FRESH BERRIES, 1 CUP | 50 |
| BABY CARROTS, 8 | 28 |
| TOTAL/WOMEN | 1,245 CALORIES |
| MEN: ENJOY MY BANANA WALNUT MUFFIN (PAGE 278) WITH ANY OF THESE 3 SNACKS | 163 |
| TOTAL/MEN | 1,408 CALORIES |

## DAY 8

| BREAKFAST | CALORIES |
|---|---|
| BLUE ON BLUEBERRY SILVER DOLLAR PANCAKES (PAGE 130) | 292 |

| LUNCH | CALORIES |
|---|---|
| FAUX-FRIED FILET O' FISH SANDWICH (PAGE 164) | 313 |

| DINNER | CALORIES |
|---|---|
| CHICKEN AMANDINE WITH GREEN BEANS AND LEMON BUTTER (PAGE 196) | 327 |

| SNACKS (3 DAILY) | CALORIES |
|---|---|
| TUNA CROQUETTES WITH DILL RELISH (PAGE 236) | 160 |
| PEAR, 1 MEDIUM | 96 |
| RED VELVET CHOCOLATE SQUARE (PAGE 263) | 106 |
| TOTAL/WOMEN | 1,294 CALORIES |
| MEN: ENJOY A CHOCOLATE MALTED MILK SHAKE (PAGE 269), WITH ANY OF THESE 3 SNACKS | 126 |
| TOTAL/MEN | 1,420 CALORIES |

## DAY 9

| BREAKFAST | CALORIES |
|---|---|
| FRENCH TOAST À L'ORANGE (PAGE 133) | 301 |

| LUNCH | CALORIES |
|---|---|
| WHITE BEAN AND KALE SOUP WITH ROSEMARY AND PARMIGIANO-REGGIANO (PAGE 152) | 234 |
| BANANA WALNUT MUFFIN (PAGE 278) | 163 |

| DINNER | CALORIES |
|---|---|
| CRISPY-ON-THE-TOP TUNA AND GREEN PEA CASSEROLE (PAGE 203) | 351 |

| SNACKS (3 DAILY) | CALORIES |
|---|---|
| COCONUT CREAM MANGO POP (PAGE 267) | 115 |
| BABY CARROTS, 8 | 28 |
| RED VELVET CHOCOLATE SQUARE (PAGE 263) | 106 |
| TOTAL/WOMEN | 1,298 CALORIES |
| MEN: ENJOY A PROTEIN BAR IN ADDITION TO THESE 3 SNACKS | 200 |
| TOTAL/MEN | 1,498 CALORIES |

## DAY 10

| BREAKFAST | CALORIES |
|---|---|
| CHERRY RED OATMEAL (PAGE 129) | 287 |

| LUNCH | CALORIES |
|---|---|
| BACON LETTUCE TOMATO ROLL (PAGE 155) | 245 |
| OATMEAL RAISIN COOKIE (PAGE 261) | 84 |

| DINNER | CALORIES |
|---|---|
| GINGER SWEET CHICKEN AND BROCCOLI STIR-FRY (PAGE 186) | 298 |
| SILKEN CHOCOLATE MOUSSE (PAGE 276) | 161 |

| SNACKS (3 DAILY) | CALORIES |
|---|---|
| ALMONDS, DRY ROASTED, 15 | 100 |
| NECTARINE, 1 MEDIUM | 45 |
| BABY CARROTS, 8 | 28 |
| TOTAL/WOMEN | 1,248 CALORIES |
| MEN: ENJOY A CHOCOLATE MALTED MILK SHAKE (PAGE 269) WITH ANY OF THESE 3 SNACKS | 126 |
| TOTAL/MEN | 1,374 CALORIES |

## DAY 11

| BREAKFAST | CALORIES |
|---|---|
| SUNRISE SANDWICH (PAGE 126) | 279 |

| LUNCH | CALORIES |
|---|---|
| BOSTON BLUE CHICKEN AND APPLE SALAD (PAGE 160) | 294 |

| DINNER | CALORIES |
|---|---|
| FETTUCCINE ALFREDO WITH SHRIMP (PAGE 207) | 374 |

| SNACKS (3 DAILY) | CALORIES |
|---|---|
| MAMA'S MINI MEATBALL BITES (PAGE 242) | 177 |
| OATMEAL RAISIN COOKIE (PAGE 261) | 84 |
| BABY CARROTS, 8 | 28 |
| TOTAL/WOMEN | 1,236 CALORIES |
| MEN: ENJOY A GREEN TEA WATERMELON SUPER PUNCH (PAGE 109) WITH ANY OF THESE 3 SNACKS | 176 |
| TOTAL/MEN | 1,412 CALORIES |

## DAY 12

| BREAKFAST | CALORIES |
|---|---|
| STRAWBERRY MALTED BELGIAN WAFFLES (PAGE 141) | 375 |

| LUNCH | CALORIES |
|---|---|
| CHICKEN AND MUSHROOM QUESADILLA (PAGE 171) | 324 |

| DINNER | CALORIES |
|---|---|
| ROAST BEEF WITH BRUSSELS SPROUTS AND BALSAMIC JUS (PAGE 179) | 246 |
| GARLIC MASHED POTATOES (PAGE 221) | 101 |

| SNACKS (3 DAILY) | CALORIES |
|---|---|
| COCONUT CREAM MANGO POPS (PAGE 267) | 115 |
| DOUBLE CHOCOLATE CHIP COOKIE (PAGE 256) | 74 |
| FRESH BERRIES, 1 CUP | 50 |
| TOTAL/WOMEN | 1,285 CALORIES |
| MEN: ENJOY A RED VELVET CHOCOLATE SQUARE (PAGE 263) WITH ANY OF THESE 3 SNACKS | 106 |
| TOTAL/MEN | 1,391 CALORIES |

## DAY 13

| BREAKFAST | CALORIES |
|---|---|
| PIZZA EGG BAKE (PAGE 121) | 251 |

| LUNCH | CALORIES |
|---|---|
| RED BEET, GOAT CHEESE, AND WALNUT SALAD (PAGE 145) | 163 |

| DINNER | CALORIES |
|---|---|
| BBQ PORK CHOPS (PAGE 212) | 398 |
| APPLE CINNAMON CRANBERRY COBBLER (PAGE 280) | 165 |

| SNACKS (3 DAILY) | CALORIES |
|---|---|
| EGGPLANT AND ROASTED RED PEPPER TORTA (PAGE 244) | 183 |
| 6 OUNCES OF SUGAR-FREE FRUIT-FLAVORED YOGURT | 60 |
| TANGERINE, 1 MEDIUM | 47 |
| TOTAL/WOMEN | 1,267 CALORIES |
| MEN: ENJOY A PROTEIN BAR WITH ANY OF THESE 3 SNACKS | 200 |
| TOTAL/MEN | 1,467 CALORIES |

## DAY 14

| BREAKFAST | CALORIES |
|---|---|
| SWEET POTATO AND BLUE CORN EGG CASSEROLE (PAGE 115) | 237 |

| LUNCH | CALORIES |
|---|---|
| RICH BEEF AND NOODLE PHO WITH LIME AND BEAN SPROUTS (PAGE 147) | 172 |

| DINNER | CALORIES |
|---|---|
| NO-BOIL MUSHROOM LASAGNA (PAGE 211) | 388 |
| TOSSED SIDE SALAD WITH REDUCED-FAT DRESSING | 50 |

| SNACKS (3 DAILY) | CALORIES |
|---|---|
| SHRIMP AND CHEDDAR TOSTADA WITH SALSA VERDE (PAGE 250) | 200 |
| FRESH BERRIES, 1 CUP | 50 |
| PITA CHIPS WITH CHARRED EGGPLANT DIP (PAGE 233) | 159 |
| TOTAL/WOMEN | 1,256 CALORIES |
| MEN: ENJOY 1 SERVING OF HOGS UNDERCOVER (PAGE 246) WITH ANY OF THESE 3 SNACKS | 189 |
| TOTAL/MEN | 1,445 CALORIES |

## NOW EAT ON THE GO!

Most of us have insanely hectic lives. Here are some tips to help you fit this plan into a busy lifestyle.

- Make your smoothie on Monday and keep the rest in the fridge for Tuesday or Wednesday. All you have to do is reblend for a few seconds.

- Dishes like the kamut part of my Apple and Cranberry Granola Cereal are great make-ahead meals. Whip it up when you have some spare time. All you have to do for breakfast is add the yogurt or skim milk and enjoy.

- Bake ahead: My muffins, cookies, brownies, and bars can be made ahead and be ready to pack as snacks or in lunches.

- Soup can be made up to a week ahead and frozen.

- Keep a stash of Coconut Cream Mango Pops in the freezer as a grab-and-go snack.

- When you cook, make enough extra food to freeze for another meal. Save time by cooking extra rice, pasta, vegetables, or whatever you are having for your evening meal, so you can use the leftovers either for lunch or as a quicker meal the next evening.

- Stock the freezer with shortcut ingredients such as individually quick frozen (IQF) fruit and vegetables.

- At the supermarket deli, look for rotisserie chicken; then pair it with simple, speedy sides like steamed vegetables, instant brown rice, or a small potato. (Remove the chicken skin prior to serving.)

- Cook items like chicken breasts and brown rice in advance to save time. Wrap the chicken breasts in foil, and place the brown rice in plastic containers. Stored properly like this, these items can keep for several days until you need them.

- Stock up on canned beans. Unlike dried beans, canned beans are presorted, soaked, and cooked, making them a great time-saver. Before using the beans, drain and rinse them—you'll wash away the excess sodium.

- Use varieties of bagged lettuce—try a different type each night—to save time.

- To keep slicing and dicing to a minimum, buy your vegetables precut. Chopped onions, peeled garlic, sliced mushrooms, broccoli slaw, cut kale, and more can be found in the produce section of many supermarkets and of course in the frozen-food section (look for no-salt-added brands).

- Have on hand portable between-meal snacks such as dried fruit, almonds, or a protein bar.

# Shopping Lists

One of the best diet habits practiced by people who've lost weight and kept it off is making shopping lists of healthy foods. So, to make that easy on you, I've put together two weeks of mistake-proof, easy-to-follow, weekly shopping lists. No more wandering the supermarket aisles, trying to figure out what to make for dinner: You'll spend less time at the store and more time enjoying your meals.

### 14-DAY FAST-TRACK PLAN

**SHOPPING LIST
WEEK 1 OF 14-DAY FAST-TRACK PLAN**

PRODUCE
3–4 heads of garlic
1 bunch of scallions
1 tomato
2 red onions
2 yellow onions
2 large Vidalia onions
1 head of romaine lettuce
1 small head of radicchio
Baby arugula (about 3 cups)
2 medium sweet potatoes
Brussels sprouts (about 2 cups)
1 package of mixed green lettuce
2 medium red heirloom tomatoes
1 package of grape tomatoes
1 cucumber
1 Hass avocado
1 medium butternut squash
Bean sprouts (about 2 cups)
1–2 heads of cauliflower

1 large head of broccoli
1 green pepper
1 container of fresh salsa
1 package of baby carrots
2 heads of kale
10 ounces of sliced cremini mushrooms
4 ounces of white button mushrooms
Celery

FRESH HERBS
1 package of tarragon
1 package of rosemary
1 package of chives
2–3 packages of basil
1 package of mint
1 bunch of cilantro
1 bunch of flat-leaf parsley

FRUIT
Fresh fruit to have on hand for snacking: grapefruit,
    apple, pear, plum, orange, tangerines, fresh berries
1 medium navel orange
Cubed seedless watermelon (about 4 cups)
Chopped fresh pineapple (1 cup)
7–8 limes
1 lemon
2 medium ripe bananas
Fresh or frozen mango chunks (about 1 cup)

DRIED FRUIT
1 package of unsweetened dried apples
1 package of dried cranberries
1 package of dried currants

FROZEN FOODS
2 packages of IQF strawberries
2 packages of IQF blueberries
1 package of frozen peas

BAKED GOODS
1 whole wheat baguette
Whole wheat hamburger buns (at least 4)
4 whole wheat split-top hot dog buns, such as
    Matthew's Salad Rolls
1 loaf of thin-sliced European whole-grain bread,
    such as Rubschlager
1 loaf of whole wheat bread

8 (6-inch) low-carb tortillas, such as La Tortilla Factory

DAIRY
3 (32-ounce) cartons of liquid egg substitute
1 carton of reduced-fat sour cream, such as
    Breakstone's
1 package of 2% reduced-fat-milk cheese, such as
    Borden's 2% Milk Reduced Fat Sharp Singles
1 package 75% reduced-fat cheddar, such as Cabot
2 packages shredded 50% reduced-fat cheddar, such
    as Cabot
1 package shredded reduced-fat mozzarella
6 large eggs
1 stick unsalted butter
At least 60 ounces (10 cartons, 6 ounces each) of
    Greek yogurt, such as Fage Total
2 quarts and 1 pint of skim milk
Reduced-fat ricotta cheese, such as Sargento (3
    cups)
2 ounces of goat cheese
Bocconcini (8 ounces)
3 cartons of grated Parmigiano-Reggiano cheese
8 ounces (1 block) of reduced-fat cream cheese

**MEAT, FISH, POULTRY**
MEAT
16 ounces 90% lean ground beef
1 (1-pound) piece plus 8 ounces of lean beef
    tenderloin
1 pound of lean pork tenderloin
8 slices (about 6 ounces) of high-quality deli ham
1 package of Canadian bacon
2 ounces of reduced-fat chorizo sausage, such as
    Wellshire Farms

FISH
Smoked salmon (at least 3 ounces)
4 (4-ounce) salmon fillets
2 sushi-grade tuna steaks (6 ounces each)
1 pound of large shrimp, peeled and deveined

POULTRY
1 pound of chicken tenders
6 ounces (about 2 cups) of chopped skinless breast
    meat from a rotisserie or roast chicken
1 pound of fresh or completely thawed boneless,
    skinless turkey breast, trimmed of all visible fat

## CANNED/PACKAGED GOODS

Kalamata olives
1 (12-ounce) can of evaporated skim milk
Light or reduced-fat coconut milk (8 ounces)
3 (15.5-ounce) cans of white cannellini beans
1 (15.5 ounce) can of black beans
1 (15.5 ounce) can of red beans
1 small can of beets (at least ½ cup)
1 can of peeled plum tomatoes (at least 1 cup)
1 jar of unsweetened applesauce
1 bottle of apple cider
½ cup (about 3.5 ounces) of jarred fried peppers,
    such as Cento Sautéed Sweet Peppers with onions,
    roughly chopped
1 cup (about 7 ounces) of jarred roasted red pepper
    strips (not oil packed), such as Cento
1 jar of reduced-fat peanut butter, such as Better'n
    Peanut Butter
1 jar of no-sugar added cranberry sauce, such as
    Steel's Gourmet Agave Cranberry Sauce
Plenty of low-fat, low-sodium chicken broth (at least
    136 ounces, or 4¼ quarts)

## CEREALS/GRAINS/PASTA

1 box of puffed millet cereal, such as Arrowhead
    Mills
1 box of puffed kamut, such as Arrowhead Mills
1 box of quick-cooking oatmeal
16 ounces of tofu shirataki noodles, such as House
    Foods
1 package of brown rice (uncooked)
1 package of whole wheat elbow macaroni
1 package of whole wheat rigatoni pasta, such as
    Bionaturae Organic
1–2 packages of whole wheat panko bread crumbs,
    such as Ian's All-Natural

## BAKING NEEDS

1 package of mini chocolate chunks
Bittersweet (60%–70%) chocolate (at least 1 ounce)
1 package of peanut butter chips
1 package of minimarshmallows
Apple juice concentrate
1 package of sliced almonds
1 package of toasted walnuts
1 package of toasted pine nuts
Whole wheat pastry flour

## OTHER

Matcha green tea powder
Hormel Real Bacon Bits
Sugar-free chocolate syrup, such as Fox's U-bet
Malted milk powder, such as Carnation
Whey protein powder, such as Designer Whey
1 packet (3 grams) of sugar-free strawberry drink
    mix, such as Crystal Light
1 packet (2 grams) of sugar-free raspberry drink
    mix, such as Crystal Light
1 package of graham crackers
1 small jar of espresso powder
1 bottle of calorie-free pancake syrup, such as
    Walden Farms
Protein bars

---

**SHOPPING LIST
WEEK 2 OF 14-DAY FAST-TRACK PLAN**

---

You may have leftover ingredients from week 1, so please
check your supplies.

## PRODUCE

2 vine-ripened tomatoes
2 medium red heirloom tomatoes
1 head of romaine lettuce
2 heads of Boston lettuce
1 pound of haricots verts or slim green beans
2 yellow onions
1 medium red onion
3 to 4 heads of garlic
3 heads of kale
1 package of baby carrots
1 Hass avocado
1 large head of broccoli
1 small eggplant
1 medium eggplant
1 large eggplant
1 pound of sliced white button mushrooms
1 bunch of shallots
3 medium sweet potatoes
2 cups Brussels sprouts
1 large russet potato
1 large head of cauliflower
4 medium red beets
6 ounces (about 4 cups) of baby arugula
Bean sprouts (about 2 cups)

10 ounces of sliced cremini mushrooms
4 ounces of white button mushrooms

FRESH HERBS

1 bunch of fresh cilantro
1 bunch of flat-leaf parsley
1 package of fresh dill
1 package of fresh rosemary
1 package of fresh chives
1 (1-inch) knob of fresh ginger
1 package of fresh oregano
1 package of fresh basil
1 package of fresh mint

FRUIT

Fresh or frozen blueberries (enough for 1½ cups)
Fruit for snacking: pear, nectarine, tangerine, fresh
   berries
1 medium navel orange
2 medium ripe bananas
1 cup of fresh or frozen mango chunks
4–6 fresh limes
3–4 lemons
2 medium Granny Smith apples
4 cups of cubed seedless watermelon
1 cup of chopped fresh pineapple
2 cups of fresh strawberries, hulled and quartered
5 golden delicious apples

DRIED FRUIT

1 package of raisins
1 package of dried cranberries

FROZEN FOODS

1 package of frozen peas
1 package of IQF cherries

BAKED GOODS

4 whole wheat hamburger buns
8 pieces of stale thin-sliced European whole-grain
   bread, such as Rubschlager
4 whole wheat, split-top hot dog buns, such as
   Matthew's Salad Rolls
Package of whole wheat English muffins (at least 4)
8 (9-inch) low-carb tortillas, such as La Tortilla
   Factory
Leftover whole wheat bread

DAIRY

2 (32-ounce) cartons of liquid egg substitute
1 dozen eggs
1 quart plus 1 pint of skim milk
1 carton of reduced-fat sour cream, such as Breakstone's
4 (6-ounce) cartons of 2% Greek yogurt, such as
   Fage Total
2 (6-ounce) cartons of nonfat Greek yogurt, such as
   Fage Total
6 ounces of sugar-free fruit-flavored yogurt
1 pint of low-fat buttermilk
4 slices (about ½ ounce each) of cheddar cheese
1 package of shredded 50% reduced-fat cheddar,
   such as Cabot
2 packages of shredded 75% reduced-fat cheddar,
   such as Cabot
2 packages of part-skim shredded mozzarella
4 slices of 2% reduced-fat cheese, such as Borden's
   2% Milk Reduced Fat Sharp Singles
1 carton of crumbled reduced-fat blue cheese, such
   as Treasure Cave
2 cups of reduced-fat ricotta cheese, such as
   Sargento
2 cartons of grated Parmigiano-Reggiano cheese
1 small jar of Romano cheese
Crumbled goat cheese (2 ounces, or about ½ cup)

MEAT, FISH, POULTRY
MEAT

4 pieces (about 2.5 ounces) of Canadian bacon
1 (1-pound) piece plus 8 ounces of lean beef tenderloin
8 thinly cut pork chops (about 2 pounds), trimmed of
   all visible fat

FISH

8 ounces of cod fillet
30 ounces of canned albacore tuna, packed in
   water, drained
¾ pound of large shrimp, peeled and deveined, tails
   removed
¾ pound of precooked large shrimp, peeled and
   deveined, tails removed

POULTRY

8 skinless, boneless chicken breasts
1 pound of skinless, boneless chicken breasts, cut
   into medium-size chunks

12 ounces of lean ground turkey breast

7 ounces (about 2 cups) of shredded skinless breast meat from a rotisserie or roast chicken

2 sweet Italian chicken and turkey sausages, such as Applegate Farms

## CANNED/PACKAGED GOODS

1 small can of beets (at least ½ cup)

1 (15.5-ounce) can of red beans

2 (15.5-ounce) cans of white beans such as cannellini

2 (12-ounce) cans of evaporated skim milk

1 jar of no-sugar-added apple butter

1 jar of sugar-free apricot preserves, such as Smucker's

2 jars of low-fat marinara sauce, such as Victoria or Trader Joe's

1 jar of tomatillo salsa

1 can of whole plum tomatoes (at least 1 cup)

1 jar of roasted red peppers, such as Cento Roasted Peppers

## CEREALS/GRAINS/PASTA

1 package of whole wheat rotini, such as Ronzoni Healthy Harvest

1 package of whole wheat fettuccine

1 box of quick-cooking oatmeal

16 ounces of tofu shirataki noodles, such as House Foods

4 ounces (about 8 sheets) of no-bake whole wheat lasagna noodles, such as DeLallo

1 box of toasted whole-grain oat cereal, such as Cheerios

1 box of puffed millet

1 package of brown rice, uncooked

## BAKING NEEDS

1 package of toasted sliced almonds

18 almonds, whole, dry roasted

12 walnut halves

1 package of chopped walnuts

8 ounces of light or reduced-fat coconut milk

2 ounces plus more bittersweet (60%) chocolate

1 package of mini chocolate chunks

## OTHER

1–2 bottles of calorie-free pancake syrup, such as Walden Farms

84 ounces (2–3 quarts) of low-fat, low-sodium chicken broth

Hormel Real Bacon Bits

12 ounces of silken tofu, such as Nasoya

Bisquick Heart Smart Baking Mix

4 ounces of baked blue corn chips, such as Guiltless Gourmet

4 ounces of whole wheat baked pita chips, such as 365 Everyday Value

6 ounces of whole wheat pizza dough, from page 166 or such as Papa Sal's

Protein bars

## SHOPPING LIST—STAPLES

2–3 bottles of agave nectar

Adobo powder

Almond extract

Baking powder

Baking soda

Balsamic vinegar

Banana extract

Bay leaves

Black peppercorns

Butter-flavored nonstick cooking spray and nonstick cooking spray

Canola oil

Cayenne pepper

2 boxes of cocoa powder, unsweetened

Coconut extract

Cornstarch

Cinnamon, ground

Crushed red pepper

Cumin

Dijon mustard

Extra-virgin olive oil

Fat-free mayonnaise

Garlic powder

Garlic-chili sauce, such as Huy Fong

Light soy sauce

Mild curry powder

Molasses

Natural red food coloring

No-sugar-added sweet relish, such as Mt. Olive

Nutmeg, whole

Onion powder

Poultry seasoning, such as the Spice Hunter

Powdered stevia, such as SweetLeaf

Red pepper flakes

Red wine vinegar

2 bottles of reduced-fat vinaigrette, such as Ken's
Light Options Olive Oil and Vinegar

1–2 bottles of reduced-sugar ketchup, such as Heinz

Salt

Turbinado sugar, such as Sugar in thē Raw

Vanilla extract

Yellow curry paste, such as Karee

## Now What?

Once you've reached the end of the 14-Day Fast-Track Plan, move on to the Now Eat This! Lifestyle Plan and follow it right down to your ideal weight. You'll eat more calories each day and continue to choose from my selection of breakfasts, lunches, dinners, desserts, and snacks.

One more thing: Be prepared to answer people when they see that you're losing weight. Expect them to ask what diet you're on and what you get to eat.

You won't be telling them celery and diet shakes. Or those puffed-rice cakes that taste like foam takeout containers. You'll be telling them you eat almost everything and anything—just not all in one sitting like you used to. As you've already discovered, not much is off-limits—except for puffed-rice cakes, celery, and diet shakes.

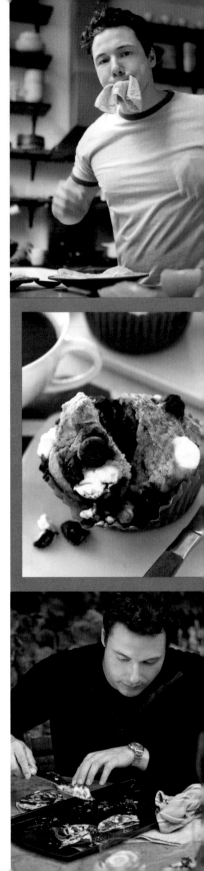

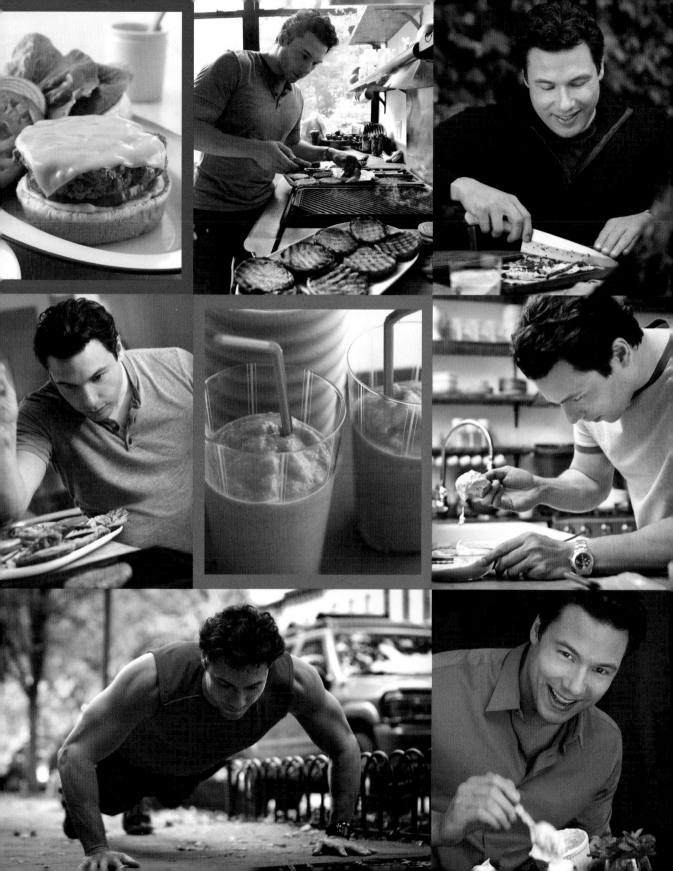

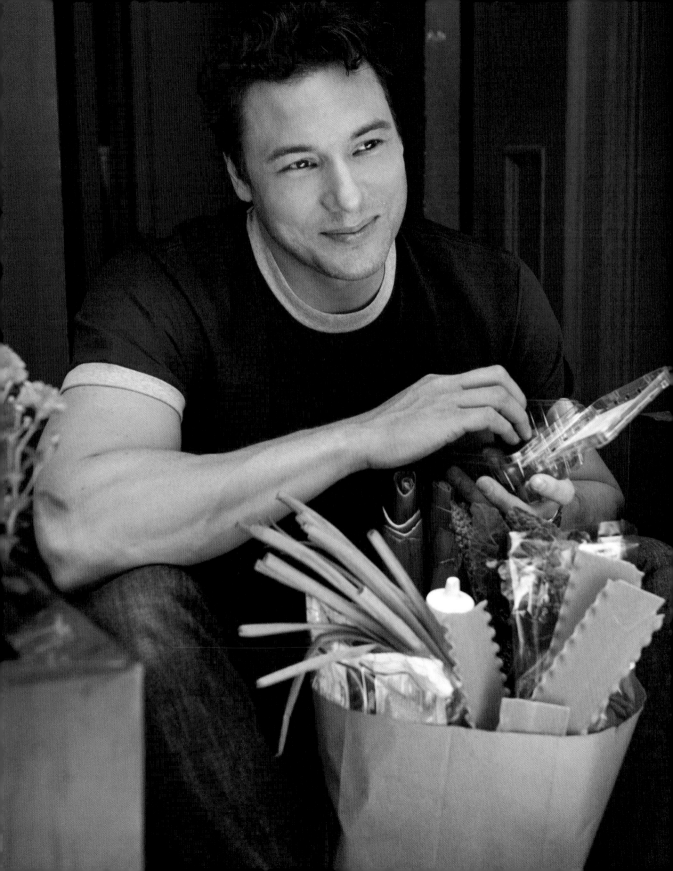

chapter

# 4

☺

# The Now Eat This! Lifestyle Plan

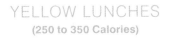

Time to talk: How did you do on the 14-Day Fast-Track Plan? What are your impressions of this new way of eating and dieting? Did you enjoy it? Are your clothes looser? Do you feel lighter?

I'm willing to bet your answers are all positive.

See? Easy—wasn't it?

You're getting the hang of my style of "dieting": a way to lose weight that feels good and tastes good. I bet you're seeing the proof in the mirror and on the scale.

Now that you've completed the 14-Day Fast-Track Plan, you're ready to continue with the Now Eat This! Lifestyle Plan. It's more liberal than the Fast-Track Plan. It increases your calories but still lets you burn off 1 to 3 pounds a week. And it gives you a foundation for a happy, healthy lifestyle.

## Day 15 and Beyond

Continue to mix and match your meals and snacks from the recipes in this book. Once again, use the recipe color codes and aim for approximately 1,400 (women) to 1,600 (men) calories a day. You should stay on this plan until you reach your best possible weight. This plan is simple and helps you automatically take in the amount of nutrients you need each day for steady weight loss. Here's how to get started:

## Planning a 1,400-Calorie Day (Women)

To my women readers: Now you can eat 1,400 calories a day. Let's look at how to plan your menus.

### YELLOW BREAKFASTS
(250 to 350 Calories)

Each morning, you'll want to eat between 250 and 350 calories. You have many options, from smoothies to baked egg dishes. Have a different breakfast every day, or stick to a few breakfasts you love.

- Any of my smoothies—Strawberry Protein Punch Smoothie (page 103), Green Tea Watermelon Super Punch (page 109), Ginger Peach Lassie (page 105), or Blueberry Vanilla Smoothie (page 107)—supplemented

with 2 slices of whole wheat toast and 1 tablespoon of all-fruit jam, or one of my muffins—a Banana Walnut Muffin (page 278) or a Blueberry Cream Muffin (page 271)

- Pizza Egg Bake (page 121)

- Apple and Cranberry Granola Cereal (page 123)

- Sunrise Sandwich (page 126)

- Cherry Red Oatmeal (page 129)

- Blue on Blueberry Silver Dollar Pancakes (page 130)

- French Toast à L'Orange (page 133)

- Rocky Road Oatmeal (page 134)

- South of the Border Scramble with Chorizo and Salsa (page 137)

- Blueberry Graham Cheesecake Oatmeal (page 138)

### GENERIC BREAKFAST SUGGESTIONS

- 1 cup of high-fiber cereal (such as All-Bran) with ½ cup of soy milk and a sliced fresh peach (Look for unsweetened cereal with at least 5 grams of fiber per serving.)

- 1 toasted whole wheat English muffin, 6 ounces of Greek yogurt, and 1 sliced fresh pear

- 1 cereal bar, 6 ounces of nonfat Greek yogurt, and 1 cup of fresh berries

- 2 slices of whole-grain toast, 2 tablespoons of reduced-fat cream cheese, 2 ounces of lox, and 1 medium orange

- 6 ounces of Greek yogurt mixed with 1 cup of high-fiber cereal and 1 cup of blueberries

### YELLOW LUNCHES
(250 to 350 Calories)

Stick to around 250 to 350 calories for lunch. Again, have a different lunch every day, or choose from a few you love. Use my lunch recipes to help you plan. Several of my snacks make delicious lunches, too. I've included other lunches that will fit your calorie budget on this plan.

- Any 250-to-350-calorie dinner as leftovers: Roast Beef with Brussels Sprouts and Balsamic Jus (page 179) with Garlic Mashed Potatoes (page 221), Lemon

Pepper Shrimp (page 185), Ginger Sweet Chicken and Broccoli Stir-Fry (page 186), Spicy-Sweet Linguine alla Vodka (page 189), or Turkey Dinner with All the Trimmings (page 191)

- A salad such as Mediterranean Tuna, Bread, and Cheese Salad (page 157) or Boston Blue Chicken and Apple Salad (page 160)

- A soup such as Beef and Orzo Soup (page 159) or Yellow Curry Shrimp and Green Pea Soup (page 162)

- Faux-Fried Filet o' Fish Sandwich (page 164)

- Individual Crispy "Loaded" Pizza (page 166)

- Chicken and Mushroom Quesadilla (page 171)

- Grilled Cheese and Ham (page 173)

- Chicken Tenders with Ranch Dressing (page 248) with a Decadent Lemon Bar (page 259) for dessert

- Shrimp and Cheddar Tostada with Salsa Verde (page 250) with a Red Velvet Chocolate Square (page 263) for dessert

- Pita Chips with Charred Eggplant Dip (page 233)—this is a great packable lunch; pack some sliced cucumbers for dipping and 2 Double Chocolate Chip Cookies (page 256) for dessert

- South of the Border Loaded Potato Skins (page 234) with a Chocolate Malted Milk Shake (page 269) for dessert

## GENERIC LUNCH SUGGESTIONS

- Brown-bag turkey sandwich: 2 slices of light whole wheat bread, 2 ounces of turkey breast, 1 teaspoon of light mayonnaise, tomato slices, lettuce or baby spinach leaves, and 1 teaspoon of mustard

- Brown-bag tuna sandwich: 3 ounces of tuna mixed with 1 tablespoon of fat-free mayonnaise on 2 slices of whole wheat bread; 1 sliced fresh tomato

- Vegetarian sandwich: 2 slices of whole wheat bread, ¼ of an avocado, mashed, a 1-ounce slice of Swiss or Jarlsberg cheese, alfalfa sprouts, and tomato slices

- Vegetable salad: 2–3 cups of mixed salad greens with tomatoes, mushrooms, onions, beets, ½ cup of chickpeas, and 1 tablespoon of light Italian dressing, and 1 piece of fruit, such as an orange, an apple, or a pear, or 1 cup of berries

- Pita sandwich: 2 ounces of turkey breast, 1 whole wheat pita pocket, ½ cup of sprouts (alfalfa or broccoli), ¼ cup of chopped tomato, and 2 teaspoons of mustard

- ½ cup of prepared hummus spread on 1 whole wheat tortilla, and 1 medium peach

## BLUE DINNERS
### (350 to 450 Calories)

Here are dinner suggestions that weigh in at 350 to 450 calories. Have a different one every day, or to save time through the week, cook in bulk and enjoy leftovers for lunch or dinner the next day. When there's caloric room, add a dessert to your dinner.

- Crispy-on-the-Top Tuna and Green Pea Casserole (page 203)

- Grilled Salmon with Curried Cauliflower (page 205)

- Fettucine Alfredo with Shrimp (page 207)

- Chicken Pesto Pasta (page 208)

- No-Boil Mushroom Lasagna (page 211)

- BBQ Pork Chops (page 212)

- Mac and Cheese with Ham and Broccoli (page 215)

- Sautéed Steak with Mushrooms (page 195) with Garlic Mashed Potatoes (page 221)

- Spicy-Sweet Linguine alla Vodka (page 189) with a Red Velvet Chocolate Square (page 263) for dessert

- Flash-Fried Chicken "Carnitas" (page 181) with a Coconut Cream Mango Pop (page 267) for dessert

- Roasted Pork Tenderloin with Butternut Squash Mash and Tarragon Gravy (page 199) with an Oatmeal Raisin Cookie (page 261) for dessert

- Ginger Sweet Chicken and Broccoli Stir-Fry (page 186) with a Fudgy Fruit and Nut Bar (page 265) for dessert

- Lemon Pepper Shrimp (page 185) with a Coconut Cream Mango Pop (page 267) for dessert

- Roast Beef with Brussels Sprouts and Balsamic Jus (page 179) with Any Berry Parfait for dessert (page 273)

## SNACKS

With breakfast, lunch, and dinner on this plan, you've used around 1,000 calories so far. That leaves you a full 400 calories for snacks. Try to incorporate 3 snacks in your meal planning each day. Here are some ideas:

## SNACKS
### (150 to 250 Calories)

NOW EAT THIS! SNACKS
Curried Chicken Skewers (page 230)
Pita Chips with Charred Eggplant Dip (page 233)
South of the Border Loaded Potato Skins (page 234)
Tuna Croquettes with Dill Relish (page 236)
Crunchy Tomato Bread (page 238)
Green Tea Watermelon Super Punch (page 109)
"Fried" Cheese Balls (page 241)
Mama's Mini Meatball Bites (page 242)
Eggplant and Roasted Red Pepper Torta (page 244)
Hogs Undercover (page 246)
Chicken Tenders with Ranch Dressing (page 248)
Shrimp and Cheddar Tostada with Salsa Verde (page 250)

FRUIT
Cantaloupe, ½ medium
Navel orange, 1 large
Grapes, 1 medium bunch
Prunes, ½ cup stewed, unsweetened

NUTS
Macadamia nuts, 7
Pecans, 20
Pistachios, shelled, 45

OTHER SNACKS
Any protein bar between 150 and 250 calories

NOW EAT THIS! SNACKS
Decadent Lemon Bar (page 259)
Oatmeal Raisin Cookie (page 261)
Red Velvet Chocolate Square (page 263)
Fudgy Fruit and Nut Bar (page 265)
Coconut Cream Mango Pops (page 267)
Chocolate Malted Milk Shake (page 269)
Chicken and Cheese Poppers (page 223)
Spicy Fried Calamari with Cherry Tomato Dipping Sauce (page 225)
Blueberry Cream Muffins (page 271)
Any Berry Parfait (page 273)

FRUIT AND DRIED FRUIT
Apple, 1 medium
Apricots, dried, 8 halves
Banana, 1 medium
Berries, 1 cup
Figs, dried, 3
Grapes, 1 cup
Guava, 1 cup diced
Mango, 1 cup diced
Orange, 1 medium
Papaya, 1 cup diced
Pear, 1 medium
Pineapple, 1 cup diced
Raisins, 1-ounce package

NUTS
Almonds, dry roasted, 20
Brazil nuts, 6
Cashews, dry roasted, 16
Mixed nuts, dry roasted, 15
Peanuts, dry roasted, 25

OTHER SNACKS
Carrot juice, 1 cup
V8 V-Fusion, 1 cup
6 ounces of yogurt (plain, nonfat, or sugar-free, fruit flavored)

## SNACKS
### (75 to 150 Calories)

NOW EAT THIS! SMOOTHIES
Strawberry Protein Punch Smoothie (page 103)
Ginger Peach Lassie (page 105)
Blueberry Vanilla Smoothie (page 107)

## SNACKS
**(under 75 Calories)**

NOW EAT THIS! SNACK
**PBJ Cookies (page 254)**
**Double Chocolate Chip Cookies (page 256)**

FRUITS
**Apricots, 2 medium**
**Cherries, 8**
**Grapefruit, ½**
**Kiwi, 1 medium**
**Nectarine, 1 medium**
**Peach, 1 medium**
**Tangerine, 1 medium**
**Watermelon, 1 thick slice**

OTHER SNACK CHOICES
**Baby carrots, 8**
**Fresh, cut-up veggies, unlimited amounts**

# Sample 1,400-Calorie Menu

Here's what a typical menu might look like if you mix and match your meals from the color-coded lists.

| BREAKFAST | CALORIES |
|---|---|
| ROCKY ROAD OATMEAL (PAGE 134) | 327 |
| LUNCH | CALORIES |
| BROWN-BAG TUNA SANDWICH | 300 |
| DINNER | CALORIES |
| CHICKEN PESTO PASTA (PAGE 208) | 385 |
| SNACKS (3 DAILY) | CALORIES |
| HOGS UNDERCOVER (PAGE 246) | 189 |
| PEAR, 1 MEDIUM | 96 |
| CHOCOLATE MALTED MILK SHAKE (PAGE 269) | 126 |
| TOTAL | 1,423 CALORIES |

# Your Daily Menu Planner

Plan your meals using the following worksheet. Using the meal lists, simply fill in what you will eat each day. Planning your meals can help you stay on track.

| BREAKFAST: | |
|---|---|
| LUNCH: | |
| DINNER: | |
| SNACK 1: | |
| SNACK 2: | |
| SNACK 3: | |
| TOTAL | 1,400 CALORIES |

# Planning a 1,600-Calorie Day (Men)

On the Lifestyle Plan, men should bump up their calories to 1,600. Here's how to do the planning:

## YELLOW BREAKFASTS
(250 to 350 Calories)

## OR

## BLUE BREAKFASTS
(350 to 450 Calories)

Each morning, aim to eat a breakfast of around 250 to 450 calories. Here are some examples:

- Sunrise Sandwich (page 126) with ½ grapefruit
- Blue on Blueberry Silver Dollar Pancakes (page 130)
- French Toast à L'Orange (page 133)
- Creamy Stuffed Crepes with Orange Butter Syrup (page 117) with a cup of fresh berries
- Rocky Road Oatmeal (page 134)
- Blueberry Graham Cheesecake Oatmeal (page 138)

- South of the Border Scramble with Chorizo and Salsa (page 137)

- Strawberry Malted Belgian Waffles (page 141)

- Pepper, Onion, and Goat Cheese Frittata (page 111) with 2 slices of whole wheat toast

- 2 Blueberry Cream Muffins (page 271) or 2 Banana Walnut Muffins (page 278) and 2 scrambled egg whites

- Green Tea Watermelon Super Punch (page 109) and 1 whole wheat English muffin

### GENERIC BREAKFAST SUGGESTIONS

- 1 cup of shredded wheat with bran, 1 cup of low-fat milk, 1 sliced banana

- 2 scrambled egg whites, 2 slices of turkey bacon, 2 slices of whole wheat toast, 1 cup of fresh berries

## YELLOW LUNCHES
### (250 to 350 Calories)

## OR

## BLUE LUNCHES
### (350 to 450 calories)

Again, have a different lunch every day, or stick to a few you love. Use my lunch recipes to help you plan. I've included other lunches that will fit your calorie budget on this plan. Here are some examples:

- Any **BLUE** dinner as leftovers such as: Crispy-on-the-Top Tuna and Green Pea Casserole (page 203), Fettuccine Alfredo with Shrimp (page 207), Chicken Pesto Pasta (page 208), No-Boil Mushroom Lasagna (page 211), or Mac and Cheese with Ham and Broccoli (page 215)

- Mediterranean Tuna, Bread, and Cheese Salad (page 157) with a Chocolate Malted Milk Shake (page 269) for dessert

- Beef and Orzo Soup (page 159) with an Oatmeal Raisin Cookie (page 261) for dessert

- Faux-Fried Filet o' Fish Sandwich (page 164)

- Individual Crispy "Loaded" Pizza (page 166)

- Chicken and Mushroom Quesadilla (page 171)

- Grilled Cheese and Ham (page 173)

- Shrimp and Cheddar Tostada with Salsa Verde (page 250) and Mexican Corn (page 229)

- Spinach and Bacon Salad (page 151) and a Coconut Cream Mango Pop (page 267) for dessert

- Yellow Curry Shrimp and Green Pea Soup (page 162) with a Decadent Lemon Bar (page 259) for dessert

- Yes, a Cheeseburger! (page 175)

### GENERIC LUNCH SUGGESTIONS

- Brown-bag turkey sandwich: 2 slices of light whole wheat bread, 2 ounces of turkey breast, 1 teaspoon of light mayonnaise, tomato slices, lettuce or baby spinach leaves, 1 teaspoon of mustard, and 1 medium pear

- Brown-bag tuna sandwich: 3 ounces of tuna mixed with 1 tablespoon of fat-free mayonnaise on 2 slices of whole wheat bread, 1 sliced fresh tomato, and 1 medium apple

- Vegetarian sandwich: 2 slices of whole wheat bread, ¼ of an avocado, mashed, a 1-ounce slice of Swiss or Jarlsberg cheese, alfalfa sprouts and tomato slices, and 1 cup of fresh berries

- Pita sandwich: 2 ounces of turkey breast, 1 whole wheat pita pocket, ½ cup of sprouts (alfalfa or broccoli), ¼ cup of chopped tomato, 2 teaspoons of mustard, and 1 banana

## BLUE DINNERS
### (350 to 450 Calories)

Here are dinner suggestions that range from 350 to 450 calories. Have a different one every day, or to save time through the week, cook in bulk and enjoy leftovers for lunch or dinner the next day. When there's caloric room, add a dessert to your dinner.

- Crispy-on-the-Top Tuna and Green Pea Casserole (page 203)

- Grilled Salmon with Curried Cauliflower (page 205)

- Fettuccine Alfredo with Shrimp (page 207)

- Chicken Pesto Pasta (page 208)
- No-Boil Mushroom Lasagna (page 211)
- BBQ Pork Chops (page 212)
- Mac and Cheese with Ham and Broccoli (page 215)
- Sautéed Steak with Mushrooms (page 195) with Garlic Mashed Potatoes (page 221)
- Spicy-Sweet Linguine alla Vodka (page 189) with a Decadent Lemon Bar (page 259) for dessert
- Turkey Dinner with All the Trimmings (page 191) with a Red Velvet Chocolate Square (page 263)
- Flash-Fried Chicken "Carnitas" (page 181) with a Coconut Cream Mango Pop (page 267) for dessert
- Roasted Pork Tenderloin with Butternut Squash Mash and Tarragon Gravy (page 199) with a PBJ Cookie (page 254) for dessert
- Ginger Sweet Chicken and Broccoli Stir-Fry (page 186) with a Fudgy Fruit and Nut Bar (page 265) for dessert
- Lemon Pepper Shrimp (page 185) with a Coconut Cream Mango Pop (page 267) for dessert
- Roast Beef with Brussels Sprouts and Balsamic Jus (page 179) with Chocolate Fondue (page 284) for dessert

## SNACKS

With breakfast, lunch, and dinner on this plan, you've used around 1,000 calories so far. That leaves you a full 400 calories for snacks. Try to incorporate 3 snacks in your meal planning each day. Here are some ideas:

## SNACKS
### (150 to 250 Calories)

NOW EAT THIS! SMOOTHIES
Green Tea Watermelon Super Punch (page 109)

NOW EAT THIS! SNACKS
Curried Chicken Skewers (page 230)
Pita Chips with Charred Eggplant Dip (page 233)
South of the Border Loaded Potato Skins (page 234)
Tuna Croquettes with Dill Relish (page 236)
Crunchy Tomato Bread (page 238)

"Fried" Cheese Balls (page 241)
Mama's Mini Meatball Bites (page 242)
Eggplant and Roasted Red Pepper Torta (page 244)
Hogs Undercover (page 246)
Chicken Tenders with Ranch Dressing (page 248)
Shrimp and Cheddar Tostada with Salsa Verde (page 250)

FRUIT AND DRIED FRUIT
Cantaloupe, ½ medium
Navel orange, 1 large
Grapes, 1 medium bunch
Prunes, ¾ cup, unsweetened

NUTS
Macadamia nuts, 7
Pecans, 20
Pistachios, shelled, 45

OTHER SNACKS
Any protein bar between 150 and 250 calories

## SNACKS
### (75 to 150 Calories)

NOW EAT THIS! SMOOTHIES
Strawberry Protein Punch Smoothie (page 103)
Ginger Peach Lassie (page 105)
Blueberry Vanilla Smoothie (page 107)

NOW EAT THIS! SNACKS
Decadent Lemon Bars (page 259)
Oatmeal Raisin Cookies (page 261)
Red Velvet Chocolate Squares (page 263)
Fudgy Fruit and Nut Bars (page 265)
Coconut Cream Mango Pops (page 267)
Chocolate Malted Milk Shake (page 269)
Chicken and Cheese Poppers (page 223)
Spicy Fried Calamari with Cherry Tomato Dipping Sauce (page 225)
Blueberry Cream Muffins (page 271)
Any Berry Parfait (page 273)

FRUIT AND DRIED FRUIT
Apple, 1 medium
Apricots, dried, 8 halves

Banana, 1 medium
Berries, 1 cup
Figs, dried, 3
Grapes, 1 cup
Guava, 1 cup diced
Mango, 1 cup diced
Orange, 1 medium
Papaya, 1 cup diced
Pear, 1 medium
Pineapple, 1 cup diced
Raisins, 1-ounce package

NUTS

Almonds, dry roasted, 20
Brazil nuts, 6
Cashews, dry roasted, 16
Mixed nuts, dry roasted, 15
Peanuts, dry roasted, 25

OTHER SNACKS

Carrot juice, 1 cup
V8 V-Fusion, 1 cup
6 ounces of yogurt (plain, nonfat, or sugar-free,
    fruit flavored)

## SNACKS
**(under 75 Calories)**

NOW EAT THIS! SNACKS
**PBJ Cookies (page 254)**
**Double Chocolate Chip Cookies (page 256)**

FRUITS
**Apricots, 2 medium**
**Cherries, 8**
**Grapefruit, ½**
**Kiwi, 1 medium**
**Nectarine, 1 medium**
**Peach, 1 medium**
**Tangerine, 1 medium**
**Watermelon, 1 thick slice**

OTHER SNACK CHOICES
**Baby carrots, 8**
**Fresh, cut-up veggies, unlimited amounts**

# Sample 1,600-Calorie Menu

Here's what a typical menu might look like if you mix and match your meals from the color-coded lists.

| BREAKFAST | CALORIES |
|---|---|
| STRAWBERRY MALTED BELGIAN WAFFLES (PAGE 141) | 375 |
| **LUNCH** | **CALORIES** |
| YES, A CHEESEBURGER! (PAGE 175) | 368 |
| **DINNER** | **CALORIES** |
| GRILLED SALMON WITH CURRIED CAULIFLOWER (PAGE 205) | 367 |
| RED VELVET CHOCOLATE SQUARE (PAGE 263) FOR DESSERT | 106 |
| **SNACKS (3 DAILY)** | **CALORIES** |
| CHICKEN AND CHEESE POPPERS (PAGE 223) | 133 |
| DOUBLE CHOCOLATE CHIP COOKIE (PAGE 256) | 74 |
| ALMONDS, DRY ROASTED, 24 | 170 |
| TOTAL | 1,593 CALORIES |

# Your Daily Menu Planner

Plan your meals using the following worksheet. Using the meal lists, simply fill in what you will eat each day. Planning your meals can help you stay on track.

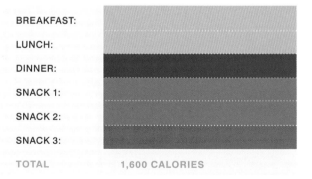

| BREAKFAST: | |
|---|---|
| LUNCH: | |
| DINNER: | |
| SNACK 1: | |
| SNACK 2: | |
| SNACK 3: | |
| TOTAL | 1,600 CALORIES |

# The Now Eat This! Lifestyle Plan—Sample Menus

If you'd rather not do much meal planning, follow my sample menus below. They give you two weeks full of delicious high-protein, moderate-carb, and moderate-fat meals. Foods rich in protein give your metabolism a boost, and that equates to improved ability to burn calories and build lean muscle. Another plus: Protein is the one to thank for that full and satisfied feeling that lasts and lasts. Carbs are the high-fiber, slow-digesting variety, with foods such as whole-grain bread, oatmeal, whole-grain cereals, and brown rice. Fruits and high-volume vegetables are featured heavily. The majority of fats are healthy fats from sources such as salmon, tuna, and olive oil.

It's a good idea to plan ahead, do your grocery shopping, and have everything on hand. This helps reinforce the idea of looking at your diet not just in terms of a single meal, but of at least a week's worth of meals. This plan is simple and helps you automatically take in the amount of nutrients you need each day for steady weight loss.

| DAY 1 | |
|---|---|
| **BREAKFAST** | **CALORIES** |
| SCRAMBLED EGGS WITH SMOKED SALMON ON TOAST | 214 |
| GRAPEFRUIT, ½ MEDIUM | 50 |
| **LUNCH** | **CALORIES** |
| YES, A CHEESEBURGER! | 368 |
| **DINNER** | **CALORIES** |
| ROAST BEEF WITH BRUSSELS SPROUTS AND BALSAMIC JUS | 246 |
| CRUNCHY TOMATO BREAD | 168 |
| TOSSED MIXED-GREENS SALAD WITH REDUCED-FAT SALAD DRESSING | 50 |
| **SNACKS (3 DAILY)** | **CALORIES** |
| DOUBLE CHOCOLATE CHIP COOKIE | 74 |
| APPLE, 1 MEDIUM | 90 |
| RED VELVET CHOCOLATE SQUARE | 106 |

| | |
|---|---|
| **TOTAL/WOMEN** | **1,366 CALORIES** |
| MEN: ENJOY CHICKEN TENDERS WITH RANCH DRESSING, WITH ANY OF THE 3 SNACKS ABOVE | 198 |
| **TOTAL/MEN** | **1,564 CALORIES** |

| DAY 2 | |
|---|---|
| **BREAKFAST** | **CALORIES** |
| TOASTED WHOLE WHEAT ENGLISH MUFFIN | 150 |
| 6-OUNCE CARTON NONFAT GREEK YOGURT | 90 |
| PEAR, 1 MEDIUM | 96 |
| **LUNCH** | **CALORIES** |
| BACON LETTUCE TOMATO ROLL | 245 |
| DOUBLE CHOCOLATE CHIP COOKIE | 74 |
| **DINNER** | **CALORIES** |
| ROASTED PORK TENDERLOIN WITH BUTTERNUT SQUASH MASH AND TARRAGON GRAVY | 343 |
| CHOCOLATE CRÈME BRÛLÉE | 158 |
| **SNACKS (3 DAILY)** | **CALORIES** |
| COCONUT CREAM MANGO POP | 115 |
| ORANGE, 1 MEDIUM | 70 |
| CHOCOLATE MALTED MILK SHAKE | 126 |
| **TOTAL/WOMEN** | **1,467 CALORIES** |
| MEN: ENJOY A PROTEIN BAR WITH ANY OF THE 3 SNACKS ABOVE | 200 |
| **TOTAL/MEN** | **1,667 CALORIES** |

## DAY 3

| BREAKFAST | CALORIES |
|---|---|
| PEPPER, ONION, AND GOAT CHEESE FRITTATA | 182 |

| LUNCH | CALORIES |
|---|---|
| SOUP AND SANDWICH: GRILLED CHEESE AND HAM | 337 |
| RICH BEEF AND NOODLE PHO WITH LIME AND BEAN SPROUTS | 172 |

| DINNER | CALORIES |
|---|---|
| GRILLED SALMON WITH CURRIED CAULIFLOWER | 367 |

| SNACKS (3 DAILY) | CALORIES |
|---|---|
| DOUBLE CHOCOLATE CHIP COOKIE | 74 |
| ORANGE, 1 MEDIUM | 70 |
| CHICKEN TENDERS WITH RANCH DRESSING | 198 |
| TOTAL/WOMEN | 1,400 CALORIES |
| MEN: ENJOY DARK CHOCOLATE–DIPPED FIGS WITH ANY 3 OF THE SNACKS ABOVE | 182 |
| TOTAL/MEN | 1,592 CALORIES |

## DAY 4

| BREAKFAST | CALORIES |
|---|---|
| ROCKY ROAD OATMEAL | 327 |

| LUNCH | CALORIES |
|---|---|
| BROWN-BAG TUNA SANDWICH | 300 |

| DINNER | CALORIES |
|---|---|
| MAC AND CHEESE WITH HAM AND BROCCOLI | 399 |

| SNACKS (3 DAILY) | CALORIES |
|---|---|
| COCONUT CREAM MANGO POP | 115 |

| | |
|---|---|
| GREEN TEA WATERMELON SUPER PUNCH | 176 |
| PBJ COOKIE | 55 |
| TOTAL/WOMEN | 1,372 CALORIES |
| MEN: ENJOY A PROTEIN BAR WITH ANY OF THE 3 SNACKS ABOVE | 200 |
| TOTAL/MEN | 1,572 CALORIES |

## DAY 5

| BREAKFAST | CALORIES |
|---|---|
| SOUTH OF THE BORDER SCRAMBLE WITH CHORIZO AND SALSA | 328 |

| LUNCH | CALORIES |
|---|---|
| YELLOW CURRY SHRIMP AND GREEN PEA SOUP | 302 |

| DINNER | CALORIES |
|---|---|
| CHICKEN PESTO PASTA | 385 |

| SNACKS (3 DAILY) | CALORIES |
|---|---|
| ALMONDS, DRY ROASTED, 15 | 100 |
| BLUEBERRY CREAM MUFFIN | 145 |
| CHOCOLATE MALTED MILK SHAKE | 126 |
| TOTAL/WOMEN | 1,386 CALORIES |
| MEN: ENJOY MY GREEN TEA WATERMELON SUPER PUNCH WITH ANY OF THE 3 SNACKS ABOVE | 176 CALORIES |
| TOTAL/MEN | 1,562 CALORIES |

## DAY 6

| BREAKFAST | CALORIES |
| --- | --- |
| 1 CEREAL BAR, 6 OUNCES NONFAT GREEK YOGURT, AND 1 CUP FRESH BERRIES | 300 |

| LUNCH | CALORIES |
| --- | --- |
| YELLOW CURRY SHRIMP AND GREEN PEA SOUP (LEFTOVERS) | 302 |
| FUDGY FRUIT AND NUT BAR | 110 |

| DINNER | CALORIES |
| --- | --- |
| NO-BOIL MUSHROOM LASAGNA | 388 |

| SNACKS (3 DAILY) | CALORIES |
| --- | --- |
| FUDGY FRUIT AND NUT BAR | 110 |
| CHOCOLATE MALTED MILK SHAKE | 126 |
| APPLE, 1 MEDIUM | 90 |
| TOTAL/WOMEN | 1,426 CALORIES |
| MEN: ENJOY A PROTEIN BAR WITH ANY OF THE 3 SNACKS ABOVE | 200 |
| TOTAL/MEN | 1,626 CALORIES |

## DAY 7

| BREAKFAST | CALORIES |
| --- | --- |
| CREAMY STUFFED CREPES WITH ORANGE BUTTER SYRUP | 239 |

| LUNCH | CALORIES |
| --- | --- |
| NO-BOIL MUSHROOM LASAGNA (LEFTOVERS) | 388 |

| DINNER | CALORIES |
| --- | --- |
| TURKEY DINNER WITH ALL THE TRIMMINGS | 323 |
| FUDGY FRUIT AND NUT BAR | 110 |

| SNACKS (3 DAILY) | CALORIES |
| --- | --- |
| CHICKEN TENDERS WITH RANCH DRESSING | 198 |
| APPLE, 1 MEDIUM | 90 |
| BABY CARROTS, 8 | 28 |
| TOTAL/WOMEN | 1,376 CALORIES |
| MEN: ENJOY AN ADDITIONAL SERVING OF CHICKEN TENDERS WITH RANCH DRESSING | 198 |
| TOTAL/MEN | 1,574 CALORIES |

## DAY 8

| BREAKFAST | CALORIES |
| --- | --- |
| BLUE ON BLUEBERRY SILVER DOLLAR PANCAKES | 292 |

| LUNCH | CALORIES |
| --- | --- |
| FAUX-FRIED FILET O' FISH SANDWICH | 313 |

| DINNER | CALORIES |
| --- | --- |
| CHICKEN AMANDINE WITH GREEN BEANS AND LEMON BUTTER | 327 |
| APPLE CINNAMON CRANBERRY COBBLER | 165 |

| SNACKS (3 DAILY) | CALORIES |
| --- | --- |
| TUNA CROQUETTES WITH DILL RELISH | 160 |
| PEAR, 1 MEDIUM | 96 |
| RED VELVET CHOCOLATE SQUARE | 106 |
| TOTAL/WOMEN | 1,459 CALORIES |
| MEN: ENJOY A CHOCOLATE MALTED MILK SHAKE, WITH ANY OF THE 3 SNACKS ABOVE | 126 |
| TOTAL/MEN | 1,585 CALORIES |

## DAY 9

| BREAKFAST | CALORIES |
|---|---|
| 6 OUNCES NONFAT GREEK YOGURT | 90 |
| BANANA WALNUT MUFFIN | 163 |
| GRAPEFRUIT, ½ MEDIUM | 50 |

| LUNCH | CALORIES |
|---|---|
| WHITE BEAN AND KALE SOUP WITH ROSEMARY AND PARMIGIANO–REGGIANO | 234 |
| BANANA WALNUT MUFFIN | 163 |

| DINNER | CALORIES |
|---|---|
| CRISPY-ON-THE-TOP TUNA AND GREEN PEA CASSEROLE | 351 |

| SNACKS (3 DAILY) | CALORIES |
|---|---|
| COCONUT CREAM MANGO POP | 115 |
| CHICKEN AND CHEESE POPPERS | 133 |
| RED VELVET CHOCOLATE SQUARE | 106 |
| TOTAL/WOMEN | 1,405 CALORIES |
| MEN: ENJOY A PROTEIN BAR WITH ANY OF THE 3 SNACKS ABOVE | 200 |
| TOTAL/MEN | 1,605 CALORIES |

## DAY 10

| BREAKFAST | CALORIES |
|---|---|
| CHERRY RED OATMEAL | 287 |

| LUNCH | CALORIES |
|---|---|
| BROWN-BAG TURKEY SANDWICH | 300 |
| OATMEAL RAISIN COOKIE | 84 |

| DINNER | CALORIES |
|---|---|
| GINGER SWEET CHICKEN AND BROCCOLI STIR-FRY | 298 |
| SILKEN CHOCOLATE MOUSSE | 161 |

| SNACKS (3 DAILY) | CALORIES |
|---|---|
| ALMONDS, DRY ROASTED, 15 NUTS | 100 |
| APPLE, 1 MEDIUM | 90 |
| ORANGE, 1 MEDIUM | 70 |
| TOTAL/WOMEN | 1,390 CALORIES |
| MEN: ENJOY APPLE AND CRANBERRY GRANOLA CEREAL AS A TRAIL-MIX-LIKE SNACK WITH ANY OF THE 3 SNACKS ABOVE | 253 |
| TOTAL/MEN | 1,643 CALORIES |

## DAY 11

| BREAKFAST | CALORIES |
|---|---|
| SUNRISE SANDWICH | 279 |
| GRAPEFRUIT, ½ MEDIUM | 50 |

| LUNCH | CALORIES |
|---|---|
| BOSTON BLUE CHICKEN AND APPLE SALAD | 294 |

| DINNER | CALORIES |
|---|---|
| FETTUCCINE ALFREDO WITH SHRIMP | 374 |
| SILKEN CHOCOLATE MOUSSE (LEFTOVER) | 161 |

| SNACKS (3 DAILY) | CALORIES |
|---|---|
| MAMA'S MINI MEATBALL BITES | 177 |
| OATMEAL RAISIN COOKIE | 84 |
| BABY CARROTS, 8 | 28 |
| TOTAL/WOMEN | 1,447 CALORIES |
| MEN: ENJOY A STRAWBERRY PROTEIN PUNCH SMOOTHIE WITH ANY OF THE 3 SNACKS ABOVE | 107 |
| TOTAL/MEN | 1,554 CALORIES |

## DAY 12

| BREAKFAST | CALORIES |
|---|---|
| STRAWBERRY MALTED BELGIAN WAFFLES | 375 |

| LUNCH | CALORIES |
|---|---|
| CHICKEN AND MUSHROOM QUESADILLAS | 324 |
| MEXICAN CORN WITH CHILI MAYO | 158 |

| DINNER | CALORIES |
|---|---|
| ROAST BEEF WITH BRUSSELS SPROUTS AND BALSAMIC JUS | 246 |
| GARLIC MASHED POTATOES | 101 |

| SNACKS (3 DAILY) | CALORIES |
|---|---|
| COCONUT CREAM MANGO POP | 115 |
| DOUBLE CHOCOLATE CHIP COOKIE | 74 |
| FRESH BERRIES, 1 CUP | 50 |
| TOTAL/WOMEN | 1,443 CALORIES |
| MEN: ENJOY A CHOCOLATE MALTED MILK SHAKE WITH ANY OF THE 3 SNACKS ABOVE | 126 |
| TOTAL/MEN | 1,569 CALORIES |

## DAY 13

| BREAKFAST | CALORIES |
|---|---|
| 2 SCRAMBLED EGG WHITES | 34 |
| 2 BLUEBERRY CREAM MUFFINS | 290 |

| LUNCH | CALORIES |
|---|---|
| RED BEET, GOAT CHEESE, AND WALNUT SALAD | 163 |

| DINNER | CALORIES |
|---|---|
| BBQ PORK CHOPS | 398 |
| APPLE CINNAMON CRANBERRY COBBLER | 165 |

| SNACKS (3 DAILY) | CALORIES |
|---|---|
| EGGPLANT AND ROASTED RED PEPPER TORTA | 183 |
| RED VELVET CHOCOLATE SQUARE | 106 |
| PEAR, 1 MEDIUM | 96 |
| TOTAL/WOMEN | 1,435 CALORIES |
| MEN: ENJOY A PROTEIN BAR WITH ANY OF THE 3 SNACKS ABOVE | 200 |
| TOTAL/MEN | 1,635 CALORIES |

## DAY 14

| BREAKFAST | CALORIES |
|---|---|
| SWEET POTATO AND BLUE CORN EGG CASSEROLE | 237 |
| GRAPEFRUIT, ½ MEDIUM | 50 |

| LUNCH | CALORIES |
|---|---|
| BEEF AND ORZO SOUP | 284 |

| DINNER | CALORIES |
|---|---|
| NO-BOIL MUSHROOM LASAGNA | 388 |
| TOSSED MIXED-GREENS SALAD WITH REDUCED-FAT DRESSING | 50 |

| SNACKS (3 DAILY) | CALORIES |
|---|---|
| SHRIMP AND CHEDDAR TOSTADA WITH SALSA VERDE | 200 |
| FRESH BERRIES, 1 CUP | 50 |
| PITA CHIPS WITH CHARRED EGGPLANT DIP | 159 |
| TOTAL/WOMEN | 1,418 CALORIES |
| MEN: ENJOY HOGS UNDERCOVER WITH ANY OF THE 3 SNACKS, ABOVE | 189 |
| TOTAL/MEN | 1,607 CALORIES |

## NEGATIVE-CALORIE FOODS

Maybe you've heard of "negative-calorie" foods. They're foods that supposedly use up more calories to chew, break down, digest, and absorb than they contain. A cup of Brussels sprouts, for example, provides 50 calories; around 75 calories are used in digestion and absorption, thus 25 calories are burned in the process. The idea of negative-calorie foods is very controversial, and most nutritionists don't put much stock in it.

Most of the foods considered as negative-calorie foods are super-healthy, full of fiber, and low in calories—and should be a part of your diet anyway.

Some examples include:

- Asparagus
- Broccoli
- Brussels sprouts
- Cabbage
- Celery
- Cucumbers
- Lettuce
- Mushrooms
- Radishes

Chewing most foods typically burns only about 5 calories an hour, but the act of digesting may require a few more. Still, for both health and weight control, avoid obsessing over negative-calorie foods. Instead, just remember that fresh vegetables are always a good choice—and that exercising will burn up far more calories than crunching down on celery or cucumbers.

# Shopping Lists

## SHOPPING LIST—WEEK 3

### PRODUCE
3–4 heads of garlic
1 bunch of scallions
1 head of romaine lettuce
2 medium red heirloom tomatoes
1 tomato
1 package of grape or cherry tomatoes
1 Hass avocado
1 package of mixed lettuce greens
1 red onion
1 yellow onion
3 Vidalia onions
2 medium sweet potatoes
Brussels sprouts (about 2 cups)
1 medium butternut squash
Bean sprouts (about 2 cups)
1 large head of broccoli
1 large head of cauliflower
1 green pepper
10 ounces of sliced cremini mushrooms
4 ounces of white button mushrooms
1 package of baby carrots
1 bunch of celery
1 container of fresh salsa

### FRESH HERBS
1 bunch of flat-leaf parsley
1 package of chives
1 package of tarragon
1 package of rosemary
2 packages of fresh basil
1 bunch of cilantro
1 package of mint

### FRUIT
1 grapefruit
2 medium oranges
3 medium apples
1 medium pear
2 mangoes
12 limes
12 medium fresh figs
Cubed seedless watermelon (8 cups)
Chopped fresh pineapple (2 cups)
2 pints of fresh berries

### DRIED FRUIT
1 package of dried currants
1 package of dried cranberries

### FROZEN FOODS
1 package of frozen peas
1 package of IQF blueberries

### BAKED GOODS
12 ounces of whole wheat baguette
4 whole wheat hamburger buns
4 whole wheat split-top hot dog buns, such as Matthew's Salad Rolls

1 loaf of thin-sliced European whole-grain bread,
    such as Rubschlager
8 (6-inch) low-carb tortillas, such as La Tortilla Factory
Package of whole wheat English muffins

## DAIRY

2 (32-ounce) cartons of liquid egg substitute
1 (4-ounce) package of reduced-fat cream cheese
1 carton of reduced-fat sour cream, such as
    Breakstone's
1 pint of low-fat buttermilk
8 slices of 2% reduced-fat-milk cheese, such as
    Borden's 2% Milk Reduced-Fat Sharp Singles
2 packages of shredded 50% reduced-fat cheddar,
    such as Cabot
1 package of shredded 75% reduced-fat cheddar,
    such as Cabot
1 package of shredded reduced-fat mozzarella
    cheese
2–3 cartons of grated Parmigiano-Reggiano cheese
2 ounces of goat cheese
Reduced-fat ricotta cheese, such as Sargento (3
    cups)
1½ dozen large eggs
1 quart of 2% milk
2 gallons of skim milk
Unsalted butter
2 6-ounce cartons of nonfat Greek yogurt, such as
    0% Fage Total
1 carton (17.6 ounces) of nonfat Greek yogurt, such
    as 0% Fage Total
2 cartons (6 ounces each) of 2% Greek yogurt, such
    as Fage Total
2 cartons (17.6 ounces each) of 2% Greek yogurt,
    such as Fage Total

## MEAT, FISH, POULTRY
## MEAT

16 ounces of 90% lean ground beef
1 (1-pound) piece of lean beef tenderloin
1 pound of lean pork tenderloin
8 slices (about 6 ounces) of high-quality deli ham
8 ounces of lean beef tenderloin, trimmed of all
    visible fat
1 package of Canadian bacon
2 ounces of reduced-fat chorizo sausage, such as
    Wellshire Farms

## FISH

Smoked salmon (at least 3 ounces)
4 (4-ounce) salmon fillets
1 (3-ounce) can of tuna
2 pounds of large shrimp, peeled and deveined

## POULTRY

1 pound of chicken tenders (about 16 pieces)
6 ounces (about 2 cups) chopped skinless breast
    meat from a rotisserie or other roast chicken
1 pound of fresh or completely thawed boneless,
    skinless turkey breast

## CANNED/PACKAGED GOODS

1 jar or other container of kalamata olives
1 (12-ounce) can of evaporated skim milk
1 (16-ounce) can light or reduced-fat coconut milk
2 (15.5-ounce) cans of white cannellini beans
1 (15.5-ounce) can of black beans
1 small can of beets (at least ½ cup)
2 cans canned peeled plum tomatoes (at least 2 cups)
1 (15.5-ounce) can of red beans
1 jar of unsweetened applesauce
1 bottle of apple cider
½ cup (about 3.5 ounces) of jarred fried peppers,
    such as Cento Sautéed Sweet Peppers with onions
1 cup (about 7 ounces) jarred roasted red pepper
    strips (not oil packed), such as Cento
1 jar of reduced-fat peanut butter, such as Better'n
    Peanut Butter
1 jar of no-sugar-added cranberry sauce, such as
    Steel's Gourmet Agave
Plenty of low-fat, low-sodium chicken broth (at least
    136 ounces or 4¼ quarts)

## CEREALS, GRAINS, PASTA

1 box of puffed millet cereal, such as Arrowhead
    Mills
1 box of puffed kamut, such as Arrowhead Mills
2 cups of quick-cooking oatmeal
1 package of whole wheat elbow macaroni
1 package of whole wheat rigatoni pasta, such as
    Bionaturae Organic
4 ounces (about 8 sheets) no-bake whole wheat
    lasagna noodles, such as Dalallo
1–2 packages of whole wheat panko bread crumbs,
    such as Ian's All-Natural

16 ounces tofu shirataki noodles, such as House Foods

1 package of brown rice (uncooked)

BAKING NEEDS

1 package of mini chocolate chunks

1 package of peanut butter chips

Bittersweet (60%–70%) chocolate (at least 3 ounces)

1 package of minimarshmallows

Whole wheat pastry flour

Whole wheat flour

2 packages of walnuts

1 package of chopped pine nuts

OTHER

1 package of ranch salad dressing and seasoning mix, such as Hidden Valley

Hormel Real Bacon Bits

Powdered gelatin

Malted milk powder, such as Carnation

1 bottle of sugar-free chocolate syrup, such as Fox's U-bet

3 protein bars

1 jar of garlic-chili sauce, such as Huy Fong

Yellow curry paste, such as Karee

Matcha green tea powder

1 package of almonds, dry roasted

1 cereal bar

1 bottle of calorie-free pancake syrup, such as Walden Farms

## SHOPPING LIST—WEEK 4

PRODUCE

3–4 heads of garlic

1 bunch of scallions

1 bunch of shallots

1 head of romaine lettuce

1 tomato

1 vine-ripened tomato

1 pound of haricots verts or slim green beans

1 head of kale

6 jalapeño peppers

2 heads of Boston lettuce

1 small eggplant

1 medium eggplant

1 large eggplant

3 yellow onions

2 medium red onions

4 ears of corn, in their husks

1 package of mixed lettuce greens

3 medium sweet potatoes

Brussels sprouts (about 2 cups)

1 large russet potato

1 large head of broccoli

1 large head of cauliflower

3 cups of cremini mushrooms

1½ pounds of white button mushrooms

1 package of baby carrots

2 large carrots

4 medium red beets

Baby arugula (about 4 cups)

1 bunch of celery

FRESH HERBS

2 bunches of flat-leaf parsley

1 package of dill

1 package of chives

1 package of rosemary

1 knob of fresh ginger

1 package of fresh basil

1 bunch of cilantro

1 package of mint

FRUIT

3–4 lemons

10 Golden Delicious apples

3 medium Granny Smith apples

3 medium pears

2 grapefruit

2 medium ripe bananas

1 medium orange

2 mangoes

2 limes

2 cups of fresh strawberries

2 pints of fresh berries

DRIED FRUIT

3 packages of dried cranberries

1 package of raisins

1 package of unsweetened dried apples

## FROZEN FOODS

1 package of frozen peas
2 packages of IQF blueberries
1 package of IQF cherries
1 package of IQF strawberries

## BAKED GOODS

4 whole wheat hamburger buns
8 (9-inch) low-carb tortillas, such as La Tortilla Factory
1 package of whole wheat English muffins

## DAIRY

3 quarts of skim milk
2 (32-ounce) cartons of liquid egg substitute
1 small carton of reduced-fat sour cream, such as Breakstone's
8 ounces (1 block) of reduced-fat cream cheese
1½ dozen eggs
4 slices (about ½ ounce each) cheddar cheese
4 slices 2% reduced-fat cheese, such as Borden's 2% Milk Reduced-Fat Sharp Singles
3 cartons of grated Parmigiano-Reggiano
1 package of shredded 50% reduced-fat cheddar cheese, such as Cabot
2 packages of shredded 75% reduced-fat cheddar, such as Cabot
1 package of crumbled reduced-fat blue cheese, such as Treasure Cave
1 pint of low-fat buttermilk
1 package of shredded reduced-fat mozzarella cheese
2 ounces of goat cheese
1 (16-ounce) carton of reduced-fat ricotta cheese, such as Sargento
Unsalted butter
2 cartons (17.6 ounces each) of nonfat Greek yogurt, such as 0% Fage Total
2 cartons (17.6 ounces each) of 2% Greek yogurt, such as Fage Total

## MEAT, FISH, POULTRY
### MEAT

2 pounds of lean beef tenderloin
1 package of Canadian bacon

### FISH

8 ounces of cod fillet

1 (12-ounce) can of albacore tuna packed in water, drained
18 ounces of canned albacore tuna, packed in water, drained
¾ pound of large shrimp, peeled and deveined
¾ pound of precooked large shrimp, peeled and deveined, tails removed

### POULTRY

8 skinless, boneless chicken breasts (4 ounces each)
A few slices of low-fat deli turkey
12 ounces of lean ground turkey breast
7 ounces (about 2 cups) of shredded skinless breast meat from a rotisserie or other roast chicken
2 sweet Italian chicken and turkey sausages, such as Applegate Farms

## CANNED/PACKAGED GOODS

1 (12-ounce) can of evaporated skim milk
1 (16-ounce) can of light or reduced-fat coconut milk
1 (15.5-ounce) can of white cannellini beans, great northern, or navy beans
1 small can of beets (at least ½ cup)
1 (15.5-ounce) can of red beans
1 jar of unsweetened applesauce
1 jar of unsweetened apple butter
1 jar of sugar-free apricot preserves, such as Smucker's
1 jar of low-fat marinara sauce
1 jar of tomatillo salsa
1 jar of roasted red peppers, such as Cento Roasted Peppers
Plenty of low-fat, low-sodium chicken broth (at least 3 quarts)

## CEREALS, GRAINS, PASTA

1 box of puffed millet cereal, such as Arrowhead Mills
1 box of puffed kamut, such as Arrowhead Mills
1 box of toasted whole-grain oat cereal, such as Cheerios
2 cups quick-cooking oatmeal
1 package of whole wheat rotini pasta, such as Ronzoni Healthy Harvest
1 package of whole wheat fettuccine
1 package of whole wheat orzo, such as RiceSelect
4 ounces (about 8 sheets) of no-boil whole wheat lasagna noodles, such as Dalallo

1–2 packages of whole wheat panko bread crumbs, such as Ian's All-Natural
1 package of brown rice (uncooked)

BAKING NEEDS
1 package of mini chocolate chunks
1 package of bittersweet (60%–70%) chocolate (at least 2 ounces)
Whole wheat pastry flour
12 walnut halves
2 packages of chopped walnuts
2 packages of sliced almonds
¾ cup Bisquick Heart Smart baking mix
6 ounces of whole wheat pizza dough, such as Papa Sal's

OTHER
4 ounces of baked blue corn chips, such as Guiltless Gourmet
Malted milk powder, such as Carnation
1 bottle of sugar-free chocolate syrup, such as Fox's U-bet
2 protein bars
1 package of almonds, dry roasted
1 bottle of calorie-free pancake syrup, such as Walden Farms
1 bottle of Ken's Light Options Olive Oil and Vinegar
French vanilla whey protein powder, such as Designer Whey
1 packet (3 grams) of sugar-free strawberry drink mix, such as Crystal Light
4 ounces of whole wheat baked pita chips (28 chips; 7 chips per serving), such as 365 Everyday Value

Experts agree on one cardinal rule of weight-loss success: Find a healthy eating plan that you feel you can live with for years to come. I believe the Now Eat This! Diet can be that plan—it's varied and interesting, so it's easier to maintain. And of course, it can really turn your weight around. The best part is that you won't feel like you're on a diet.

## FUEL YOUR BODY FOR EXERCISE

To get the most out of your workouts, incorporate snacks into your meal planning. These may include pre-exercise snacks, postexercise snacks, or both. Here are some guidelines.

- If you prefer to exercise in the morning on a mostly empty stomach, know that consuming a small snack at least 15 minutes prior to beginning a morning workout can be beneficial. This may mean grabbing a half cup of dry cereal like my Apple and Cranberry Granola Cereal (page 123), or eating a small piece of fruit.

- If you prefer to spend your lunch hour at the gym, be sure to eat a regular balanced breakfast like the ones I suggest. Then about a half hour before your workout, eat a small carbohydrate-rich snack. Again, this could be a small piece of fruit.

- Refuel after your workout. This is the most critical time. Because glycogen (carbohydrate stored in the muscles) is often depleted after strenuous exercise, it should be restored within 30 minutes after you work out. This is best achieved with a small snack containing carbs and protein. Any of my smoothies will do the trick, or have 6 ounces of yogurt with a serving of nuts. Protein and carb snacks also help repair damaged muscle tissue.

## THE BADDEST OF THE BAD

Don't kid yourself: There are plenty of bad foods out there. Here are my top 10 worst foods (in no particular order) if you're trying to lose weight and improve your health, according to recent studies. The following foods are so bad for your body that there is not much reason to eat them. Not only do they have lousy nutritional value, but they also give your body a dose of toxins, which should make the idea of eating them really hard to swallow. I don't list any brand names, but you'll know which stuff to steer clear of next time you're making the rounds in the grocery store.

### SOFT DRINKS (Carbonated or not, sugar sweetened or artificially sweetened)

- Diet sodas contain artificial sweeteners, which can have potential ill effects.
- Many soft drinks contain Red 40, the most widely used food dye, which can cause allergic reactions.
- Diet sodas may increase cravings for real sugar.
- Regular soft drinks are high in sugar (1 can of regular soda has about 10 teaspoons of sugar, about 150 calories).
- Soft drinks can be high in caffeine (30 to 55 milligrams of caffeine per 1 can of soda).
- They're loaded with artificial food colors and sulfites.
- They have been linked to bone weakening, obesity, tooth decay, and heart disease.

### NON-BAKED POTATO CHIPS

- Potato chips are filled with added fat as well as lots of salt.
- They contain a chemical called butylated hydroxyanisole (BHA). The U.S. Department of Health and Human Services states that BHA can be "reasonably anticipated to be a human carcinogen."

### WHITE FLOUR, BREAD, AND ROLLS

- White flour, bread, and rolls are void of nutrition, including fiber.
- They are metabolized like sugar in the body. This means these foods spike insulin levels, resulting in greater fat storage.
- They contain an additive called bromate, used to increase the volume of bread. Bromate causes cancer in animals and has been banned worldwide, except in the United States and Japan. Look for breads that say "bromate free" on the label.

### MARGARINE

- Margarine is loaded with empty calories. Just 1 tablespoon of margarine contains 101 calories, 12 grams of fat, and 93 milligrams of sodium.
- It's packed with trans fat, which is the worst type of fat to consume, implicated in cancer and heart disease.
- It increases Lp(a) lipoprotein, a type of LDL cholesterol found in varying levels in the blood. Researchers have found that elevated levels of this form of cholesterol can increase your odds of developing heart disease by 70 percent.
- It raises triglyceride levels.
- It is linked to illnesses such as cardiovascular disease, high cholesterol, and cancer.

### DOUGHNUTS

- Doughnuts are full of trans fat (store-bought doughnuts contain 35 to 40 percent trans fat).
- They're high in sugar (an average doughnut contains about 300 to 400 calories, mostly from sugar), and 12 grams of fat.
- Most varieties are full of nutritionally empty white flour.

### FRENCH FRIES

- French fries are high in free radicals, which are harmful to the body.
- A large order of fries contains 539 calories, 29 grams of fat (half of which is trans fat and saturated fat), and 328 milligrams of sodium.
- French fries are high in acrylamide, a potent toxic chemical formed as a result of frying the starch in the potatoes.

### PACKAGED FRIED SHELLFISH (SHRIMP, CLAMS, OYSTERS, AND LOBSTERS)

- Packaged fried shellfish is high in trans fat.
- It contains carcinogenic acrylamide.
- It may be high in toxic mercury.
- It can be contaminated with parasites and microbes.

### GRANOLA (STORE BRANDS)

- Store-brand granola can be high in white sugar, corn syrup, or both.
- It's high in calories (400 to 550 calories in 1 cup).
- It's high in fat (unless it's specifically a low-fat brand)—around 12 grams of fat in 1 cup.

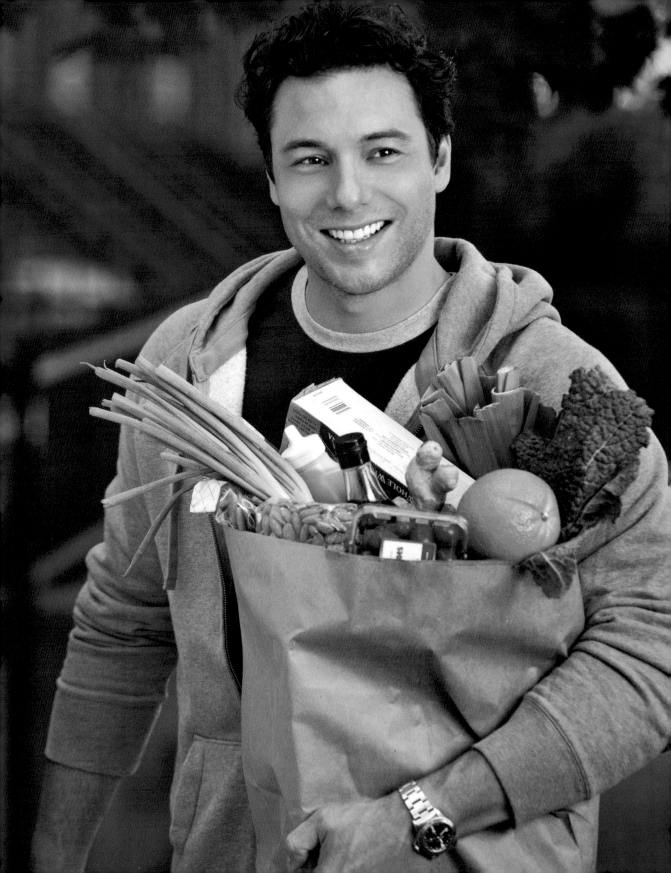

chapter

# 5

☺

# Gotta-Have Ingredients

Food has got to taste good, or you won't eat it. Wow, what a concept. I've known this since age one, when I turned my little nose up at anything that wasn't my favorite flavor: orange.

Real-deal flavor is the secret to successful weight loss—so every dish has to be high in taste and quality. I didn't compromise on either when I created the recipes in this book; I wanted combinations that are exciting and magical. There are so many ways to make that happen.

One reason is that we now have access to a global food fair. Pasta used to be elbow macaroni and spaghetti and red sauce. Now it's pappardelle, rigatoni, tortellini, and two dozen others on every menu in America. Chanterelles, morels, line-caught bass, diver sea scallops, organic beef, artisanal cheese, and curiosities like truffle oil and yuzu are all widely available—and all outrageously delicious.

All foods taste different. Have you ever wondered why? You have about ten thousand tiny taste buds on your tongue that act like text messages telling your brain what flavors you're sampling. You can taste many different flavors, but they are really a combination of four basic tastes: salty, sweet, sour, and bitter. The salty taste is found in foods like cheese, nuts, celery, and meats. It is a baseline flavor that really stirs the appetite.

The sweet taste imparts satisfaction and comfort while providing balance. The sources of the sweet taste are many: most fruits, many vegetables, nearly every grain, as well as eggs, dairy products, and of course, sugar and honey.

The sour taste, the predominant flavor in lemons, limes, vinegar, yogurt, and fermented foods, gives food tension and helps promote digestion. Many chefs' favorite flavor enhancers are sour: lemon, orange, and vinegars including white wine, apple cider, and balsamic.

The bitter taste provides complexity. Bitter flavors are the chords versus the notes; they help cross the t's and dots the i's in food. Without them, everything would taste like lollipops. Bitter is found in leafy green vegetables such as broccoli, spinach, kale, and mustard greens, as well as in coffee, chocolate, and charred foods. In Indian cuisine, foods with predominantly bitter flavor are considered to be natural detoxifiers with particular benefit to the liver.

Researchers at Rutgers University discovered that when it comes to how people experience food, there are supertasters and there are nontasters. Supertasters love the bitter flavors in broccoli and other foods, and they tend to be thinner than others. People who are nontasters like foods that are fattier and sweeter. This finding makes a great deal of sense to me. If you love vegetables and eat fewer sweets, you'll probably be thin and fit—and you have your predilection for the rich complexity of bitter flavors to thank.

In reality, each of the four flavors needs to have a presence in meals, but none can dominate. A squeeze of sour lemon or lime juice on fried shrimp will cut through the excessive fatty quality of fried food; a sprinkling of salt on charred steaks off the grill will enhance the beef's sweetness. Adding a tad of good sugar to a bitter food, like cocoa, makes the food not only edible, but alluring. Well, it makes it . . . chocolate!

With the recipes in this book, I've instinctually worked to use the four flavors in various combinations to play off each other and make bad-rap dishes more interesting, palatable, satisfying, and healthy.

The following ingredients help make that happen, and I can't live—or cook—without them. They're easy to find, come in a variety of brands, and are loaded with flavor. These are my gotta-have ingredients:

## AROMATICS

I cook with plenty of scallions, bulb onions, ginger, garlic, and lemongrass—an ingredient group called aromatics. The name says it all. Without adding a single calorie they add flavor and aroma to food, big-time.

## BAKED TORTILLA CHIPS

Baked tortilla chips save you fat calories and taste great, making standard fried tortilla chips obsolete. Several of my recipes call for baked chips, and I love using them. Not only are they delicious, but they also add tremendous texture to a dish. Oh, and just in case you don't think it matters what kind of chips you use, let's do the math: 12 regular tortilla chips have around 140 calories and 7 grams of fat; 12 baked chips, 118 calories and 1.6 grams of fat. So have only baked chips on hand (but try not to gulp down the whole bag).

## BALSAMIC VINEGAR

If you haven't discovered balsamic vinegar, your taste buds are in for a real treat. Its sweet-tart, wood-aged blend of flavors add a special accent to salad dressings, marinades, pastas, and meats with virtually no trace of fat or calories.

Balsamic vinegar is made from the unfermented juice of white grapes. I use it in many recipes in this book. Because it has a syrupy consistency right out of the bottle, balsamic vinegar makes a wonderful sauce base. It keeps the calories down, offers a great flavor profile, and imbues a perfect light brown color that makes all sauces so appetizing.

## CAULIFLOWER

If I fired the word *cauliflower* at you and asked you to say the first thing that came to mind, you'd probably say "ugh." Yet this unsung cooking hero is versatile and delicious; it's one of my favorite vegetables. I use mashed cauliflower as a stand-in for part of the potatoes in my Garlic Mashed Potato recipe on page 221. This cuts the carbs and calories considerably, but none of the taste. Normally, a side order of garlic mashed potatoes will run about 369 calories. Mine are only 101 calories a serving! I hope this gives you a new outlook on this underrated vegetable. Enjoy—and go dig out your skinny clothes.

## CORNSTARCH

Cornstarch is a fat-free thickener—great for giving body to low-fat gravies, soups, sauces, dressings, and fillings that could normally require lots of cream and butter. It has about twice the thickening power of flour and a fraction of the calories. I rely on it to provide the same thickness and creaminess that we associate with foods like cream and butter. But I use so little of it that you don't have to worry about too many carbs sneaking into a dish.

## DIJON MUSTARD

Nothing wakes the palate and perks up the flavor in food like a touch of Dijon mustard. We think of it as something to be passed from limousine to limousine, like in that 1980s television commercial, but at only 15 calories a tablespoon, I like to use it generously. I brush it lightly over fish fillets before broiling them and use it in marinades. Dijon mustard is a flavor detonator. It can blow up a dish (in a good way) like crazy.

## EGG SUBSTITUTE

One of the easiest ways to get high-quality protein is to turn to eggs. But if you're trying to outlaw fat and cholesterol from your diet, regular eggs may have more cholesterol than you'd like to eat. Liquid egg substitutes to the rescue.

Made primarily from egg whites, egg substitutes retain all the protein but none of the fat and only a fraction of the cholesterol of regular eggs. Going yolkless also spares you a lot of calories. There are 30 calories per serving of egg substitute, compared to 75 calories for 1 large egg.

I use egg substitutes in many baked dishes, including frittatas. A frittata is a traditional Italian dish (I was practically weaned on them) with eggs, vegetables, and herbs. Egg substitutes work great for frittatas, but I also use them in other egg dishes, such as my Pizza Egg Bake or South of the Border Scramble with Chorizo and Salsa.

## EGG WHITES

Whipped egg whites are my secret weapon in "faux frying." The protein in the egg whites binds beautifully to breading. Add just a tiny bit of fat, and you've got chicken, fish, onion rings, or fries that taste like they just emerged from a deep-fat fryer.

## EVAPORATED SKIM MILK

I indulge without the fat by substituting evaporated skim milk for cream in certain dishes. As a topping, it whips almost as well as heavy cream, but not quite, so store an unopened can of evaporated skim milk in the refrigerator until it is very cold; then whip it. For added richness, sweeten it with a drop of vanilla extract. Serve over fresh berries or atop one of my dessert bars. Who said eating right was hard to do?

## ESPRESSO POWDER

Most people have a love affair with chocolate. Mine is with coffee—espresso powder to be exact. When you add it to any chocolate dish—from a chocolate milk shake to chocolate chip cookies, it intensifies and brings out the chocolate flavor.

## FRESH HERBS

Fresh herbs can make the difference between a dull dish and a spectacular one. My favorites are chives, tarragon, cilantro, basil, rosemary, mint, and flat-leaf parsley. Use these on meats and vegetables, and there's no need to add flavor that comes with fat. If you must use dried herbs in a pinch, understand that they pack more concentrated flavor, so for every ¼ cup of fresh herbs, use 1 teaspoon of dried herbs where applicable. Don't even bother with dried parsley, cilantro, or basil; there is no substitute for the fresh item.

## FRESH-SQUEEZED LEMON/CITRUS

It's gotta be fresh! Some people try to use bottled lemon or lime juice in their cooking. Trust me; it doesn't work.

You'll taste too much lemon or too much lime or too much preservative—and nothing else. This throws the whole dish off. Acid is a hugely important tool to make food taste good, and the tension between sweet and sour is what makes so many of our favorite dishes so flavorful. If you want to perk up your vegetables without extra fat or sodium, a squeeze of fresh lemon or lime juice will do the trick. Besides, refrigerated lemons and limes can last for weeks.

## GARLIC

Health experts say garlic works like magic to reduce your risk of scary diseases. I don't know all the medical science there, but I do know that this vegetable works like magic in cooking. When used properly, garlic is one of the very best friends a cook can have. Garlic stimulates the palate and can substitute for salt. And it has almost no calories. Using fresh garlic is best, and now you can find fresh peeled garlic in most supermarkets. Stay away from the chopped garlic in jars. It stinks—and not in a good way.

## GREEK YOGURT

Greek yogurt is a miracle ingredient. It replaces butter or cream in most recipes at almost a one-to-one swap. You save a ton of calories with this tangy, naturally thick ingredient. Consider: Butter has 1,600 calories a cup, and cream, 800. Full-fat Greek yogurt (Fage Total is my favorite brand): just 300 calories a cup! You can downsize the calories in recipes even more by using 2% Fage Total Greek yogurt at only *148 calories per cup*, or 0% Fage Total Greek yogurt at just 90 calories in a six-ounce carton, or 120 calories in a full cup.

For a baked potato, Greek yogurt is a great substitute for sour cream and butter. Greek yogurt differs from the usual gelatin-thickened, artificially flavored slop we think of as yogurt in that it's just milk and yogurt cultures; no sugar, no fruit on the bottom, no thickeners or artificial flavors. The difference is huge.

## IQF FRUIT

I learned how to use IQF (individually quick-frozen) fruit from a trainer I knew who made great smoothies. He told me to get the blueberries, and I rooted around for them in the refrigerator section forever. Finally he said, "Hey, knucklehead, they're in the freezer!"

IQF fruit such as strawberries, blueberries, blackberries, and raspberries rivals fresh-picked fruit in taste and nutritional content. It contains no added sugar or preservatives and very few calories. The fruit is delicious, and I use it in smoothies and breakfast syrups all the time. You can buy IQF fruit in bulk at any food club, and organic IQF is also available. Organic products contain no preservatives—a critical factor in nutritional health.

## LOW-SODIUM, LOW-FAT CHICKEN BROTH

Good stock is like the foundation of a building. It lays the groundwork for a delicious soup, stew, or pan sauce. Trouble is, many versions are drowning in sodium (often 1,000 milligrams per cup). Low-sodium, low-fat chicken broths, canned or boxed, have considerably less, usually between 140 and 450 milligrams per cup. You get a caloric bargain with these products, too. A cup contains between 5 and 10 calories, whereas a cup of regular broth has around 80 calories. I recommend low-fat, low-sodium versions.

## LOW-SODIUM SOY SAUCE

For sodium-restricted diets, you can't beat low-sodium soy sauce. A little bit goes a long way, and you can't tell the difference between it and its much-saltier version. If you really want to slash sodium, consider using Bragg's Liquid Aminos, available at health-food stores. It has about 60 percent of the sodium of regular soy sauce.

## MATCHA

Ask any chef the difference between a good dish and a great one and the answer is often a single, out-of-the-ordinary (but not necessarily hard-to-find) ingredient. Enter matcha. This superfood was revealed to me only recently (Buddhist monks have been enjoying it for nine hundred years). Matcha is a natural green tea powder, prepared by milling specially cultivated green tea leaves under very low temperatures. All of the antioxidant and weight-loss benefits of green tea are preserved. I use matcha powder in my Green Tea Watermelon Super Punch, but you can add it to any beverage. Look for matcha powder at any high-end grocery store, Asian markets, or online. Think of it as a turbo-charged version of green tea.

## NO-BOIL WHOLE WHEAT LASAGNA NOODLES

I had heard about "no-boil" lasagna recipes for some time, but frankly, I was skeptical. While I was growing up, lasagna was one of those special pastas because it was labor- and love-intensive. I thought of no-boil lasagna noodles as cheating. How could you layer sheets of raw pasta into a lasagna pan without boiling them first? It didn't seem right—or Italian. Now I know better. These special "no-boil" noodles are manufactured differently, and the texture is softer than a traditional noodle's. And they're so convenient; they make preparing lasagna a real possibility instead of a scoff. I've never looked back.

## NONSTICK COOKING SPRAY

Nonstick cooking sprays come in basic oil flavors: Canola, olive, and butter are common and are a must for low-fat cooking. Normally we use fat to keep food from sticking, and we generally use way too much—which is why nonstick cooking spray is ingenious. You can also use it to create "you'd-never-believe-it's-low-fat" oven-fried foods. Spray breaded fish, chicken, or onion rings for 3 seconds with the spray; then bake at high heat to give the food a crunchy, tasty coating and a moist interior. You'll like it better than fried food! A 1-second spray of Pam Original or Pam Olive Oil cooking spray contains less than a gram of fat, compared to almost 14 grams of fat in 1 tablespoon of oil—and they do the same amount of work.

## PARMIGIANO-REGGIANO CHEESE

Now, here's a cheese that really rocks. In Italy, Parmigiano-Reggiano cheese is the king of cheeses. The people who make it dedicate their lives to making the perfect cheese. And then they wait. And wait. Parmigiano-Reggiano cheese is aged longer than any other cheese in the world: a minimum of two years, in fact. It's easier to digest than any other cheese, too. In fact, Italian mountain climbers pack chunks of Parmigiano-Reggiano cheese instead of energy bars for quick energy, since the body can absorb the protein from Parmigiano-Reggiano in 45 minutes, four times faster than it can absorb the protein from other cheese. And because it's made with part-skim milk, it also has a lower fat content than most other cheeses. If you want to be extremely clever, try Grana Padano instead of Parmigiano-Reggiano because in Grana all the milk is skimmed, whereas in Parmigiano only half is. This makes Grana Padano a little less fatty than Parmigiano-Reggiano. How about that piece of food knowledge for a game of Trivial Pursuit?

## REAL BACON BITS

I love bacon. It's the greatest taste treat on the planet. I'd wash my breakfast down with the drippings if I could. Yes, I know it's not that great for your health. Fatty bacon stands at the head of the diet cops' hate list. So when I bring home the bacon these days, it's a product by Hormel called Real Bacon Bits. It's a low-fat alternative to cooking your own artery-popping bacon. And I like it much better than turkey bacon. Here are the stats: 3 ounces of real bacon bits has 30 calories and 1.5 grams of fat. Comparatively, 3 ounces of cooked bacon slices has 458 calories and 35 grams of fat. And 3 ounces of turkey bacon? That's 213 calories and 15 grams of fat. Got it? 'Nuff said.

## REDUCED-FAT BLUE CHEESE

You just can't beat blue cheese for Cobb salads, as a dipping sauce for hot wings, stuffed inside juicy hamburgers, and all that good stuff. Unfortunately it's so damn fat and calorie laden. Recently, I discovered reduced-fat blue cheese. It has the flavor but not the fat. My favorite is made by Treasure Cave. Available in practically every supermarket, it's easy to use in any recipe that calls for blue cheese—and it's great tasting. I defy you to tell the difference.

## REDUCED-FAT CHEDDAR CHEESES, 50% AND 75%

Who doesn't love a sharp bite of cheddar cheese? Every morsel offers an amazing culinary experience—along with enough artery-clogging saturated fat to make you think twice about indulging. Good news, though: You can have your cheese and eat it, too. There are some great reduced-fat cheeses out there. My favorite is Cabot 50% Reduced-Fat Cheddar because it doesn't taste low fat. One ounce contains just 70 calories and 4.5 grams of fat. Cabot also makes a 75% Reduced-Fat Cheddar with only 60 calories and 2.5 grams of fat. Compare this to 1 ounce of regular cheddar at 114 calories and 9.4 grams of fat.

## REDUCED-SUGAR KETCHUP

Ketchup is such an integral part of American cuisine that most people are reluctant to give it up. I haven't had "regular" ketchup in years, though it's what I grew up on. I'm a convert to reduced-sugar ketchup, and I can't taste a difference. Most traditional ketchup has more sugar in it per ounce than ice cream, resulting in 15 calories per tablespoon. The sugar is high-fructose corn syrup, that rather nasty sweetener that has been implicated in obesity and other diseases. Heinz's reduced-sugar variety has 75 percent less sugar and two-thirds fewer calories. It does contain an artificial sweetener, so using this product is a philosophical decision you have to make. If you don't like artificial sweeteners in your foods or condiments, agave ketchup is a good alternative.

### SALSA, FRESH AND JARRED

I'd put salsa on ice cream if I could. It's great stuff, perfect as a topping for fish and chicken, as well as a wonderful dip. But be sure to check the jarred variety to make sure no sugar or fat has been added. I also love store-bought fresh salsa and use it all the time. This chunky, spicy relish injects a lot of flavor and texture into food without the fat. Salsa, which has only 6 calories per tablespoon, often can be used to replace fattening, sugar-laced condiments. If you want to get creative, try making your own salsa. Just combine some seeded tomatoes, chopped celery, green peppers, garlic, diced onion, jalapeño pepper, lime juice, and perhaps crushed red pepper and salt to round out the taste.

### SALT AND SALT SUBSTITUTIONS

I know all too well that many people are on salt-restricted diets. After my mom had heart surgery in 2005, she was told "no salt or sodium of any kind." I had to get up to speed fast on salt-free diets. After experimenting, we made two amazing discoveries: first, that the less sodium you consume the less you crave it, and second, that big flavors like lemon and lime juice; good vinegars; spices like cayenne, crushed red pepper, and curry powder; and aromatics like garlic and fresh herbs go a long way to make a dish taste great without all the salt. There are a number of good salt substitutes out there, too, such as Morton's Salt Substitute (sodium-free) and Morton's Light Salt (50 percent less salt than table salt). For anyone not bound by sodium restrictions, use kosher salt or sea salt in dishes to arouse maximum flavor.

### SHIRATAKI NOODLES

How would you like to stuff yourself with a plateful of pasta with barely any calories? This is no fantasy. It's shirataki, delicious and filling noodles made from yam flour (konjac) or tofu. The former has no calories and the latter packs all of 20 calories per 4-ounce serving. Compare that to about 200 calories for, say, ziti. The konjac variety is available only online at miraclenoodle.com, and don't worry—the more readily available soy-based noodles taste nothing like tofu. They have the body and taste of a light egg noodle and come in three shapes—fettuccine, spaghetti, and angel hair. Try some other healthy pasta choices, too, such as whole-grain pastas, legume-based pastas, and quinoa pasta, as well as spaghetti squash. Now you can eat pasta, and plenty of it.

### SPICES

People trying to lose weight say the food they eat is blah. I combat blah by using spices. Some of my favorites are curry powder, hot sauce, nutmeg, adobo, and crushed red pepper—all used extensively in this book. Cooking with spices can actually help whittle your waistline. Spiced food is infinitely more satisfying and flavorful. And spicy foods contain an active component called capsaicin. It irritates the nerves in the mouth so they swell up and make you think you're eating something rich, so you eat less. When your mouth's on fire, you're not as likely to go back for seconds. Plus, spicy foods fire up your metabolism—so don't be afraid to spice it up!

### SRIRACHA (ROOSTER SAUCE)

If there's a bottle of hot sauce on a restaurant table or grocery shelf, particularly one I haven't tried, you can bet I'm going to introduce myself. Sriracha (pronounced SEE-rah-chah), which hails from Thailand, is one of those sauces. I first met it at a Vietnamese joint. Sriracha is made mostly with red chili peppers, salt, vinegar, garlic, and too little sugar to count, and has a hot, sour, and sweet flavor going on. I use it as a base for barbecue stir-fry sauces, and it performs beautifully in that capacity. And because it's thick it saves a lot of sauce-making time, too.

### SUGAR-FREE RELISH

To me, discovering new ingredients is like going on a treasure hunt and finding a 50-carat diamond. One of my recent gems is sugar-free relish—great in salad dressings or on tuna salads or sandwiches. It has 0 to 5 calories per tablespoon, compared to 20 calories for regular sweet relish.

### WHOLE WHEAT BREAD AND BUNS

Bread lovers, rejoice. Now you can eat bread on your diet. Besides the obvious—that bread is what makes a burger a burger, and who can eat pasta without garlic bread?— bread, in its whole-grain form, is actually good for you. And whole grain is what I'm recommending here. Okay, what does that mean?

A little Bread 101 here: When grain is refined, most of the fiber, about 25 percent of the protein, and at least seventeen key nutrients are lost. Sure, refined flour is enriched with vitamins and minerals, but whole grains provide more protein, more fiber, and many more vitamins and minerals. With more fiber, there's a slower release of carbs into the bloodstream and, long story short, less weight gain. Look for labels that say 100 percent whole wheat or 100 percent whole grain, rather than "made with whole grain," or "wheat bread." (Even white bread is made from wheat, and some products calling themselves "wheat" breads are just darker-colored white bread.)

## WHOLE WHEAT PANKO BREAD CRUMBS

Almost anything that's traditionally coated in crumbs, such as chicken or fish, can be faux-fried in the oven. Instead of traditional bread crumbs, I use whole wheat panko bread crumbs, lightly sprayed with cooking spray. The effect is a crisp coating that seals in the juices and tenderness. Panko is a Japanese bread crumb that is lighter and crisper than the typical American-style bread-crumb coatings. I use panko in dishes such as Chicken Tenders with Ranch Dressing (page 248) and Spicy Fried Calamari with Cherry Tomato Dipping Sauce (page 225)—both better than the original, not just because of taste but also because your hands don't get greasy. Look for Ian's All-Natural panko bread crumbs in the bread section of your grocery store, or right next to traditional bread crumbs.

## WHOLE WHEAT PASTRY FLOUR

Here's another miracle ingredient. To create the breakfast recipes for this book, I had to break the flour code. Regular flour just wouldn't fit the bill. It's too caloric and has no nutritional value. Whole wheat flour is too heavy in protein. It's fine for the elastic structure required in bread baking, but it's the last thing you want for fluffy pancakes and waffles. Whole wheat pastry flour has half the protein of whole wheat flour, plus a fine texture, so it's perfect for the delicate, light texture I love in pancakes and waffles. Whole wheat pastry flour: Stock up on it. Find it in the natural foods section of stores. Batter up, baby!

Cooking can help you get fat, but it can also help you get fit. Keep a low-fat kitchen, stock it with high-quality, flavorful ingredients, let your experimental spirit run wild, and trust me—this time your diet will last longer than half of Monday.

## SWEETENERS

| TYPE | CALORIC CONTENT | NUTRITIONAL BENEFIT | COOKING TIPS |
|------|-----------------|---------------------|--------------|
| AGAVE NECTAR | 20 CALORIES PER TEASPOON | Contains a natural fiber called inulin that helps prevent blood sugar elevations | In recipes, use ¼ to ⅓ cup of agave syrup for each cup of sugar. In baking, reduce liquid in recipes by 2 tablespoons for each ¼ cup of agave liquid used. |
| SWEETLEAF | 0 CALORIES | Balances blood sugar levels, reduces cravings, and contains antioxidants | In baking, use 1½ tablespoons powdered (or 1 teaspoon liquid) stevia for 1 cup sugar. |
| TRUVIA | 0 CALORIES | Won't alter blood sugar | In recipes, ⅓ cup + 1 tablespoon is the same as 1 cup of sugar. |
| SPLENDA GRANULAR | 0 CALORIES | Seems to work best in pie fillings, cheesecakes, sweet sauces, marinades, and glazes | In recipes, 1 cup is the same as 1 cup of sugar. |
| SPLENDA SUGAR BLEND | 20 CALORIES PER TEASPOON | Contains sucralose and sugar and helps baked goods brown, rise, and retain moistness—more like those made with sugar, but with fewer calories | In recipes, ½ cup is the same as 1 cup of sugar. |

# Fake and Bake:
## Natural and Artificial Sweeteners

Creating healthy, low-sugar desserts is a tough act. I know the flavor profile I want before I even start: natural sweetness with no weirdo aftertaste from artificial sweeteners. My desserts typically go through more drafts than any other low-calorie dish, and they take weeks to nail down.

The challenge is always to cut the sugar in a recipe, not only because of the calories but also because sugar is right up there with criminals on the most-wanted list. It's blamed for a lot of things—the evil source of flab, temper tantrums in kids—and may end the human race as we know it. I wouldn't be surprised if before long we see a package of sugar on a poster in the lobby of the post office. Ha!

We just eat far too much of this stuff, causing a host of health problems (hypertension and diabetes, to name just two). Some studies say that sugar acts like a fertilizer to cancer, providing energy to cancerous cells.

Most people can shed about 5 pounds simply by cutting processed sugars from their diets. That's what I did. So it's not a bad idea to watch your sugar intake, even if you don't have a medical condition.

One way to curb sugar intake is to use artificial sweeteners. But even those have been demonized. Get this: A well-publicized study by Purdue University researchers showed that artificial sweeteners can make you fat. Basically, artificial sugars end up stimulating your appetite. You get hungry, you overeat, and you gain weight.

Even if sugar substitutes don't make you fat, at one time or another they have been linked to cancer, reproductive disorders, and immune breakdown—claims all denied by the manufacturers. I don't know about you, but news like that scares the living hell out of me. If I want to make a sugar-free cake, I have to sort out numerous studies that have been done on artificial sweeteners and decide whether I want to protect myself against diabetes or get cancer.

I get it that you may have to try artificial sweeteners if you can't have sugar. However, don't let anyone kid you. Recipes cooked with artificial sweeteners will turn out good, but not the same as they would if they're cooked with sugar. Sugar not only provides sweetness; it helps brown a crust, it tenderizes, and it keeps items moist. Artificial sweeteners can't do that. You may end up with a drier, tougher product that doesn't brown very well. That's why some low-sugar recipes still call for a little raw sugar or molasses to help with browning and flavor. I have devised recipes that are great regardless.

I hear from people who are concerned about the safety of these sweeteners, and I've even had a shift in consciousness about sugar substitutes, so I try to temper my use of them in recipes.

All that being said, let me emphasize that I'm far from being an expert on these products. However, I have experimented with them in recipes. Like any cook, I have my favorites. (By the way, aspartame—aka NutraSweet or Equal—isn't among them. It's the worst for baking. Let's just skip it altogether.)

### Agave Nectar
At the top of my list is agave nectar. Although this honeylike sweetener might be new to some cooks, it's not really new at all. In fact, folks in Mexico have used it for thousands of years. Unlike honey, agave nectar is metabolized very slowly. This slow metabolizing explains its health benefits.

Agave also contains inulin (not insulin). This is a carbohydrate high in indigestible fiber. It feeds friendly bacteria in the digestive tract, reduces cholesterol, and blocks fat absorption in the intestines. In this way, agave can play a small but significant part in your diet, as long as you don't eat large quantities.

I learned about this sweetener and its benefits while working with *The Biggest Loser*. I wasn't allowed to use any artificial sweeteners for desserts; the only sweetener I was allowed was agave nectar, so I had to get up to speed on it fast. I'm glad I did. Its carbohydrate content is similar to that of sugar, but because it's about three times sweeter, you can use less.

Agave nectar comes from the "juice," or sap, of a plant that looks like a gigantic aloe vera. It grows in the desert and gets a lot of sun. Sun and soil equal flavor in any fruit or vegetable. Tequila is made from the same plant. In fact, the nectar is basically tequila before it's distilled. If you like tequila, you will definitely like agave nectar. I use it in desserts, sauces, and salad dressings. Its advantages are unmatched by any sugar or sugar replacement. You can buy it at whole-foods-type stores, higher-end supermarkets, and gourmet shops.

Here's a tip: Before pouring agave nectar into a measuring cup or spoon, spray the cup or spoon with a little cooking spray so all the syrup will come out. Otherwise, a significant amount will stay in the cup or spoon.

## SweetLeaf Stevia

I discovered SweetLeaf recently, and I am in love. This is a 100 percent natural sugar substitute made from stevia, a calorie-free herb said to be up to three hundred times sweeter than sugar. Stevia is natural in the sense that it is not a chemical concocted in a lab. It's a natural extract from the stevia plant, found mostly in Paraguay.

Stevia has been used in Japan for decades and in South America for centuries. It's actually good for you. It doesn't raise blood sugar, it's filled with antioxidants, and it might even cut your cravings for sweets.

Finally, a sugar substitute that doesn't scare me!

## Truvia

Truvia is another stevia-derived sweetener. It also contains erythritol, a sugar alcohol. Sugar alcohols aren't sugar and won't make you drunk. They're made by adding hydrogen atoms to sugars. Erythritol comes in granulated and powdered forms and occurs naturally in fruit, mushrooms, and fermented products like soy sauce. Erythritol has a minimal effect on blood sugar,

has no calories, and is low in carbs. It also doesn't tend to produce intestinal distress like other sugar alcohols.

Truvia is now sold in bulk for baking. No more tearing open and dumping dozens of little packages into the mixing bowl.

## Sucralose (Splenda)

I've done a lot of cooking and baking with sucralose—and taken a lot of heat for it. In the world of sugar-free, people think sucralose is a badass sweetener. Questions about its safety linger, and you don't know who to believe.

Sucralose is six hundred times sweeter than sugar on average and is marketed as a "no-calorie sweetener," even though it contains 96 calories a cup. Billed as a natural sweetener because it's sugar based, sucralose is actually a processed product formed by treating sugar, or sucrose, with chlorine (a gas). This changes the molecular structure so that the human body no longer recognizes it as something to be metabolized. Most of it passes straight through the digestive tract without leaving any calories behind.

As for cooking with this stuff, sucralose bakes well. Substitute it in the same measurement that is listed for sugar, but be careful with your baking time. Sucralose tends to make things cook faster.

If you can't stand the aftertaste, try combining two different sweeteners, like sucralose and some sugar or brown sugar. This blending helps impart more sweetness and less artificial taste.

As to which is better: That is up to you and your God. A dessert with a natural sweetener, artificial sweetener, or a combo—that's a personal choice. I'm not a nutritionist or a scientist, nor did I ever play a doctor on TV; I'm just giving you a few facts as I understand them. Think of any recipe as a suggestion rather than a command. With a little experimentation, you can adjust it to fit your preference, budget, diet, or nutrition philosophy.

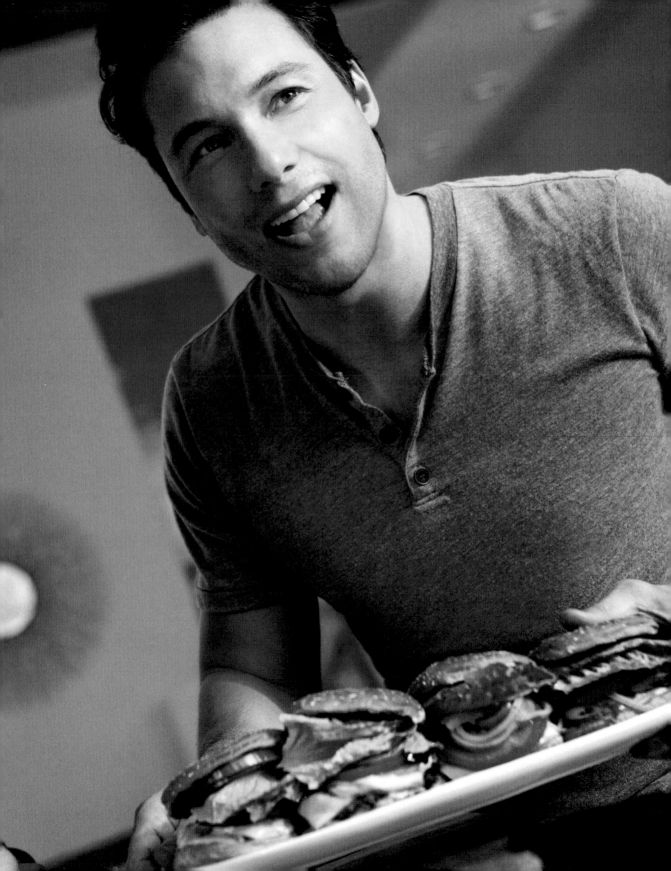

chapter

# 6

☺

# Let's Cook

Think you can't cook? Well, you're wrong! Try this simple experiment with me. All you need is a can of low-sodium chicken broth and a can of black beans.

Open both cans and pour them into a saucepan. Stir everything together with a large spoon and bring the mixture to a boil.

Voilà—you have just made black bean soup.

If you can do that, you can do everything that I will ask you to do in this book.

There's no question in my mind that everyone on this planet can cook. If you have ever put something in a microwave, pressed the button, and waited for it to heat up, you have cooked. If you have steeped a tea bag in a cup of hot water, you have cooked. If you have slathered peanut butter between two slices of bread, you have cooked.

One of the first things I made as a child was a sandwich. A big sandwich. I took a loaf of Italian bread and filled it with about two pounds of meat, along with cheese and pickles, and ate the whole thing. You know, in Italy a good eater is a good son. And I was always a huge eater. Ask my mom.

The cooking you'll learn in this book is almost as simple. It doesn't take an enormous amount of time or a lot of complicated ingredients. You can whip these recipes up fast—30, 20, or 15 minutes, or even less, especially if you keep your kitchen well stocked—with items like canned beans, broth, tuna, low-fat pasta sauces, tomato products, condiments (like salsas and mustards), vinegars, oil, herbs and spices, whole-grain pastas and rice, and much more. You don't have to learn advanced culinary skills, only some very basic techniques. And I guarantee you'll be able to prepare successful meals every day, and in the process you'll relax, unwind, and bring pleasure to life.

## Your Most Important Cooking Skill

My great romance with food started when I was very young, in my mother's kitchen. I paid attention to what my mom cooked and I was curious all the time. I was always intrigued with the beautiful colors, aromas, and flavors. It seemed she had special powers over food. She never messed up, never burned anything, and never came across a food she didn't know what to do with. There was nothing bland, no overcooked vegetables or watery sauces. At the same time, things were never overseasoned or greasy. She knew how to combine different ingredients to make a beautiful dish. Nothing was ever haphazard, even if it was thrown together at the last minute. I learned that hers was not a supernatural power; it was not memorization of recipes and techniques; the food was so good because she knew how it should taste and feel, and she tasted it often. Her food was great because her palate told her so.

Your palate—that sense of taste—is the most fundamental skill in cooking. It was formed over the course of your lifetime—through your childhood, ancestry, culture, the place you grew up, the places you've lived, your family's holiday traditions. All of these life experiences swirl together to become your palate. All you need to do is cook to please your palate, and you are on your way to becoming a cook. This is why I advise people to taste frequently and at every stage of cooking. Your taste buds are your best friend. Tasting the food you make while you are making it is paramount to producing a great dish.

Taste every part and don't wait until the end. Let's say the black bean soup you made in the experiment above is a little bland. Sweet potatoes or butternut-squash chunks are great with black beans. Check the vegetable drawer of your fridge, or your freezer, for cabbage, corn, okra, green beans, onions, squash, and so forth. Add them with enough time to cook them through. Taste and adjust seasonings for salt, pepper, and hot pepper. Add fresh herbs toward the end of cooking.

Not everyone has the same personal taste. The person who created the recipe you are following might not have liked as much sugar or black pepper or lemon juice as you do. On the flip side, maybe they like too much. This is why it is important to taste a dish as you cook and adjust the flavors to your own liking.

So find your taste equilibrium as you cook. Flavor brings food to life.

The rest of cooking is simple trial and error. And, like putting together a toy for your child at Christmas, there is some assembly required. Simply follow the recipe, step by step, to get the most out of it.

## Recipe for Love

There is something I want you to remember as you begin to prepare meals: The main ingredient in cooking is love. This is true and always has been, from the beginning of time. Think about it: You were lovingly fed by your mother from the moment you were born. The supply of food is the first thing to bind us to other human beings.

When you cook for someone, you let them know that they mean something to you. I discovered this my very first day on the job at a Queens pizzeria when I was eleven years old, and to this day, nothing makes me happier. As chefs, we burn ourselves, shop, prep, and wash dishes, and the reason we do all that is so we can have people come into our lives and enjoy our food, and we can enjoy their energy.

I could talk about different types of salts and olive oils for days, but what's really important is that cooking is a sacred, social experience. The food is the means to the end: The end is enjoying the company of other people. And a man cooking for a woman is the ultimate gesture of love, care, and generosity. When a man cooks, it shows his maternal, nurturing, and sensitive side.

Yes, going to a nice restaurant and enjoying a good meal is nice. But I believe it is even more special for me to share my cooking with a meal that I have personally prepared. It creates an intimate atmosphere because it is something I can do for others. I know my food makes them feel cared for and nurtured. And that is what you can do for your friends and family: Make them live happier and healthier.

Eating may mean staying alive, but cooking makes staying alive meaningful. Never reduce cooking to a chore; it is one of life's gifts that nourish the soul as well as the body.

## Overcoming Obstacles to Cooking

I feel, too, that cooking is a life skill we should all have—and a skill we should teach our children. I know parents who have taught their kids how to escape from a car trunk, but they wouldn't know how to make a peanut butter and jelly sandwich if you put the bread in their hands. There's a big problem here: I'm sure we would all like nice, tasty, healthy meals, but most of us wouldn't know how to make one, even if given the ingredients. It's amusing, and alarming, that we know so little about one of the most vital aspects of our lives. But if we want to change our diets and get healthier, the obvious thing is to cook ourselves nice, balanced meals. That said, I know you face obstacles

when it comes to home cooking—and there are five big ones I hear about all the time. Let's talk about them now.

### TIME

The first obstacle is time. How many times have you said, "I don't have time to cook"? Sound familiar? I'll concede that time is at a premium for Americans, divided and hurried through work, school, sports, and meetings.

Getting a healthy dinner on the table is a challenge and can often seem like a chore. But if you consider the importance of what you're really doing, it's the best investment you could make for your family.

All you need is 30 minutes to prepare most meals, and even less time if you prepare foods in advance, making use of freezing and leftovers. The recipes in this book are designed to help harried, time-crunched cooks prepare real meals and dinners quickly, with real food, in very little time.

If you think about it, 30 minutes isn't that much time. Analyze your day. How much time do you spend driving your children to dance class, soccer practice, baseball, recital, on and on and on? Maybe it is time to reprioritize, give up just one of those activities, and make cooking a family affair—a time to talk about what you've been doing all day and forge family bonds. Your own kitchen—the spiritual center of the American home—is a much better place to communicate with your family than in a sometimes noisy, hectic restaurant.

Cooking is as important a skill to learn as any sport, dance, or science. As a matter of fact, cooking is cross training for all those endeavors and more because it teaches many life skills. It's a chance to teach kids how to follow instructions, tell time, learn the value of teamwork, even how to do math fractions. It's a chance to help them develop their palates, too, since kids are more likely to taste something they've made themselves and learn to like it for the future. Plus, cooking is so popular now, with all the cooking shows on TV, that it is a great way to immerse your kids in today's popular culture.

There's just no downside to cooking at home. Even the tiniest effort will make a difference in the health and longevity of your family. So if you find yourself saying, "I didn't have time to prepare healthy food," let me ask you this: Would you have found time if your life and the lives of your loved ones depended on it? Well, they do.

Also, think about how much time you sit around with your spouse, girlfriend, boyfriend, or family, deciding where and what to eat. It's a dialogue that goes something like this:

You: *"I'm hungry. Where do you want to eat?"*

Spouse/partner: *"I don't know. Where do you want to eat?"*

You: *"I don't know. I'm up for anything."*

Spouse/partner: *"Okay, how about sushi?"*

You: *"No, we had sushi the other night."*

Spouse/partner: *"But you said you were up for anything."*

You: *"Yeah, except for sushi."*

I've had these conversations myself, and they take up a good 30 minutes of nonsense. But that's not all. If you order takeout, there's the tedious call to the restaurant, explaining what your preferences are, being misquoted, and giving them your credit card, expiration date, and security code. Next, there's the wait, and finally, the arrival, plus the unpacking and eventual disappointment that the order isn't right. It's a maddening process—one that cumulatively takes up about 2 hours of your time, resulting in an experience with which no one is happy. In that same time period, I could have prepared an amazing meal, and so could you. So, I rest my case: We all have time to cook, if we just make the time.

## MOTIVATION

The second obstacle is motivation. The sad fact is that the thing that prevents us from cooking healthy meals is often the same thing that made us fat in the first place: sheer laziness. Inside everybody I feel there is a great body—and a great cook—just waiting to climb out. It's not easy to change old habits, and some people just won't do it, even with the clear understanding that they may be harming themselves by failing to change. Fair enough. Still, improving your health and your chances for a longer life doesn't have to be an all-or-nothing proposition, nor does it have to happen at once. Just try a few of these recipes and see what you think. I'm willing to bet that they will get you started on some new healthy habits.

If you're not motivated by the desire to live a longer, healthier life for yourself, then at least think about your family, friends, children, and loved ones. There are at least a few people who would like you to take better care of yourself and a few people you should take better care of.

Let's not forget, too, that bad habits begin in childhood. Children's menus in American restaurants seem to be made up of fried foods, hamburgers, fried chicken fingers, and fat-laden macaroni and cheese. Restaurants will say that it is because that's what kids like. I say that's what parents are teaching their children to eat.

Let's teach our children to appreciate good food and the pleasure we can take from eating leisurely together as a family. They'll be less likely to overdose on junk food and suffer the consequences of bad health later. If that's not motivation, I don't know what is!

## LACK OF CONFIDENCE

The third obstacle is lack of confidence. A lot of people believe they can't cook, or if they try, they'll screw up a dish so royally that it's an embarrassment. And far too many people think that when they cook, the dish has to be as perfectly prepared as they see on television.

First of all, when you cook, you should only make something that you like. You don't have to impress others or worry that your roast pork won't stand up to your mother-in-law's standards. Nor do you have to aspire to be a top chef someday. All of those things that you see us do on TV are for the purpose of entertainment and not necessarily what you should be trying to accomplish in your effort to create healthy meals.

Aim high, but don't let your aspirations get in the way of cooking for your family. Cooking at home is not about showing off new cookware, your wine collection, or pretty tablescapes; it's about making sure your family knows they matter to you, that you care enough to hand make the nutrition they live on. Start trying the recipes in this book. They are as confidence building as they come.

Cooking should not be feared. It should be a source of pleasure and well-being. So sauté a little sliced garlic in a bit of extra-virgin olive oil until it sizzles, add some plump tomatoes and a handful of diced onions, cook for 15 to 20 minutes, stir in some fresh basil, and toss with a little pasta. Then sit down with your family and enjoy one of life's simple pleasures together.

## GET COOKING WITH A HEALTHY DINNER CLUB

Enjoying a fine meal with friends is one of life's pleasures. But, sadly, it's a pleasure often overlooked in our busy lives.

One solution to the problem: Start a dinner club. And make it a *healthy* dinner club. The idea is to eat good meals and have fun doing it. It's a great way to sample new dishes.

Invite eight to ten friends who would enjoy preparing and tasting healthy meals. Assign recipes from this book, my previous book, *Now Eat This!*, or other healthy cookbooks, and have everyone bring their assigned dish. Rotate the location each time. The idea is to have fun, learn how to cook with less fat and calories, and gain confidence in the kitchen.

I think a dinner club is a wonderful way to share great conversation and delicious food. It's also an opportunity for you to build bonds around food, friends, and fun.

### MONEY

The fourth obstacle is money. Lots of people think fresh foods are more expensive, but that's a myth. Pound for pound, unprocessed whole foods are always less expensive because you have to do the work. And if you follow my instructions, the work you do will produce a healthier end result.

Science backs me up on all this. Switching to a diet of mostly low-sugar, low-fat foods can shave up to $600 a year off your family's grocery bill, according to a study in the *Journal of the American Dietetic Association*.

When I was asked by *The Biggest Loser* to create healthy, low-calorie, low-fat meals, I was also challenged to prepare meals that would fit the average weekly budget for a family of four. That's around $219, according to the the USDA Center for Nutrition Policy and Promotion. I found that the only way to do this was to buy raw, unprocessed ingredients as close as possible to their natural state—and of course, that's the healthiest food you can have. The less done to your food, the less expensive it is.

Strive to buy healthy foods instead of, not in addition to, junk food. That means your shopping cart should be filled with whole-grain products and fruits and vegetables. The potato chips and cookies will have to stay on the store shelves.

Maybe right now you're thinking you can't live without your favorite junk foods. I understand; I used to think that way, too. Very few people know this, but even though I'm a multistarred chef, I once had a problem with junk food. While I was growing up, my father forbade me to eat candy, candy bars, and all types of junk food. He wouldn't even allow that stuff in our house. So naturally, when I grew up, I wanted what I couldn't have. I ate heavy doses of sugary and fatty junk food, and I bought it in bulk. I found ridiculous pleasure biting into the silky-smooth, tempting seductress, otherwise known as chocolate.

But I got smart after realizing this junk was turning my brain and body into junk. I walked into my kitchen one day, gathered it all up, and tossed it out.

### EQUIPMENT

The fifth obstacle is equipment. Does anyone really need an artichoke stand, a strawberry huller, a shrimp peeler, an iced tea brewer, a popcorn machine, a 4-quart collapsible salad spinner, or a blender with a motor that can puree steel beams? (Well, maybe keep the powerful blender.) The answer is no. We don't need more than a dozen pieces of equipment to cook just about everything. Sure the gadgets are nice sometimes, but not necessary.

I think it's ridiculous that so many people run out and stock their kitchens with enough stuff to run the Culinary Institute of America. I blame myself and every chef like me, who for years emphasized the wrong things, like fancy equipment and exotic ingredients. It was wrong, and I should have known better. For my whole life I watched my mother and grandmother cook with the bare essentials: a Magic Chef four-burner stove (electric for my grandmother!), a big pot (Grandma used the same one for many years), a paring knife (with no tip), and an old cast-iron skillet (with the handle broken off); not even a cutting board, because they cut foods like bread against their bodies in their hands.

You don't need all the stuff! It's a myth that you need state-of-the-art equipment to be a great cook. All you need are some basic, inexpensive pieces of equipment, and you're on your way. Here's a list (and I bet you own most of it already):

- Two sharp knives—a big one and a small one: a chef's knife and a paring knife; make sure they stay sharp, and you can cut anything from tomatoes to bread to steaks and even a tin can with either one of these knives.

- Two pots—a big one (5–6 quarts) and a small one (1–2 quarts), both with tight-fitting lids. In these two pieces of cookware you can do everything from blanching vegetables to cooking pasta to making soups and stews.

- One large skillet, frying pan, or sauté pan. If you want it to be maintenance free and cheap, get a cast-iron pan. If you want to go a step up, get an all-stainless-steel pan. If you want to cook with less fat, get a heavy nonstick coated pan. Just stay away from uncoated aluminum. Whatever pan you get should be at least 10 inches in diameter so you can fit four portions in it.

- Baking pans. You can use disposable aluminum if you really want to, or you can invest in an oven-safe glass baking dish. One oval or large rectangular baking dish (about 3 quarts) will roast a chicken, a leg of lamb, or a small roast and cook a casserole or a recipe of lasagna. If you like, add an 8-inch square glass casserole for the brownies and a 9-inch glass pie plate, which can bake quiches or serve as a small casserole. Both are inexpensive.

- One 12 x 18-inch sheet pan.

- One wire rack to fit in that pan. Many of my recipes call for a wire rack. It elevates meat or poultry to keep it out of its juices (and grease) and allows air circulation for even cooking and browning. Placing some liquid, such as water or chicken broth, in the pan below the rack adds humidity to your oven, so meats come out tender and moist.

- One large cutting board. Wood or hard rubber is the best. Glass, thermoplastic, and even your counter top will ruin your knives.

- One set of measuring cups and measuring spoons.

- A colander for draining vegetables, pastas, and other items cooked in water.

- One flexible slotted spatula for turning meat, fish, or anything you don't want to touch with your hand.

- One stainless-steel whisk—about 10 inches long.

- One large stirring spoon and two tablespoons for tasting and stirring.

- One food processor.

- One blender. Here's where to splurge if you can. My favorite blender is a Vita Prep 500 if your budget allows. If not, a $20 glass bar mixer is just fine.

# Fat Out, Flavor In

To get the most flavor from the fewest calories, I experimented with a lot of different cooking methods. Nothing influences the flavor of food more than how it's prepared. I discovered that you'll get the best results from the following techniques—all easy to do.

### ROASTING

Roasting uses hot, dry oven air to cook food, usually meats and poultry. It seals the outer surface of the food so that the inner juices cook the inside of the food. Roasting is one of the best ways to cook vegetables such as onions, garlic, squash, or eggplant. The high heat brings out their natural sweetness as the carbohydrates in them caramelize, so that they take on a whole different flavor and texture.

### BAKING

Baking is similar to roasting, but it involves oven cooking ingredients used in bread, cake, pie, brownie, quiche, casserole, and cookie recipes. However, fish, vegetables, and fruit can be successfully baked, too.

### GRILLING

I would grill year-round if I could. I love the way an open fire intensifies the flavor of food, but without a lot of fat. Indoors or out, grilling is more versatile than you might think. You can grill meat, fish, and poultry; toast bread; steam vegetables in foil; or smoke pork chops. You heat up the grill until it's burning hot and toss your food on it until it's done. Grilling is simply the best way to brown, char, and caramelize food without using a lot of fat. For a smoky flavor, you can add certain types of wood chips. Away from the heat, blast your grill rack with cooking spray before you grill to keep food from sticking.

### BROILING

One of the simplest of all cooking methods, broiling cooks by exposing food to radiant heat in an electric or gas oven. It renders the same results as grilling, but in grilling the heat comes from below, while in broiling it

# Chopping 101

Ninety percent of cooking happens with a knife and a cutting board. If you know how to use a knife, any cooking project is a cinch. So let's do a short cooking lesson on one of the most common kitchen tasks: chopping an onion. This is not how pro chefs do it, but it's the easiest way to do it at home.

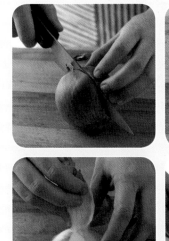
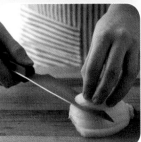

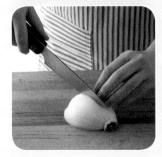
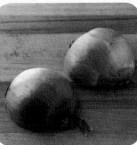

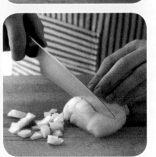

① Place the onion on a cutting board. Use a sharp knife to slice the onion in half vertically, through both the root and the stem ends.

② Place each half cut side down.

③ Peel the outer skin off each half, and leave the root (this holds the onion together).

④ Chop one onion half by drawing the knife through the onion three or four times horizontally, then three or four times vertically.

⑤ Repeat with the other onion half.

SHORTCUT:

If you're pressed for time, buy prechopped onions from the produce section in the grocery store.

*let's cook*

comes from above. During broiling, you do not get the interplay of juices and fire, but you do get a nice, crispy texture that is delicious.

## STEWING

Stewing involves slowly simmering pieces of food (meat or vegetables) in liquid. If you wish, this liquid will eventually become the stock or sauce that is served with the food. Stews make a complete meal on their own.

## SAUTÉING

Sautéing involves cooking meat or vegetables in a skillet containing butter, oil, or another fat. The French word sauté means "jump," and it comes from that fancy-looking move a chef makes when he moves a pan quickly back and forth across a burner to toss the food slightly up in the air. (I don't recommend this unless you want your food to fly all over the place. Actually, go for it! It's fun, and when you get it right, it's impressive and makes food taste better.) Normally, you need a relatively small amount of fat to sauté, but even a few sprays of cooking spray will do the trick—plus slash the fat and calories considerably.

I like to heat the pan first. When it's visibly hot and not a second sooner, you move it away from the stove, for safety, and add the cooking spray or oil and let it spread. (Never add the spray near an open flame.) You might need to do the spreading. Just pick the pan up and roll the liquid around; then place it back on the heat. When the fat is hot, then you add your goodies and get them moving so they won't burn. Use a spatula or a large spoon to get them moving. The goal is to get all sides of your food nicely browned and cooked through.

## POACHING

With poaching, you submerge food in a flavored liquid such as wine or chicken broth. The food takes up the flavor of the cooking liquid and then gives flavor back, so the liquid can be reduced to make a sauce. When poaching, there should be little to no bubbles on the surface; 160 to 170°F is a good range to poach in. Be careful to not let the liquid reach the boiling point because high heat can actually dry the food. Plus, the vigor of boiling can damage delicate foods that are traditionally poached, such as fish, eggs, chicken breasts, and pears. Poach only in highly flavored liquids, and add as much spice and as many aromatics as you can.

## STEAMING

Steaming is, simply, cooking food in an enclosed environment surrounded by superheated water vapor. Steam has more heat energy than boiling water, and when you add pressure (like from a lid), you cook foods much faster. Because you don't submerge foods in water, you aren't leaching out any nutrition. You can steam in a variety of ways: My favorite is the $3 Chinese bamboo steamers that stack on top of a pot. Steaming cooks fast and preserves flavor, eliminating the need for added fats during preparation. It also preserves nutrients better than any other cooking method except microwaving. It's perfect for fish and shellfish because it doesn't dry out the delicate flesh. Halibut, cod, and snapper steam really well, and so do vegetables.

## MICROWAVING

When you microwave a food, you are essentially steaming it from the inside out. Like steaming, microwaving lends itself to low-fat or no-fat cooking. Foods that microwave well include vegetables, because they retain their color along with their nutrients, and fish and chicken, which plump up well compared to beef and pork.

## FAUX FRYING

This is my signature style of "frying"—something I developed specifically for calorie reduction and weight loss. It is one of the best ways to turn comfort food into health food, and the results are amazingly delicious. I start with a slightly modified breading procedure and ingredients: white flour is replaced with 100 percent whole wheat flour, whole eggs are replaced with whipped egg whites, and bread crumbs are replaced with whole wheat panko bread crumbs. Whatever is being breaded is placed on a baking rack, sprayed with cooking spray, and baked in a very hot oven. The result is a crisp crust that tastes just like it was deep-fried. You'll love it, and you won't miss deep-fried foods.

## FLASH FRYING

Flash frying lasts roughly 30 seconds at about 400 degrees, as opposed to 8 or 9 minutes for deep-frying at the same heat. With flash frying, food spends very little time in the oil, meaning much less fat is absorbed into the food, whereas in deep-frying, cups of oil are absorbed. Flash frying cooks only the outside of the product, and fixes the breading to give a feather-light crunch.

# Now You're Ready

There are just two parts to cooking: the "prep," which includes food planning and grocery shopping, and the actual cooking. I've provided extensive shopping lists for you which is 75 percent of the work; all you need to do is go to the grocery store or order online once a week and stock your pantry and refrigerator accordingly. Some tips:

- Take your list to the grocery store on paper or in your PDA and make sure you include everything. A missing ingredient could make a difference in the taste of what you prepare.

- Once you're ready to prepare a recipe, make sure you have enough room to work. So clear off your counters and tabletops. It will make life in the kitchen a whole lot easier.

- Read through the entire recipe at least once before making it.

- Assemble your ingredients. Chefs call this *mise en place*. It's a French phrase that means "to put in place," referring to having all the ingredients for a dish prepared and ready to combine up to the point of cooking. Prepping and assembling the ingredients saves a ton of time and reduces confusion and stress when the moment comes to put it all together.

- Gather your equipment—whatever the recipe calls for.

- Wash your hands thoroughly with soap before you start and throughout the steps, and especially after handling meat, chicken, or poultry.

Cook—then enjoy!

## TAKE CHARGE OF YOUR WEIGHT WITH THESE TIPS

Once you get your basic moves down, take your culinary skills a little further by applying these flavor-enhancing, calorie-busting tips. They'll help you make over your favorite recipes.

- Skin your chicken breast after cooking it. You'll retain moisture yet still strip away 148 calories and 13 grams of fat.

- Substitute egg whites for some of the whole eggs in recipes. Replacing each egg with 2 egg whites will save you 5 grams of fat.

- Use butter-flavored cooking spray, not a tablespoon of margarine or butter, to make grilled cheese sandwiches and egg dishes.

- Cook chicken or fish fillets in tightly wrapped foil. The foil lets the fillets steam in their own juices, increasing flavor without adding fat-filled oils. You can also pour a tablespoon of broth or wine over each fillet and lightly season with herbs of your choice. Place on a baking sheet and cook in a preheated, 400°F oven for 20 minutes, or until the fillets are opaque.

- If a baking recipe calls for oil, try replacing a third of the oil with buttermilk or unsweetened applesauce. (Increase the baking powder by about ¼ teaspoon.)

- Substitute lesser amounts of extra-sharp, reduced-fat cheese for mild cheddar cheese for more flavor, less fat.

- Add vegetables to your favorite spaghetti sauce; mix in bite-size amounts of broccoli, cauliflower, and carrots for extra nutrition.

- Splash herb-infused vinegars on roasted veggies, grilled fish, grains, and salads.

- Grated rind, especially the zest (flavorful outer rind), gives a tang to poultry, vegetables, salads, and sauces.

- Season your foods with hot sauce or chili peppers (if you like spicy foods). Both are high in capsaicin, which may help curb your appetite. A study in the *British Journal of Nutrition* revealed that people who had a hot sauce on their food ate 200 fewer calories in the next 3 hours than did those who ate their meal plain.

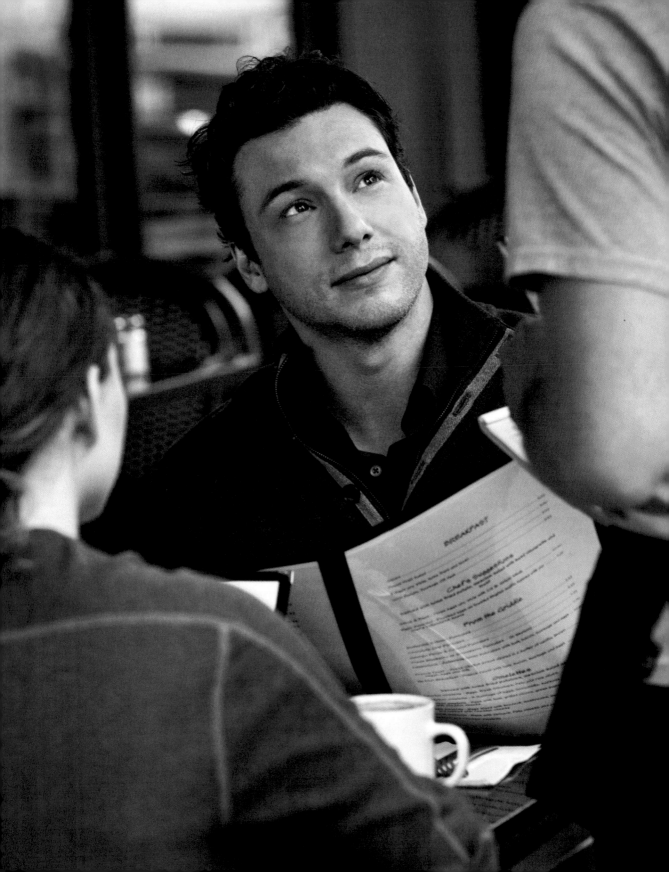

chapter

# 7

☺

# Now You Can Eat Out

Have you ever felt timid or reluctant to ask for exactly what you want in a restaurant? Well, don't. As a former restaurant owner, I know firsthand that people in the restaurant business exist to make you happy—they live for it—and they love to grant special requests. So you shouldn't feel bad or shy about asking for anything special if you're on a special diet for weight loss, health, or other reasons. As a guest in a restaurant, you should command what you eat and how it's prepared.

Even though I was in the restaurant business, I didn't always believe this or even honor my customers' wishes. My modus operandi was: What the chef says, goes. An unusual experience changed that attitude forever.

On an early Saturday evening in 1998, a seventy-something man walked into Union Pacific restaurant at 111 East Twenty-second Street in New York City, where I was part owner and executive chef. He had clear blue eyes behind his thick black-framed glasses, and his hair was streaked with gray. Wearing a tweed suit jacket and a bolo tie, he walked like he was strung together with wires. His cheeks were sunken and deeply lined. He asked to be seated under the skylight so he could see the menu better.

The old man was shown to his table by a waiter who was pleasant and polite and presented him with our menu, which overflowed with choices. Once ready to order, he began firing questions like a game-show host.

"What's this? What's that? Can I have my tuna well done?" he fired away in a low, raspy voice.

"Er . . . well, the chef prefers it served medium-rare," said the waiter.

"What about the sauce? Can I have a different sauce?"

"No . . . the chef prepares it with this sauce only."

"Can I substitute a baked potato for the asparagus? Can you do that?"

The now-exasperated waiter seemed a little irked at having to pay attention to the old guy's demands.

"We don't have any baked potatoes tonight, sir."

And so it went. Whatever the customer asked for, there were rules that applied and had been imposed by the chef, who of course was me.

But I was also the old man in the tweed jacket and bolo tie, disguised on purpose by a very accomplished makeup artist. I was on a secret mission to see what it was like to dine in my own restaurant.

I used to rely on "secret diners," the restaurant version of secret shoppers, to go to my restaurant, experience the food, the service, and the ambiance, and report back to me. But I finally realized that I would never truly know what the experience was like until I went myself—and did so incognito. So that's what I did. None of my staff even recognized me. Nor did the doorman at my apartment building. That's how cleverly disguised I was.

My undercover experience evoked an epiphany deep within my chef's soul. Until that day, I was one of those cocky, snobbish, annoying chefs who never wanted to accommodate any special requests. I felt that my personal preference was more important than the customer's. I knew how to cook the tuna, grill the steak, and dress the salad. I had so many rules that I made the dining experience oppressive and unpleasant for both my waiters and my customers.

The day after my masquerade, I announced to my partners and staff that the rules were changing. They never found out why, but they were thrilled. From that point on, there were no more rules—except for one: Whatever the customer wants, the answer is yes.

Most chefs are very accommodating and are always happy to grant special requests, but you must ask. So I want to talk to you about how to do that in most restaurants. Let's start at the very beginning of the restaurant experience: before you even get there.

## Take Control Ahead of Time

I suggest that you call ahead and talk to the reservations manager. Explain to this person that you're on a restricted diet, per your doctor's instructions, and you can't eat high-calorie foods. Ask if the restaurant can accommodate you. If they hedge, stammer, or debate, move on. There are plenty of other places to go. As a diner you've got plenty of choices for dining out. There are nearly one million restaurants in the United States, according to the National Restaurant Association.

Calling ahead is smart. Time is a precious resource in a restaurant. Chefs have a very limited ability to change their system on the fly, but if they know a customer's needs ahead of time, they'll be more willing to help you.

Check the restaurant's menu well before you go (most restaurants post their menus online these days) and see what the choices are. Let's say the restaurant serves an Almond Chicken. Fax the chef my recipe for Chicken

Amandine and request that he or she prepare it this way. You can do this with just about any low-cal recipe, especially if the restaurant has a similar but higher-calorie version on its menu.

Alternatively, let the restaurant know you can't eat more than 500 calories per meal. The chef should be able to do the math and work with you.

Once you get to the restaurant, remind them of who you are and what you requested. The bottom line is to take control of your dining experience right from the beginning.

Take control with confidence. You are the customer, and the customer is the most important person in the restaurant equation. Remember that, and you can eat out—anywhere—and stay true to your diet.

## Don't Go Hungry

It wouldn't be a bad idea to munch on one of your snacks before you go out to eat. If you're ravenous when you get to the restaurant, you're in a weakened state and are setting yourself up for diet failure. Hunger is one of the most powerful evolutionary urges there is. The server could put a hot bowl of chicken grease in front of you and you would slop it down because you're so hungry. So don't be too hungry when you arrive; it's like walking into battle with an unloaded weapon. You're apt to inhale the bread—and the basket it's served in.

## Ask Your Server to Decode the Menu

Restaurants have so many different items on the menu that you can get old and gray while choosing. And of course, many are soaked in hidden fat. Your intentions may be good when you order grilled chicken and steamed vegetables, but you can't be certain that your meat is truly low fat unless you ask if the chicken can be prepared without oil and the vegetables free of butter. By the way, at a quality restaurant, assume that butter is in everything, because it is.

Sauces with cream, cheese, or butter are obviously heavyweight. Sauces that cling to the food are likely to add more fat to your body than those that run off the food. Be cautious with nut sauces, peanut sauces, tahini, hollandaise, mayonnaise, sour cream, crème fraîche, olive

sauces, or guacamole, or anything made with avocado. These are all loaded with fat.

In better restaurants, be specific about how you want your food prepared. Tell your server, for example, that you want your fish poached in chicken stock, or your vinaigrette made with 1 part oil and 3 parts balsamic vinegar instead of 3 parts oil and 1 part vinegar.

Order items with these descriptions: fresh, boiled, steamed, roasted, in wine sauce, in its own juice, baked, vegetable-based sauce, grilled, and poached. Avoid items that read: fried, crispy, with butter, creamy, in gravy, hollandaise, au gratin, casserole, stewed, cream or cheese sauce, battered, or breaded. See my Restaurant Primer below to get up to speed on food-preparation methods in restaurants.

## ROCCO'S RESTAURANT PRIMER

| LOWEST-FAT OPTIONS | LOW-FAT BUT HIGH-SODIUM OPTIONS | HIGH-FAT OPTIONS |
| --- | --- | --- |
| AU JUS (IN ITS OWN JUICES) | BARBECUED | ALFREDO |
| BROILED | BLACKENED | AU GRATIN (WITH CHEESE) |
| FLAME-COOKED | CREOLE SAUCE | BATTER-DIPPED |
| GRILLED | IN BROTH | BÉARNAISE |
| PARBOILED | MARINATED | BEURRE BLANC |
| POACHED | MUSTARD SAUCE | BREADED |
| ROASTED | PICKLED | CREAMY |
| STEAMED | SMOKED | CRISPY |
| | WITH SOY SAUCE OR MSG | EN CROÛTE |
| | TERIYAKI | ESCALLOPED |
| | | FLAKY |
| | | FRIED |
| | | HOLLANDAISE |
| | | PARMIGIANA |
| | | POT PIE |
| | | PRIME |
| | | TEMPURA |

Ask for things on the side. If the entrée comes with a sauce, ask for it on the side so you can control the amount used. Same with salads. Opt for the healthy oil-based dressing and get it on the side.

Substitute bad for good. It might cost you a little more on the bill, but your body will thank you. Get fruit instead of fries or ask for extra veggies, for example. Anytime a restaurant offers low- or no-fat versions of a dish, go for it.

## Alcohol Smarts

The beginning of the meal usually means the beverage. Alcohol, as appealing and relaxing as it may be, is the epitome of empty calories (calories that have no nutritional value). So if you care, switch to fizzy water—club soda, seltzer, or mineral water—and enliven it, if you like, with a wedge of lime, a dash of bitters, or a spritz of orange juice.

Wine can be an important part of any meal. It makes the food taste richer and better. But don't go overboard, because wine contains roughly 120 calories per glass. Try cutting your wine with sparkling water—a wine spritzer.

Resist the urge to order a bottle of wine. Though it's more expensive per ounce to buy by the glass, you'll probably drink less and there is no pressure to finish the bottle. Overall, after you sip your wine, drink some water. Alternate like that through the evening. This not only cuts your calories for the evening; it helps ward off a hangover by keeping you hydrated.

If you're watching your calories and carbs, fermentation and distillation make hard alcohol, such as vodka, rum, gin, and whiskey, a great choice—but without the high-calorie, high-sugar mixers. Mixed drinks really pour on the calories. With a little forethought, you can substitute most cocktail mixers with something less caloric: tomato juice, club soda, sugar-free lemonade or iced tea, diet sodas, and the like, thus keeping calories reasonable. Or have hard liquor over ice, without the mixers. Get familiar with the calorie counts of other alcoholic drinks, and make lower-calorie choices. (See the chart.)

In general, watch your alcohol intake while losing weight—for three reasons. First, calories in alcohol are used before stored fat calories. Second, people who are overweight actually gain weight more easily when they drink alcohol. Third, calories from alcohol tend to be stored in the gut. This gives *six-pack* a whole new meaning.

| ALCOHOLIC BEVERAGE | CALORIES |
|---|---|
| BEER (12 FLUID OUNCES) | |
| REGULAR BEER | 140 |
| LIGHT BEER | 110 |
| LOW-CARB BEER | 95 |
| NONALCOHOLIC BEER | 70 |
| WINE (5.1 FLUID OUNCES) | |
| CHAMPAGNE | 85–95 |
| CHARDONNAY | 120 |
| FLAVORED WINES (ARBOR MIST, WILD VINES) | 80 |
| MERLOT | 119 |
| PINOT GRIGIO | 114 |
| PINOT NOIR | 117 |
| BURGUNDY, CABERNET | 127 |
| SAUVIGNON BLANC | 122 |
| NONALCOHOLIC WINE | 50 |
| SAKE (RICE WINE) | 194 |
| SHIRAZ | 116 |
| WHITE ZINFANDEL | 108 |
| ZINFANDEL | 123 |
| SPIRITS/LIQUORS (80 PROOF—1.5 FLUID OUNCES, OR 1 SHOT) | |
| BOURBON | 100 |
| GIN | 96 |
| RUM | 97 |
| SCOTCH | 103 |
| TEQUILA | 97 |
| VODKA | 103 |
| LIQUEURS AND CORDIALS (1.5 FLUID OUNCES, OR 1 SHOT) | |
| AMARETTO | 120 |

| | |
|---|---|
| BENEDICTINE | 133 |
| COFFEE LIQUEUR | 165 |
| COINTREAU | 140 |
| CRÈME DE CACAO | 148 |
| CRÈME DE MENTHE | 158 |
| CURAÇAO | 140 |
| DRAMBUIE | 120 |
| FRANGELICO | 106 |
| GRAND MARNIER | 112 |
| KAHLÚA | 135 |
| SAMBUCA | 148 |
| SCHNAPPS | 151 |
| TIA MARIA | 133 |
| TRIPLE SEC | 110 |
| POPULAR MIXED DRINKS | |
| BLOODY MARY (10 FLUID OUNCES) | 125 |
| BOURBON AND SODA (STANDARD COCKTAIL GLASS) | 110 |
| COSMOPOLITAN (4 FLUID OUNCES) | 213 |
| DAIQUIRI (4 FLUID OUNCES) | 211 |
| GIN AND TONIC (6 FLUID OUNCES) | 143 |
| LONG ISLAND ICED TEA (10 FLUID OUNCES) | 300 |
| MAI TAI (STANDARD COCKTAIL GLASS) | 260 |
| MANHATTAN (STANDARD COCKTAIL GLASS) | 130 |
| MARGARITA (10 FLUID OUNCES) | 464 |
| MARTINI (STANDARD COCKTAIL GLASS) | 135 |
| MOJITO (10 FLUID OUNCES) | 428 |
| PIÑA COLADA (8 FLUID OUNCES) | 437 |
| SCREWDRIVER (STANDARD COCKTAIL GLASS) | 180 |
| SEX ON THE BEACH (STANDARD COCKTAIL GLASS) | 240 |
| TEQUILA SUNRISE (10 FLUID OUNCES) | 348 |
| TOM COLLINS (STANDARD COCKTAIL GLASS) | 120 |
| WHISKEY SOUR (STANDARD COCKTAIL GLASS) | 125 |
| WHITE RUSSIAN (STANDARD COCKTAIL GLASS) | 284 |

## Stay in the No-Dessert Zone

Let's say you've just finished your dinner and you've ordered coffee. Suddenly you hear something squeaking toward your table. It's the dessert cart. You don't want to look, but you can't help it.

Turtle cheesecake. Flans. Triple-decker carrot cake. Chocolate mousse with shaved white chocolate. Massive chunks of tantalizing, gooey, scrumptious-looking concoctions loaded with more calories than you've eaten this year.

Escape is not an option. In a moment of weakness, you order one of everything. Sound familiar?

First of all, wave off the dessert cart before it starts rolling anywhere near your direction. Do the same with the dessert menu. Ask the server for fresh fruit. If it's not available, sip your coffee in silence and be proud. You were nearly seduced, but you resisted and taught those mouthwatering morsels a serious lesson: No dessert can tempt you!

Honestly, there's really no dessert that you can order in a restaurant if you're trying to shed flab. And don't even try a bite or two. No one has that kind of control, so why even risk it?

And don't be fooled into ordering sorbet. It's mostly sugar.

## ROCCO'S RULES OF ORDERING

I wouldn't be a chef if I didn't love food. My job requires me to eat, whether I'm hungry or not. And I have to taste a lot of food. When I go out to eat, the chefs are always bringing me lots of different foods to sample, including gooey desserts—so I have to be very careful. Here are some of my personal techniques and tips:

- Choose a restaurant that meets your needs. Patronize places likely to offer healthful choices. Don't expect a rib joint to carry low-fat food. Forget all-you-can-eat places, too, or else you'll be circling the table with a clean plate in hand for round 3.

- Ask the server to remove the bread basket (after your companions have served themselves).

- Be the first to order. Waiting until everyone in your party has ordered can weaken your resolve to eat right.

- Make special requests. Don't be shy. Ask for mustard instead of mayo, salsa instead of butter for baked potatoes, broccoli instead of coleslaw.

- Practice portion control. Request a doggy bag at the start of your meal; don't wait until the end, or you may be tempted to clean your plate. Or split your entrée with a friend; I do this all the time. Sharing food may also create a more intimate mood.

- Drink several glasses of water while dining. It helps fill you up. Gulping down one small reservoir at your meal should do.

- Fill up on filling appetizers. Skip high-fat choices. Order tomato juice, a fruit cup, a vegetable tray, or a clear, broth-based soup. Having soup will fill you up, and you'll eat less of the main course.

- Bring a bottle of Tabasco and shake it on certain foods. Tabasco contains capsaicin, a chemical irritant that inflames a nerve inside of your mouth. The net effect is that your food feels richer.

- Ask for salad dressing on the side. Then use the fork-dip method: Dip the tines of your fork in the dressing and spear your salad. Another option: Bring your own mister with a little oil and balsamic vinegar inside, or pack a salad spritzer in your purse. Ask for an undressed salad and dress it yourself.

- Be adventuresome. Try new, healthy foods that you might not prepare at home, such as quinoa, broccoli rabe, pork tenderloin, wild striped bass, chilled burdock root, Japanese sweet potato, lentil salad, tuna tartare, Moroccan-spiced loin of lamb . . . I could go on and on!

## Savor the Experience

Perhaps another secret to staying trim and healthy is to not only to adopt a delicious diet but also its attitudes, which include enjoying and savoring the experience of food and the company of those with whom we break bread. As an Italian kid growing up, I can tell you we never ate in a hurried fashion, nor until we exploded. Our meals lasted for two hours, mostly for chatting, and maybe only twenty minutes for chewing. Take a trip to Italy and you'll see that there are not a lot of obese Italians.

Unfortunately, as the pace of life increases and the need for efficiency rules, the culture of eating is one of the first things to erode. Some restaurants nurture neither the soul nor the body. Easy-to-prepare packaged food numbs the palette. On-the-run eating dulls the art of conversation.

I advocate a return to the intimate, social aspects of dining. The reason we go to restaurants is not just to eat, but to enjoy the company of our friends. Friends sharing a meal tend to share stories—about life, love, family, and work. There is a level of intimacy hard to find elsewhere. The experience makes you feel alive and human. It's one of the few times during the day when you can let yourself relax and not do, or worry about anything else. And the more you talk, the less you'll eat. Eating more slowly helps you feel full faster.

Food is so much more than physical survival. Sharing food can be many things: romantic, nurturing, socializing, and celebratory.

So as you dine out with your friends and family, savor the experience. Give each other the precious gift of time, and celebrate life.

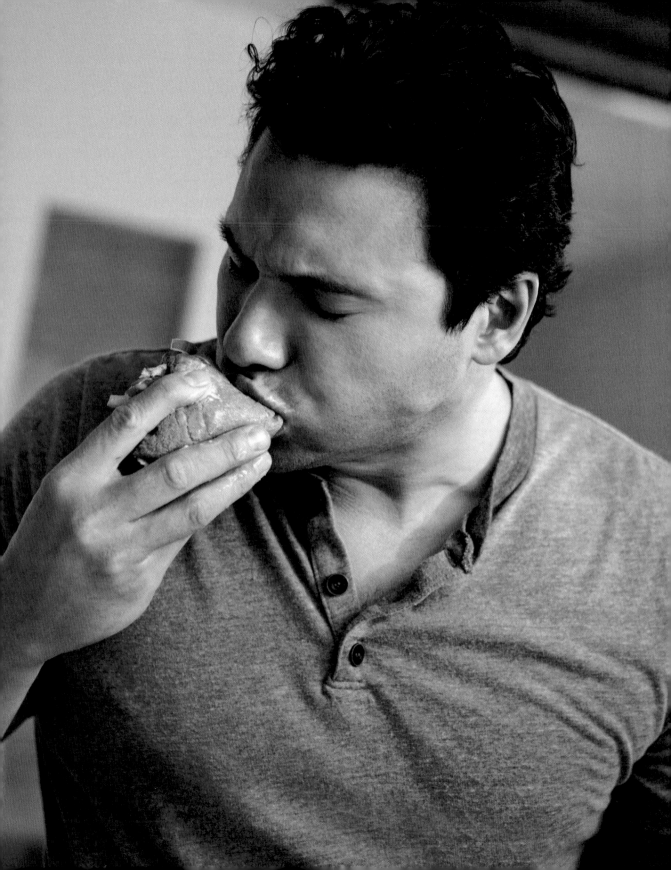

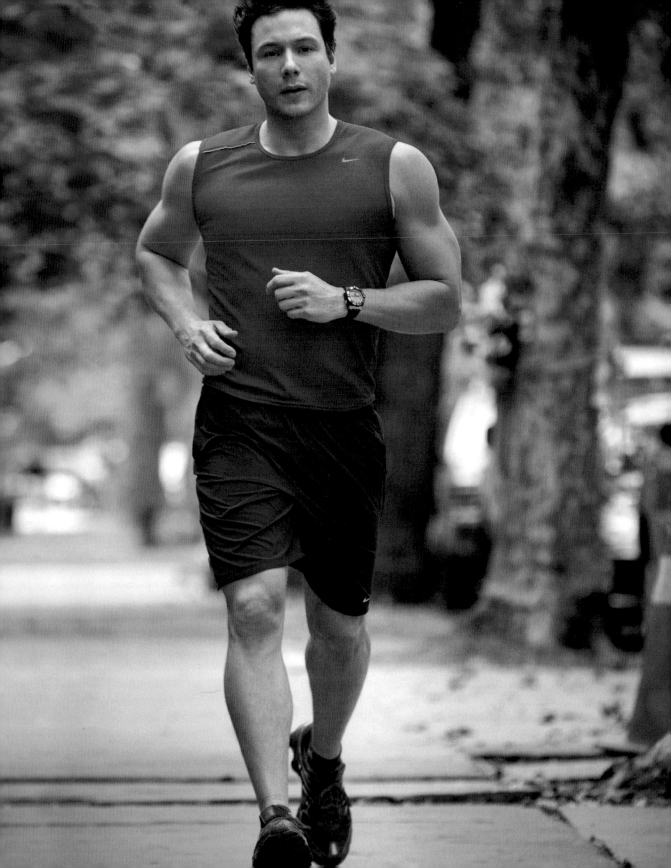

chapter

# 8

☺

# The Exercise Recipe

If you really want to shed pounds and inches on this diet, now you've got to exercise.

A confession: I was never much into exercise. I toyed with it, but I never made it a huge priority in my life.

One reason was I had major back problems that had plagued me my whole life. I knew eventually I wouldn't be able to stand at the stove anymore, or stand anywhere, period. My health was getting in the way of my life and my livelihood.

Fortunately, I got a good recommendation from a trainer I knew and found a chiropractor who worked wonders. He put me back on my feet, pain-free.

But he did something else, too: He got me much more active—which would ultimately help me change my diet and lose weight.

I've often told this story, but it bears retelling. One day I walked into my chiropractor's office for my regular adjustment, and he asked me if I would participate in a triathlon for charity. Chefs are suckers for charities, so I said, "Sure, how many portions of tuna do you need? What kind of scallops do you want?"

"Cook? I want you to compete!" he said.

I thought he was kidding. Here I was with serious back issues, and he wanted me to compete in a triathlon? Me? I had never been in anything organized unless it involved mass quantities of food as part of the competition.

A triathlon sounded intimidating. It would mean three grueling events to train for—swimming, biking, and running. But I was game—I always say yes when it comes to charity—but I had to get in shape. I hooked up with a trainer to help me. I couldn't walk a mile, much less run 3, 6, 13 miles. I couldn't even swim when I started. Actually, I was afraid of deep water.

Gradually, I went from walking, to walking and jogging, eventually getting to the point where I could almost run. Despite challenges, my swimming and cycling also steadily progressed.

One day after training, I remember coming home, lying on the couch, and thinking, "This is just too hard. I don't I think can do it." I would lie awake in bed picturing the different ways I would drown or how I might collapse before reaching the finish line.

But I got focused anyway, doing cardio training—twice a day, six days a week. In June 2006, I competed in my first triathlon.

The day of the race I stood on the starting line hyped up on a mixture of terror and excitement. I swam. I biked. I ran. I loved every second of it.

After training for months to complete this triathlon, I didn't care where I finished. I just cared that I finished and preferably not on a stretcher, crawling, puking, or after everybody else had left for the day.

And as I ran the last leg, I realized, "A few more yards and I'm a triathlete!" I almost burst into tears. I crossed the finish line, feeling shock, awe, and pure exaltation. Me, a triathlete! I wanted to pinch myself, even though I was sore.

I finished dead last, far behind a pack of sixty-year-old women who passed me in the water like I was standing still. But I didn't care. I think it was the sense of accomplishment that hooked me. That feeling of knowing that even though something is hard, you can keep pushing to achieve it.

Competing opened up a whole new world for me. Before that week was over, I was looking at a race schedule to see what the next one would be. I've gotten seven triathlons under my belt since that first one, including the Ironman 70.3 World Championship in Clearwater, Florida, in 2009. That entailed swimming 1.2 miles, biking 56 miles, and running 13.1 miles against more than fifteen hundred elite athletes from around the world. I endured six hours straight of pure pain, but I achieved a personal best of over 1 hour and 30 minutes faster than my last one, and I loved every bit of it. You are out there racing with a big group of people, but in the end, you are really just competing against yourself. I wasn't going to give up. I'm an absurdly stubborn guy.

I like the feeling of accomplishment. I also like the feeling of sore muscles the day after the race. It's my body telling me that my chunk of flesh and flab has worked hard and is maybe building some muscle.

I will keep doing triathlons. No question about it.

Oh—and I like to share my triathlon experiences in the hope that they might inspire others to get more active. Hey, I'm a flat-footed chef with a bad back. If I can start exercising, anyone can.

# The Calorie Burn

I'm not saying you have to train for triathlons or marathons (unless you've set your sights on those goals). But if you want to get in better shape, exercise is key. With just 5, 10, 15, 20, or 30 minutes of exercise a few days a week, you can convert your own metabolism (the rate at which you burn calories) from a smolder to a blaze. Unless your physical activity burns more calories than you consume, you will gain weight no matter what you eat. It's the concept of iso-caloric balance: Calories in have to equal calories out to maintain weight, and calories in have to be less than calories out to lose weight. A very smart woman once told me to eat less and move more; that's all we are talking about here.

Sure, you can lose weight without exercising. People do it all the time. But the ones who manage to keep off lost weight for at least a year are involved in a regular exercise program. By comparison, a substantial number of people who lose weight through diet alone gain it back after a year, with interest.

No matter how healthy your diet is, you're going to put on a few pounds if you don't work out to burn those calories. While there are a few tricks out there in terms of diet, this is a universal truth.

## Translate Calories into Exercise

Most people worry about variables like duration (how long you work out), intensity (level of effort), and frequency (how many times a week you exercise). All are important, but I've got a better idea: Translate calories into exercise.

To lose a certain amount of weight, you've got to know the amount of time you need to engage in a certain physical activity.

Suppose you want to burn 1,750 calories in a week to help you lose an extra ½ pound. What would that take to burn off by exercising?

Look over the following chart. Like my diets, the following chart is color-coded according to calories burned, on average, in 1 hour.

To burn 1,750 calories, you could do:

3 **BLUE** activities (1,200 calories)

1 YELLOW activity (300 calories)

1 **GREEN** activity (200 calories)

1 **PURPLE** activity (50 calories)

So if you walked very briskly 3 times a week, had sex for an hour one night, cleaned your house, and took a nap, you'd burn ½ pound in 1 week. It's pretty easy to lose weight if you translate calories into exercise.

What I suggest is that you set a goal each week for how many calories you want to burn; then plan your activities accordingly.

## 400 ACTIVITIES THAT BURN CALORIES AN HOUR ☺

Aerobics, low impact

Ballroom dancing, fast

Cycling, 10–11.9 mph, light

Hiking, cross-country

Mowing the lawn, walking, using a power mower

Playing basketball, nongame

Playing racquetball

Running, 5 mph (12 minute mile)

Stationary cycling, moderate

Swimming leisurely, not laps

Taking an exercise class

Tennis, doubles

Walking 4.0 mph, very brisk

Weight lifting, body building, vigorous

## 300 ACTIVITIES THAT BURN CALORIES AN HOUR ☺

Ballet, jazz, tap

Cycling, under 10 mph, leisure bicycling

Golf, walking and carrying clubs

Painting

Raking lawn

Riding a horse, general

Sex
(30 minutes of foreplay, 30 minutes of intercourse)

Stationary cycling, light

Yoga

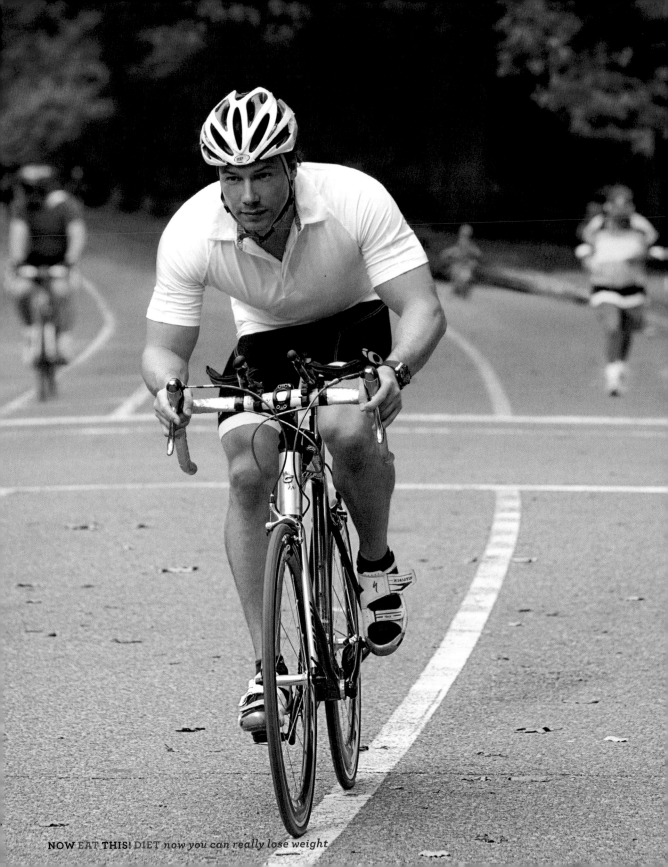

NOW EAT THIS! DIET *now you can really lose weight*

# 200 ACTIVITIES THAT BURN CALORIES AN HOUR ☺

Ballroom dancing, slow

Calisthenics, light

Frisbee playing, general

General cleaning

Golf, using power cart

Stationary cycling, very light

Walking 3.0 mph, moderate

Weight lifting, light workout

# 100 ACTIVITIES THAT BURN CALORIES AN HOUR ☺

Walking, under 2.0 mph, very slow

Watering lawn or garden

# 50 ACTIVITIES THAT BURN CALORIES AN HOUR ☺

Reading

Sleeping

Calculations are based on research data from *Medicine and Science in Sports and Exercise*, the official journal of the American College of Sports Medicine.

# Tack on Extra Food

On the days you work out harder, say, walking briskly or lifting weights, add half the calories you burned off to your allotted intake on the Now Eat This! Diet. This rule of thumb will give you the extra energy you need to sail through a sweat session but won't undo all your hard work. So if you walked briskly one day and burned off 400 calories in an hour, eat an extra snack that is—or is close to—200 calories. Some examples:

Green Tea Watermelon Super Punch (page 109)

Red Velvet Chocolate Square (page 263)

Dark Chocolate–Dipped Figs (page 282)

Chicken Tenders with Ranch Dressing (page 248)

"Fried" Cheese Balls (page 241)

Hogs Undercover (page 246)

Shrimp and Cheddar Tostada with Salsa Verde (page 250)

The key to successful weight loss is to reduce your calories by limiting the amount of food that you eat, exercising to burn calories, or using a combination of the two.

# Now You Can Eat More of What You Want

My favorite benefit of exercising is that you earn the right to eat a little more. Once I got into better shape, I could do this because I was burning 3,000 to 4,000 calories a day by training for triathlons. It was actually hard to keep weight on. Among my favorite things to eat (only rarely) is a dark chocolate chocolate chip cookie from the Levain Bakery in New York City. It's my desert island dish, my food epiphany, my food addiction at its most lustful. In other words, it's one hell of a cookie. The owners invented this 6-ounce über-caloric cookie because they, too, were training for triathlons and couldn't keep their weight on. That's how great exercise can be.

Still, I ate what all the smart diet experts out there tell us to eat: lean protein, fruit, vegetables, and good carbs (carbs with fiber). Days before a race, I would carbo-load, and during a race I'd consume mostly carb-laden foods like apples, energy bars, and fruit gels to power up the carb-consuming machine that is a triathlete.

Once you start exercising, even if it is walking 30 minutes a day, you don't want to eat just anything. You'll want to eat mostly foods that are good for you. But if you do want to splurge, you can work it off.

## If You're Not an Exerciser . . . Yet

For the athletically challenged, like me, working out can seem daunting, but it doesn't have to be. Nobody says you have to sweat a puddle, either. Exercising can be as simple as taking a walk around the block, playing catch with your kids, walking the dog one more time a day, volunteering for chores instead of loathing them, or getting dressed up in your finest white polyester suit and going dancing. Even everyday activities like raking leaves, doing housework, or pushing a stroller can help get you healthier.

If you haven't been very active, I'd suggest you start by walking. That's what I did. After all, you've been doing it since you were about a year old. You have perfected it so much by now that you don't even think about how to walk anymore. It's an easy exercise: no new rules to learn, no special clothes and equipment to drag around, no club membership to buy, no court to reserve. You don't have to gather a team together. All you have to do is get up off your butt and walk. Anything helps—even 2 minutes—it's all worthwhile. If you want to get a little more serious, start walking briskly for an hour at least 3 times a week to start. That will burn 1,200 calories a week. And in 1 year the walking alone will help you lose nearly 18 pounds.

There's more good news about walking: It's ready when you are. You can walk whenever you have the time, whether it be squeezing in a walk before work or during your lunch hour. And the locale is up to you, too. Walking outside on a track, around your own block, or indoors in a local shopping mall are popular choices. Just slide into some appropriate walking shoes and you're off.

And there are amazing benefits to walking. A pile of research studies show that walking:

- Lowers the risk of heart disease
- Helps control weight
- Improves HDL, the good-guy cholesterol
- Slows osteoporosis by strengthening your bones
- Improves your mood
- Relieves stress

If you're just starting a walking program, most experts will tell you to begin the first week by walking 20 minutes 3 times a week. For the next few weeks, increase your time to 30 minutes. As you feel more energetic and fit, add an extra session or two to your weekly walking program. Try to work up to 5 sessions a week, for 45 to 60 minutes each time, especially if you're trying to pare off fat pounds. The important thing here is that you're moving. Any amount you do is a positive, so start small and just gradually build from there, like I did.

Start your walking routine with a warm-up that includes 5 to 10 minutes of slow walking, and gradually build up to your normal pace. Warm up your body with dynamic movements such as rolling your shoulders and neck or marching in place. Don't forget this part, because even the best walkers may get sore or injured if their muscles aren't warmed up. And, although stretching exercises are important for maintaining flexibility, do them after your walk. Stretching prior to exercise has been debunked quite a bit in the last few years. It's more important to do a slow warm-up to increase the temperature of the muscle versus stretching it out beforehand. So, when you're finished walking, it's okay to stretch. Stretching your muscles will increase your flexibility and keep you from getting sore muscles.

Walking requires proper form and the right posture to avoid injury and maximize benefits. Move your arms and shoulders freely to help propel you. If possible, keep your arms bent at a 90-degree angle, or swing your arms at your sides and build up to 90 degrees. Hold your head high, with your chin parallel to the ground and your back and neck as straight as possible, all the while gently tightening your abdominal muscles and taking normal-size steps.

Keep safety in mind. Carry your cell phone when you walk, and program your local emergency services number for quick retrieval, as well as your doctor's number.

Map out your walking routes and let someone know where you're going. Walk a circular route so you're never too far from home. And, if you feel dizzy or short of breath or suffer chest pain or any unusual sensation while walking, stop and call for help.

One more thing: Look the part. Your sneakers should be walking shoes, designed to handle the specific terrain you've chosen. You don't want to be caught walking in tennis shoes.

have a new body basically, from the inside to the outside." His words kept me motivated.

Be patient and forgiving. Change will come, but it takes time. Remember, losers fall down and stay down. Winners fall down but get up. Remind yourself that you're a winner.

## Fun Ways to Get Fit

Walking is only one of many ways to get in shape. If it doesn't appeal to you, try something else—especially something you feel is fun, not a bore or a chore. Recapture the kid in you. When you see exercise as enjoyable rather than something you're guilted into doing, it's a whole lot easier. Try taking up a team sport you may have enjoyed as a child, like basketball or softball, or try roller-skating or swimming. Choose activities that interest you so you will be more likely to stick with them, and don't repeat the same activity day after day, if exercise bores you. There are hundreds of possibilities.

And add variety. If you like sightseeing, walk, bike, jog, or skate your way around town. If you enjoy picnics in the park, round up the family for a game of tag or touch football before you eat.

Keep trying different fitness activities that spark your interest: ice skating, salsa dancing, racquetball. Try new things until you find something you like. After all, experimenting is the fun part.

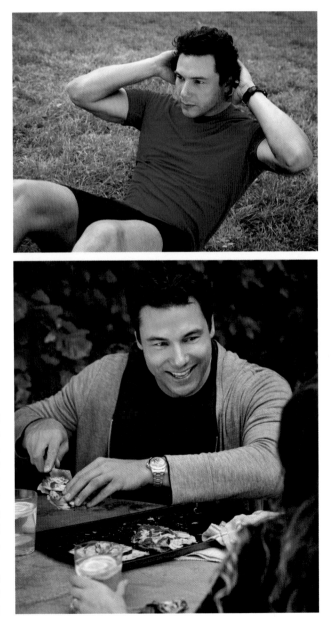

## Stay Focused and Positive

Your muscles may do all the work when you exercise, but your mind provides the momentum. A positive attitude gets you off on the right foot to fitness and keeps you there. Get your mind primed for fitness by visualizing how good your body will look and feel. Set realistic goals, and reward yourself when you reach them. Stay psyched for fitness by linking up with a fitness partner—someone who provides company, can push you when you need that extra motivation, or can keep tabs on you to make sure you stay on track.

Triathlon training is basically solo work, and so I thrive on encouragement from others. I remember a few years ago, my doctor said: "Wow, you've rebuilt yourself. You

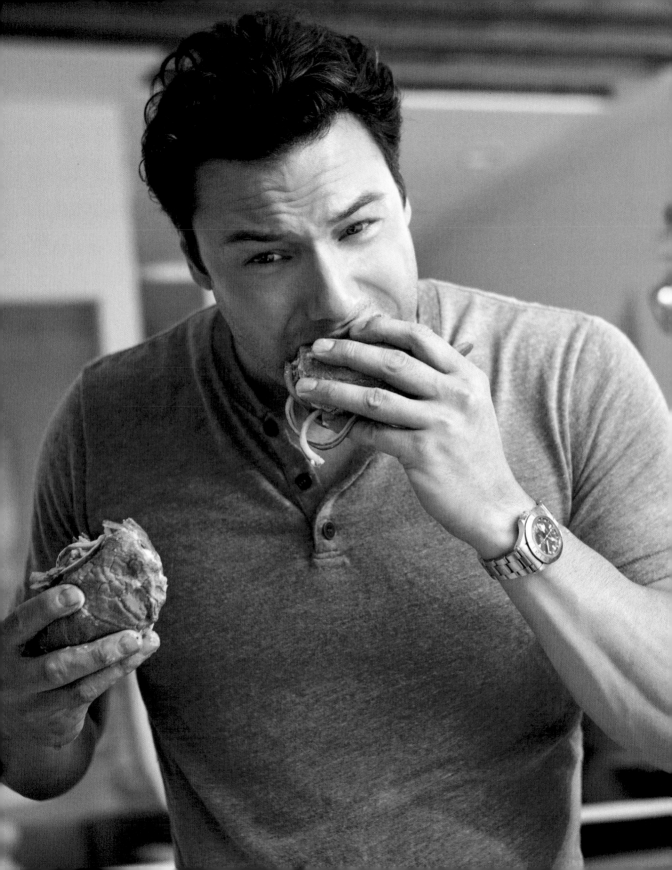

# PART TWO

## Now Eat This! Diet Recipes

You are about to take the foods you love and turn them into low-fat and low-calorie masterpieces. They're going to be delicious, and you're not going to feel deprived.

Every recipe comes with a nutritional breakdown provided by a board-certified dietitian. This breakdown includes calories, carbs, fat, protein, fiber, and sodium. And just in case you're counting points, I've added those as well. I call them Food Value Points. The recipes are meant to be more healthful versions of the originals; they trade some of the saturated fat for unsaturated fat and increase fiber.

You'll also find a comparison of fat and calories for the traditional preparation of a dish versus my version. I used the following online sources: calorieking.com, food.com, and recipezaar to come up with the average calorie and fat counts for the traditional recipe comparisons.

For example, traditional crème brûlée weighs in at around 400 calories and 31 grams of fat. My version (page 274) contains 158 calories and only 2 grams of fat per serving. Both taste wonderful, but mine won't make you have to test the tensile strength of your jeans.

Please make these recipes your own, too. To me, a recipe is not an exact formula. It should empower you, especially to do something you've never tried before. Use your sense of taste and your personal dietary goals to determine any changes you'd like to make to these recipes. Take it even further: Use what you learn here and a little of your own ingenuity to make over your family's favorite recipes.

This book shows you not only how to modify your favorite recipes, but also how to build them into meal plans that make healthy eating a part of, not an option in, your life. This plan is so uncomplicated and flavor oriented that it won't send you headfirst into a gallon of rocky road ice cream.

This isn't a diet; it's a lifestyle, and I hope you make it a part of yours. I've kept the recipes low in calories, fat, sugar, and bad carbs, while using real ingredients that are easily accessible and found just about anywhere. I've held true to this principle for years: that the more natural and real your ingredients are, the easier it is to accomplish and keep up as a lifestyle. I've already said a lot of this, but it bears repeating.

The most important thing is to make healthful, nutritious food an important part of your day. Time spent planning and cooking well-balanced meals is a wise investment. Take care of your body and it will take care of you.

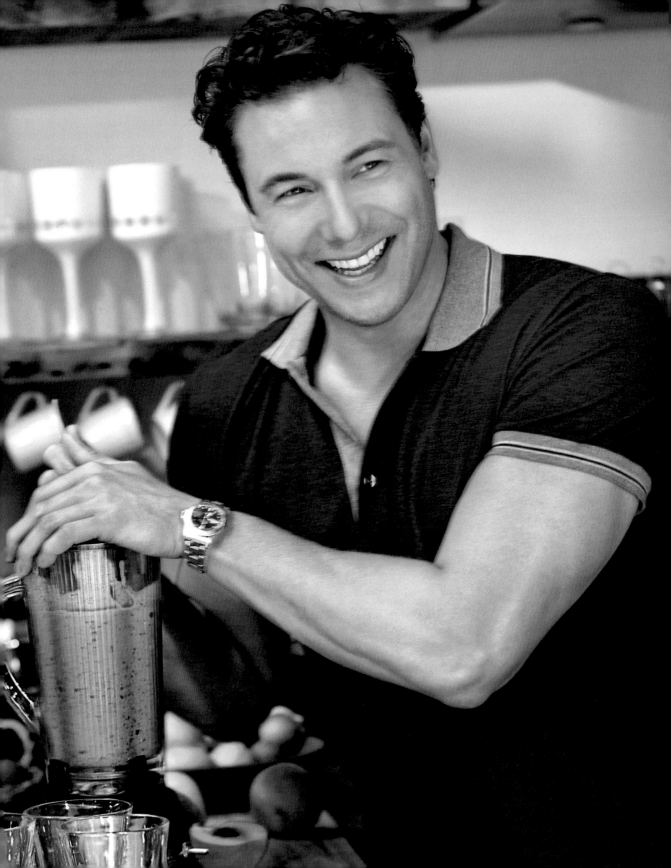

chapter

# 9

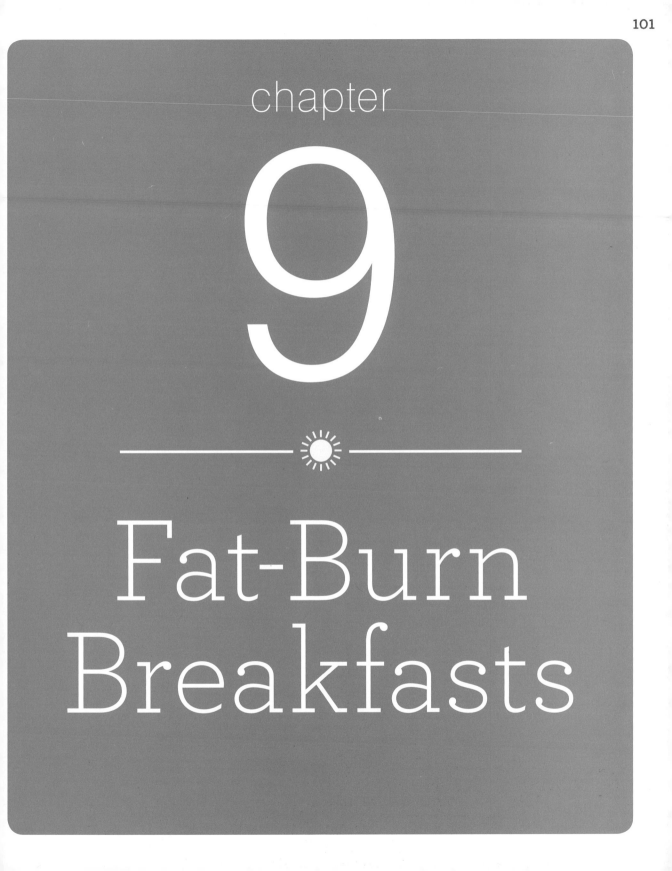

# Fat-Burn Breakfasts

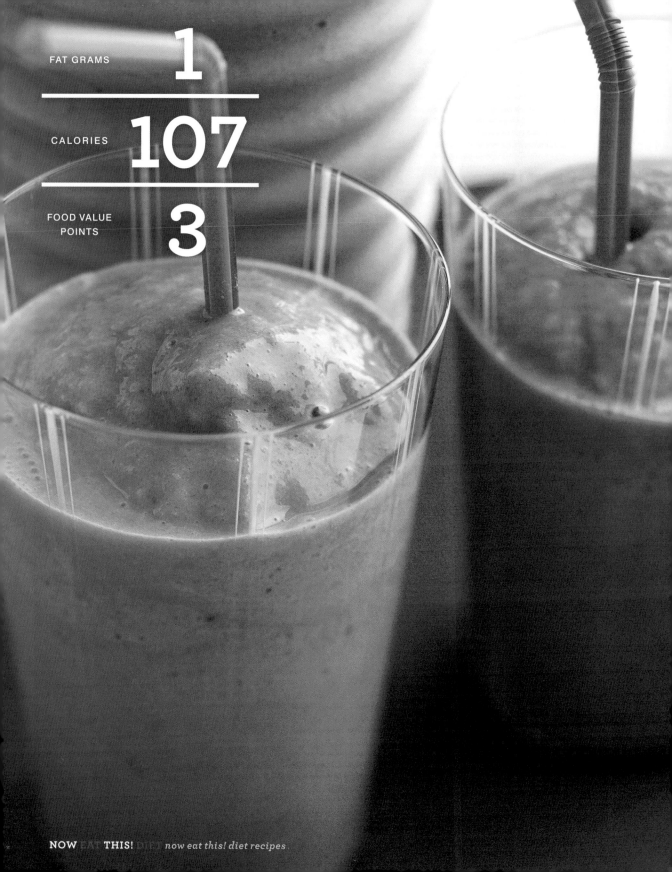

FAT GRAMS **1**

CALORIES **107**

FOOD VALUE
POINTS **3**

# Strawberry Protein Punch Smoothie

SERVES 2
(24 ounces each)

**GOT STRAWBERRIES,** whey protein powder, and a blender? Then you've got a great, no-fuss, nutritious breakfast. I like to pump up my smoothies with immune-boosting whey. It's a great substitute for dairy in a smoothie, in case you can't tolerate milk. Blend your smoothie for at least 5 minutes. According to a Pennsylvania State University study, people who drank a breakfast smoothie mixed to twice its initial volume ate about 100 fewer calories at lunch than when they drank the same smoothie at its original volume. The extra air makes you feel fuller, say researchers.

## INGREDIENTS

2 cups ice

1 scoop French vanilla whey protein powder, such as Designer Whey

12 ounces water

2 cups unsweetened frozen strawberries

1 packet (3 grams) sugar-free strawberry drink mix, such as Crystal Light

## METHOD

1 Toss all ingredients into a blender and blend for at least 5 minutes to increase volume.

2 Serve in glasses with a straw.

PER SERVING
**107**calories **1g**fat ( **0.5g**sat / **0g**mono / **0g**poly )
**27.5mg**cholesterol **33mg**sodium
**15g**carbohydrate **3g**fiber **10g**protein

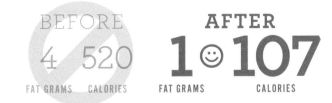

BEFORE
4 520
FAT GRAMS  CALORIES

AFTER
1 ☺ 107
FAT GRAMS  CALORIES

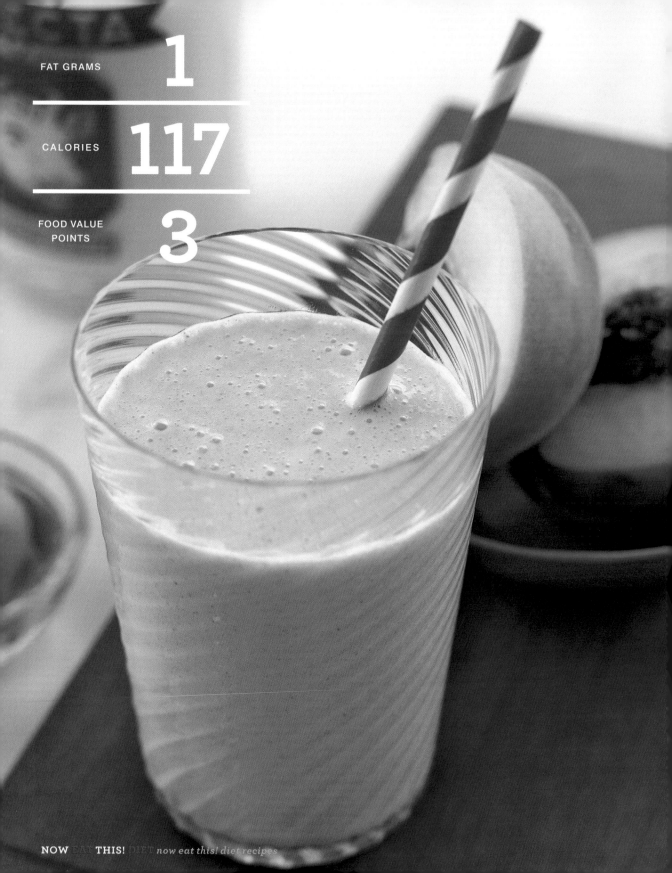

FAT GRAMS **1**

CALORIES **117**

FOOD VALUE POINTS **3**

# Ginger Peach Lassie

**HAVE YOURSELF A SMOOTHIE,** and I'm not talking about the Hollywood type with the ability to charm. I'm talking about the kind you drink—those blender beverages made with whatever you want to toss in, like I did here. This is a true health drink, thanks to the addition of fresh ginger. Far more than a seasoning, ginger has a long résumé of impressive health benefits: It improves digestion, prevents and manages stomach ulcers, protects against symptoms of colds and flu, stimulates blood circulation, works as an aphrodisiac, lowers cholesterol, and acts as an antioxidant. Other than all that, it really gives this smoothie a zing.

---

### 5 More Reasons to Love This Smoothie

I've spiced this smoothie up with turmeric, too. It's a spice we should all get a little more intimate with. The Indian spice blend we know as curry powder owes its golden color to turmeric. Turmeric contains a powerful compound called curcumin that has been the focus of some recent research. Studies have found that curcumin may:

- Suppress the spread of cancer cells
- Decrease cholesterol levels
- Improve morning stiffness, walking time, joint swelling, pain, and discomfort in people with arthritis
- Provide respiratory benefits
- Work as an antidepressant

---

## INGREDIENTS

| | |
|---|---|
| 2 | cups ice |
| 1 | scoop French vanilla whey protein powder, such as Designer Whey |
| 12 | ounces water |
| 2 | cups unsweetened frozen peaches |
| 1 | packet (about 4 grams) sugar-free lemonade drink mix, such as Crystal Light |
| ½ | teaspoon grated fresh ginger |
| ½ | teaspoon ground turmeric |

## METHOD

1 Toss all ingredients into a blender and blend for 5 minutes to increase the volume

2 Serve in glasses with a straw.

PER SERVING
**117** calories **1g** fat ( **0.5g** sat / **0g** mono / **0g** poly )
**27.5mg** cholesterol **40mg** sodium
**17g** carbohydrate **2g** fiber **10g** protein

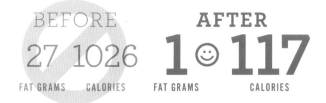

BEFORE
27 1026
FAT GRAMS    CALORIES

AFTER
1 ☺ 117
FAT GRAMS    CALORIES

*fat-burn breakfasts*

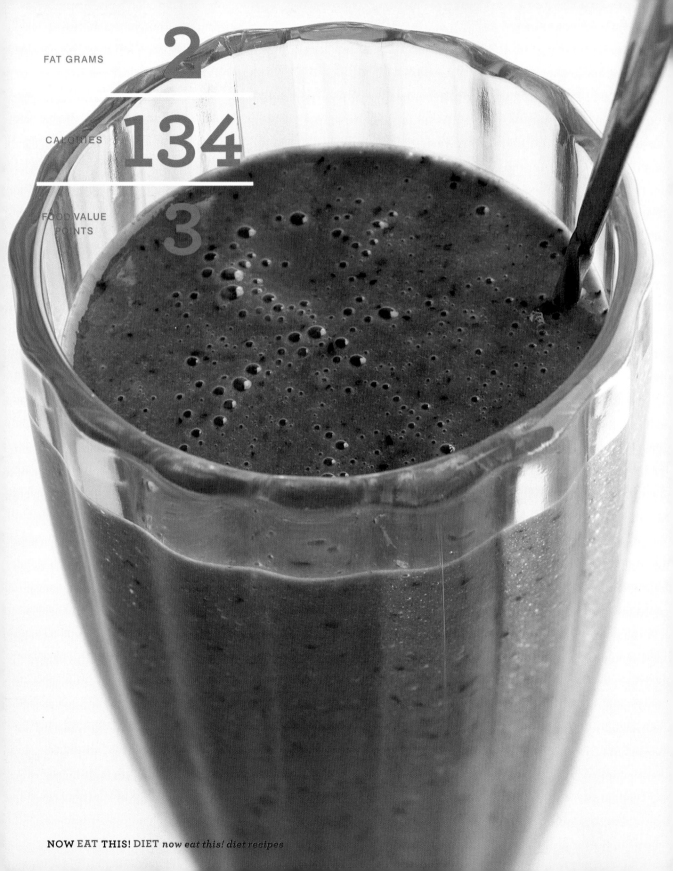

FAT GRAMS **2**

CALORIES **134**

FOOD VALUE POINTS **3**

# Blueberry Vanilla Smoothie

SERVES 2
(24 ounces each)

**IF YOU EVER FEEL** like making a Crisco and potato chip smoothie, come to your senses now and make this one instead. It's sugar- and fat-free. Plus, the frozen fruit makes this thick and icy.

Incidentally, smoothies have been with us since at least 1946. That's when someone actually discovered a torpedo-shaped cylinder that was made to be filled with ice cream and fruit and powered by $CO_2$.

## INGREDIENTS

2   cups ice

1   scoop French vanilla whey protein powder, such as Designer Whey

12  ounces water

2   cups unsweetened frozen blueberries

1   packet (2 grams) sugar-free raspberry drink mix, such as Crystal Light

## METHOD

1  Toss all ingredients into a blender and blend for 5 minutes to increase volume.

2  Serve in glasses with a straw.

PER SERVING
**134** calories **2g** fat ( **0.6g** sat / **0g** mono / **0g** poly )
**28mg** cholesterol **47mg** sodium
**20g** carbohydrate **4g** fiber **10g** protein

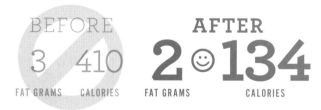

BEFORE
3   410
FAT GRAMS   CALORIES

AFTER
2 ☺ 134
FAT GRAMS   CALORIES

*fat-burn breakfasts*

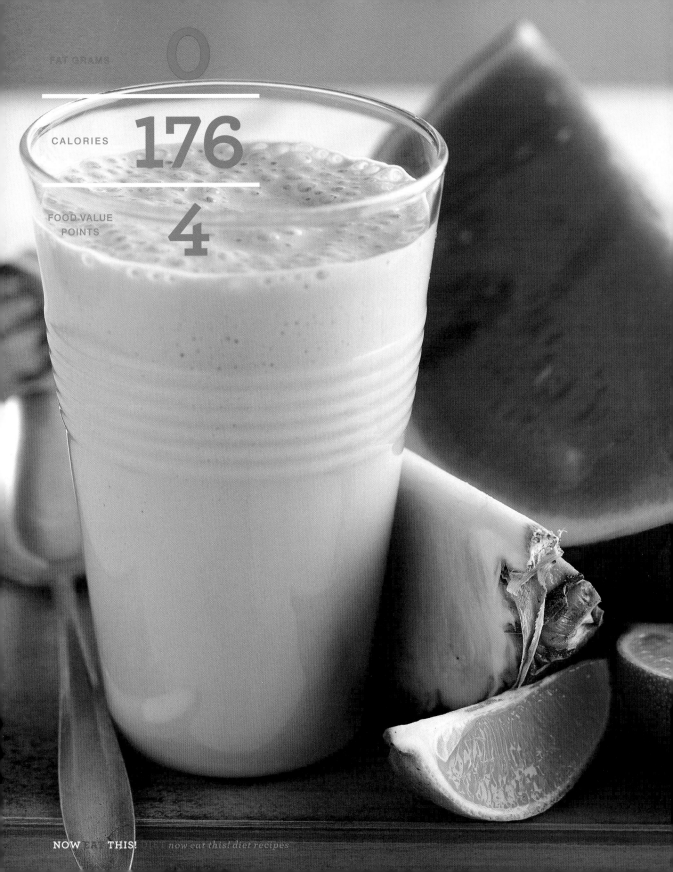

FAT GRAMS 0

CALORIES 176

FOOD VALUE POINTS 4

# Green Tea Watermelon Super Punch

**I CRAVE SMOOTHIES.** I have 2 to 3 a day. Did I mention I'm forming a support group? This smoothie is one of my favorites. It's souped up with high-antioxidant matcha (green tea powder). This one is made with yogurt, too—a wonderful probiotic food that has been shown in studies to help with fat burning. Oh, and if you suspect you've been unintentionally overdosing on smoothies, get help.

## INGREDIENTS

| | |
|---|---|
| 2 | **cups ice** |
| 4 | **cups cubed seedless watermelon** |
| 1 | **cup nonfat Greek yogurt, such as 0% Fage Total** |
| ¼ | **cup fresh lime juice** |
| ¼ | **cup agave nectar** |
| 1 | **cup chopped fresh pineapple** |
| 4 | **teaspoons unsweetened matcha green tea powder** |

## METHOD

1 **Toss all ingredients into a blender and blend for 5 minutes to increase volume.**

2 **Serve in glasses with a straw.**

PER SERVING
**176**calories **0g**fat ( **0g**sat / **0g**mono / **0g**poly )
**0mg**cholesterol **22mg**sodium
**37g**carbohydrate **1g**fiber **6g**protein

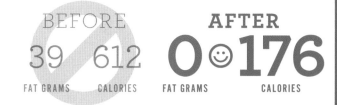

BEFORE
39 612
FAT GRAMS    CALORIES

**AFTER**
0 ☺ **176**
FAT GRAMS    CALORIES

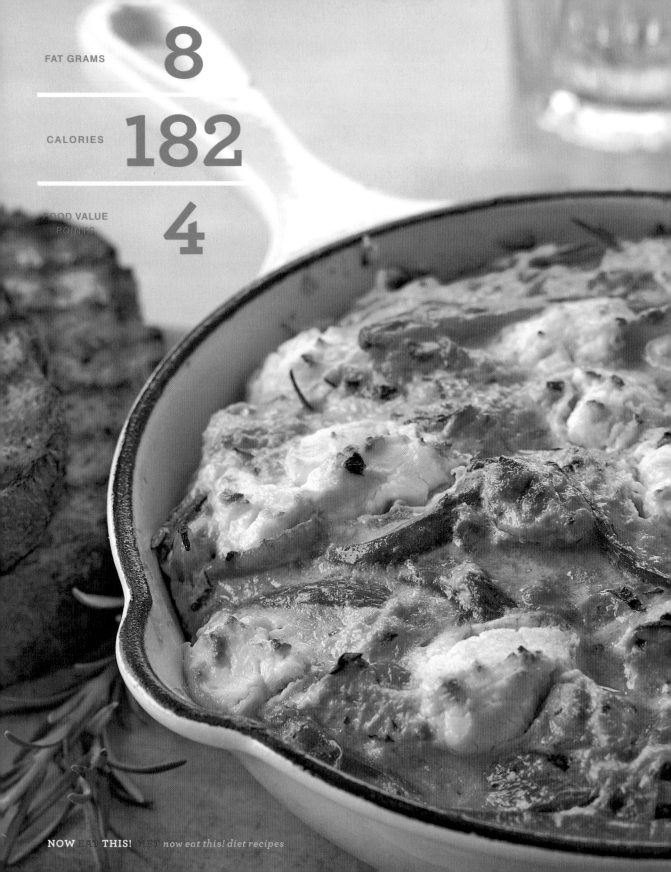

FAT GRAMS **8**

CALORIES **182**

FOOD VALUE POINTS **4**

# Pepper, Onion, and Goat Cheese Frittata

SERVES 4

**A FRITTATA** is an Italian omelet, only with the ingredients mixed throughout the eggs instead of folded in the middle. Frittatas are a great way to use up bits and pieces of leftover meats, vegetables, and cheeses you may have on hand. This frittata is made with peppers, onions, goat cheese, and fresh herbs. Starting your day with a frittata will keep you satisfied all day long. That's because eggs (in the form of egg substitutes) are loaded with protein.

## INGREDIENTS

| | |
|---|---|
| 1 | tablespoon extra-virgin olive oil |
| ½ | medium yellow onion, sliced |
| 2 | cloves garlic, minced |
| 1 | teaspoon roughly chopped fresh rosemary |
| ½ | teaspoon red pepper flakes |
| ½ | cup (about 3½ ounces) jarred fried peppers, such as Cento Sautéed Sweet Peppers with onions, roughly chopped |
| 1 | cup (about 7 ounces) jarred roasted red pepper strips (not oil packed), such as Cento |
| 2 | tablespoons chopped fresh flat-leaf parsley |
| | Salt |
| | Freshly ground black pepper |
| 2 | cups liquid egg substitute |
| 2 | ounces goat cheese |

## METHOD

1. Preheat the oven to 475°F. Adjust the rack to the top third of the oven.

2. Heat a 10-inch nonstick ovenproof pan over medium-high heat. When hot, add the olive oil and onion. Sauté the onion until it is soft, about 3 minutes. Add the garlic and cook for another 2 minutes. Add the rosemary, red pepper flakes, peppers, and parsley. Stir until combined, and season with salt and pepper to taste.

3. Meanwhile, in a medium bowl, add the egg substitute and season with salt and pepper to taste.

4. Pour the egg mixture into the pan. Using a heatproof rubber spatula, stir the eggs until they begin to solidify. Incorporate half of the goat cheese into the eggs. Dot the remaining goat cheese over the eggs, and then transfer the pan to the oven.

5. Bake the eggs for 5 to 6 minutes or until the eggs are completely set and the cheese is browned.

6. Remove the pan from the oven and run a heatproof spatula around the perimeter and bottom of the eggs. Tilt the pan and carefully slide the eggs onto a plate. Cut into quarters.

PER SERVING
**182** calories **8g** fat ( **2.6g** sat / **3g** mono / **0.5g** poly )
**7mg** cholesterol **612mg** sodium
**10g** carbohydrate **3g** fiber **16g** protein

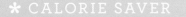

**＊ CALORIE SAVER**

Omit the goat cheese and fried peppers and save **60** calories a serving.

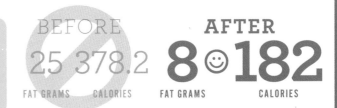

BEFORE
25 378.2
FAT GRAMS   CALORIES

**AFTER**
**8** ☺ **182**
FAT GRAMS   CALORIES

*fat-burn breakfasts*

FAT GRAMS   5

CALORIES   214

FOOD VALUE
POINTS     5

# Scrambled Eggs with Smoked Salmon on Toast

SERVES 4

**IF I WAKE UP** to a loud noise, it's either my dog snoring or my stomach growling. Maybe both. But if it's the latter, I've got to eat something fast. This ultrasavory breakfast does the trick. You can whip it up in just 5 minutes. Few ingredients are as luxurious as smoked salmon, rich, decadent, and a relative calorie bargain for the flavor benefits. Olives pose a triple threat to bad health: they are rich in vitamin E a fat-soluble antioxidant that neutralizes damaging free radicals, and full of polyphenols and flavonoids, which have anti-inflammatory properties. Sorry—no canned pitted olives here. It just wouldn't be the same.

## INGREDIENTS

| | |
|---|---|
| 2 | garlic cloves |
| | Nonstick cooking spray |
| 2 | cups liquid egg substitute |
| | Freshly ground black pepper |
| 8 | kalamata olives, roughly chopped |
| 1 | tablespoon chopped fresh flat-leaf parsley |
| 2 | tablespoons chopped chives |
| 3 | ounces sliced smoked salmon |
| 4 | ounces whole wheat baguette |
| ¼ | cup reduced-fat sour cream, such as Breakstone's |

PER SERVING
**214**calories **5g**fat ( **2g**sat / **1.7g**mono / **0.5g**poly )
**10mg**cholesterol **796mg**sodium
**19g**carbohydrate **3g**fiber **22g**protein

## METHOD

1 Mince one of the garlic cloves and set aside.

2 Heat a large nonstick sauté pan over medium heat. When hot, remove it from the stove just while you coat it with cooking spray. Add the minced garlic and cook till lightly brown, about 1 minute.

3 In a small bowl, add the egg substitute. Season with pepper to taste. Pour the egg mixture into the pan. Using a heatproof rubber spatula, stir the eggs occasionally until large curds form. When the eggs are still wet, fold in the olives, parsley, chives, and salmon. Season with pepper.

4 Cut the baguette into slices and toast in the toaster oven. Rub the toasted pieces with the remaining clove of garlic.

5 Serve the eggs with a dollop of sour cream and the garlic bread.

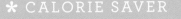

**★ CALORIE SAVER**
Omit the bread and save **87** calories a serving.

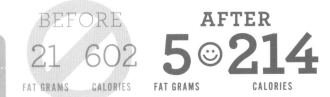

BEFORE
21 602
FAT GRAMS CALORIES

AFTER
5 ☺ 214
FAT GRAMS CALORIES

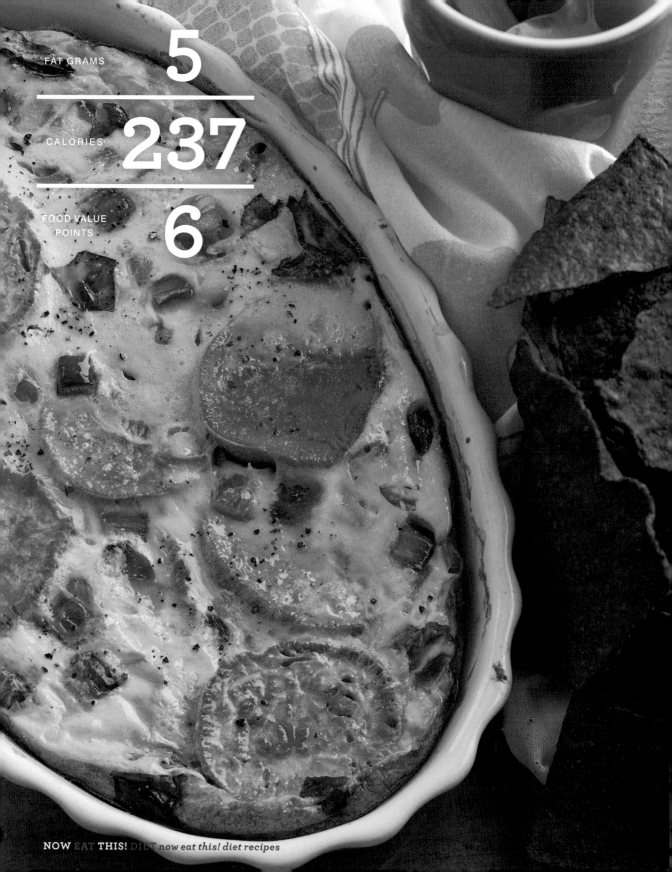

FAT GRAMS
**5**

CALORIES
**237**

FOOD VALUE
POINTS
**6**

# Sweet Potato and Blue Corn Egg Casserole

SERVES 4

**YOU SAY SWEET POTATO.** I say superfood. It's arguably the most healthy vegetable on earth. The sweet potato's orange color is a dead giveaway of its high vitamin A content (in the form of beta-carotene). Plus, it's loaded with potassium, vitamins C, folic acid, and fiber. With a lower rating on the glycemic index than white potatoes, sweet potatoes are an excellent substitute if you're watching your weight or trying to control your blood sugar levels. ✱TIP: Microwaving, steaming, or baking sweet potatoes preserves more nutrients than boiling them in water. Vitamins can leach out into the water. Leave the skin on the potatoes if you like.

## INGREDIENTS

Nonstick cooking spray

1 medium sweet potato

1½ teaspoons extra-virgin olive oil

1 medium red onion, cut into small dice

Salt

Freshly ground black pepper

1 garlic clove, minced

2 cups liquid egg substitute

1 tablespoon chopped fresh basil

4 ounces baked blue corn chips, such as Guiltless Gourmet

### PER SERVING

**237** calories **5g** fat ( **0g** sat / **1.4g** mono / **0g** poly )
**0mg** cholesterol **504mg** sodium
**35g** carbohydrate **3.5g** fiber **16g** protein

## METHOD

1 Preheat the oven to 475°F. Spray an 8 x 8 x 2-inch baking dish with cooking spray, and set it aside.

2 Prick the skin of the sweet potato with a fork and microwave on high till it is soft and tender, about 5 minutes, turning halfway through. Allow to cool.

3 Heat a large nonstick sauté pan over medium-high heat. When hot, add the olive oil to the pan. Add the onions and cook until the onions begin to soften, about 5 minutes. Season with salt and pepper to taste. Add the garlic and cook for another 2 minutes. Set aside.

4 In a small bowl, add the egg substitute and season with salt and pepper to taste.

5 Remove the skin of the sweet potato and slice it crosswise into ½-inch-thick slices. Layer the potatoes into the bottom of the prepared baking dish. Spread the onions on top, and then pour the egg substitute into the dish. Scatter the basil on top.

6 Transfer the dish to the oven and bake until the eggs are completely set, about 15 to 18 minutes. Serve with baked blue corn chips.

✱ CALORIE SAVER

Omit the chips and save **122** calories per serving.

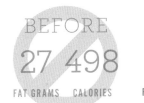
BEFORE
27 498
FAT GRAMS CALORIES

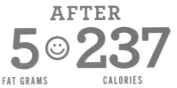
**AFTER**
5 ☺ 237
FAT GRAMS CALORIES

*fat-burn breakfasts*

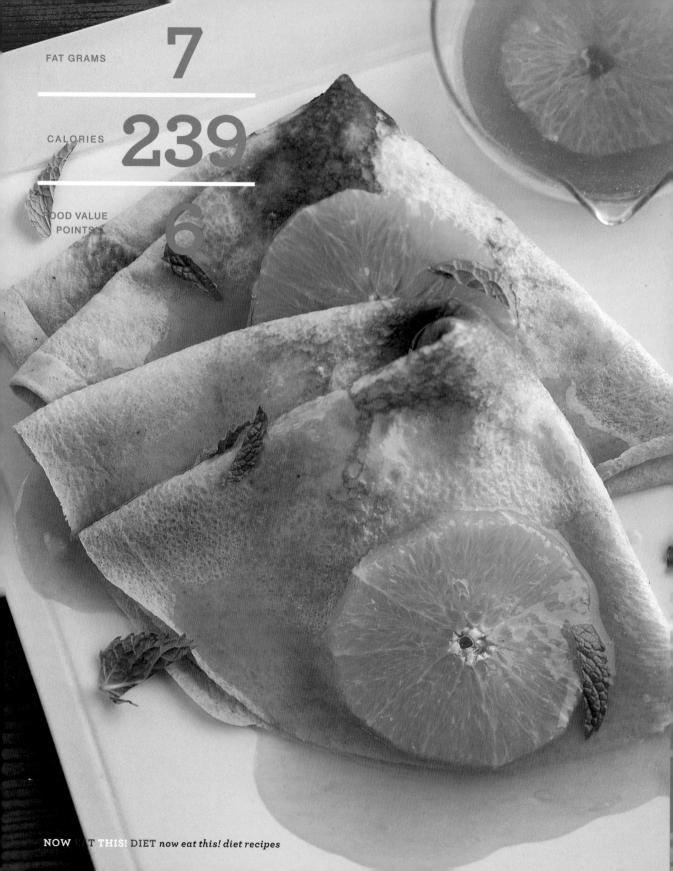

# Creamy Stuffed Crepes with Orange Butter Syrup

SERVES 4

**CREPES ARE PAPER-THIN PANCAKES,** really, and they have many things going for them. First, crepes are easy to make and everyone loves them. Second, they transform leftovers into meals—simply stuff, cover, and bake. Third, crepes aren't just for dessert anymore. You can serve them for breakfast, too. My version is filled with creamy low-fat ricotta cheese and topped with an orange syrup that will make your mouth do somersaults. ✱TIP: If possible, get whole nutmeg and use a microplane or rasp to grate it. The flavor and aroma are superior to those of powdered nutmeg.

## INGREDIENTS

| | |
|---|---|
| 1 | cup whole wheat pastry flour |
| ¼ | teaspoon salt |
| ¾ | cup liquid egg substitute |
| 1 | cup skim milk |
| 2½ | teaspoons vanilla extract |
| 1 | tablespoon canola oil |
| 8 | ounces low-fat ricotta cheese |
| 2 | grates of a whole nutmeg |
| 1 | medium navel orange |
| ½ | cup calorie-free pancake syrup, such as Walden Farms |
| | Butter-flavored nonstick cooking spray |
| 1 | tablespoon chopped fresh mint |

PER SERVING
**239** calories **7g** fat ( **2.2g** sat / **2.4g** mono / **1g** poly )
**19.5mg** cholesterol **446mg** sodium
**29g** carbohydrate **3g** fiber **16g** protein

## METHOD

1 In a large bowl, whisk together the flour and salt. Create a well in the center of the bowl, and whisk in the egg substitute, milk, ½ teaspoon vanilla, and canola oil. Blend until smooth. Set aside.

2 In a small bowl, combine the ricotta, the remaining vanilla, and 2 grates of nutmeg. Stir together until well blended. Set aside.

3 Cut off the top and bottom of the orange. Position the orange so that the flat bottom end is resting on the cutting board. Using a sharp paring knife, cut the skin and white pith off in a downward curving motion. Continue cutting around the orange so that it is no longer surrounded by the skin and pith. Cut the orange crosswise into ¼-inch slices.

4 Transfer the orange slices to a small saucepan over low heat. Add the pancake syrup, and stir to combine. Simmer for 5 minutes, and then turn off the heat and set aside.

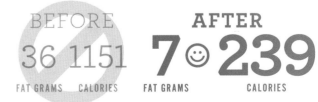

BEFORE
36 1151
FAT GRAMS   CALORIES

**AFTER**
7 ☺ **239**
FAT GRAMS   CALORIES

## METHOD

5  Heat a large nonstick sauté pan over medium-high heat. When hot, remove the pan from the stove just while you coat it with cooking spray. Pour a quarter of the batter into the pan. Immediately begin to tilt the pan to spread the batter so that it evenly coats the bottom of the pan. Cook about 30 seconds on one side, and then flip the crepe with a heat-resistant spatula. Cook for another 20 seconds or until the crepe is golden brown. Transfer the crepe to a plate. Repeat with the remaining batter. (The batter should make 4 large crepes.)

6  Spread the ricotta filling in each crepe, and then fold the crepe into quarters.

7  Serve the crepes with the orange syrup. Scatter the mint on top of each crepe.

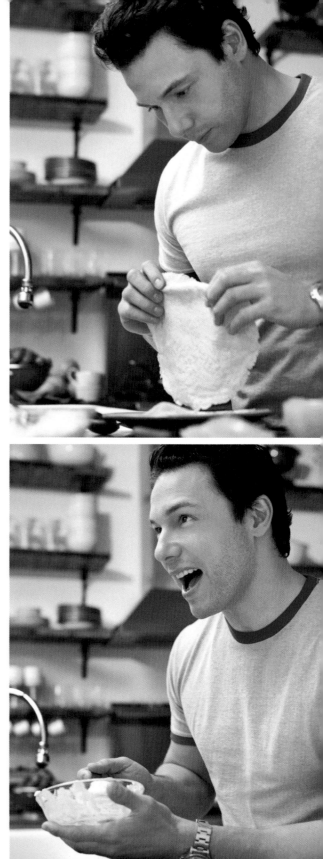

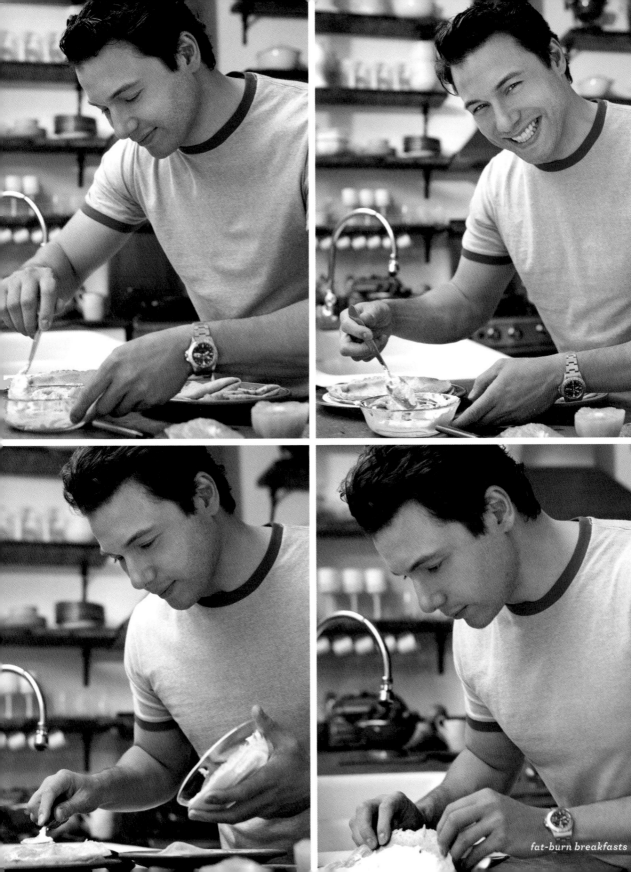

fat-burn breakfasts

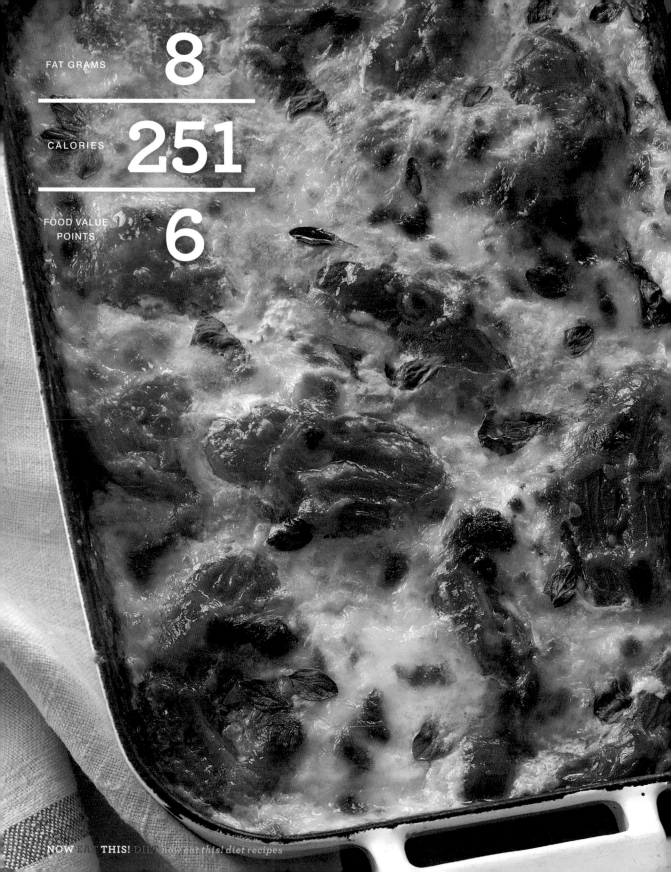

# Pizza Egg Bake

SERVES 4

**OKAY I ADMIT IT:** Leftover pizza has long been one of my favorite breakfasts. Hey, some foods are so good that you dream about them and wake up wanting to eat the leftovers for breakfast . . . so I got to thinking: Why not a pizza with eggs? It may sound unusual, but this pizza-inspired breakfast bake is as scrumptious as it sounds. Now I dream of my Pizza Egg Bake. *TIP: Most people don't know this, but canned plum tomatoes have a more intense and concentrated flavor than vine-ripened tomatoes.

## INGREDIENTS

2   cups liquid egg substitute

1   garlic clove, minced

1   cup drained canned, whole plum tomatoes, roughly chopped

1   tablespoon chopped fresh oregano

1   tablespoon chopped fresh basil

    Salt

    Freshly ground black pepper

    Nonstick cooking spray

4   ounces part-skim shredded mozzarella

¼   cup grated Parmigiano-Reggiano

4   ounces whole wheat bread, cut into 4 slices

PER SERVING
**251** calories **8g** fat ( **4g** sat / **1.8g** mono / **0g** poly )
**20mg** cholesterol **737mg** sodium
**20g** carbohydrate **2g** fiber **24g** protein

## METHOD

1   Preheat the oven to 475°F. Adjust the rack to the top third of the oven.

2   Heat a 10-inch nonstick ovenproof pan over medium-high heat.

3   In a medium bowl, combine the egg substitute, garlic, tomatoes, oregano, basil, and salt and pepper to taste. Mix well with a fork.

4   Away from the heat, spray the pan with cooking spray. Pour the egg mixture into the pan. With a heat-resistant rubber spatula, stir the egg mixture in the sauté pan. Continue to stir as the eggs begin to solidify. When there are large curds but the mixture is still wet, scatter the cheeses over the eggs, and then transfer the pan to the oven.

5   Bake the eggs for 5 to 6 minutes, or until the eggs are completely set and the cheese is brown and bubbly.

6   Meanwhile, toast the bread in the toaster oven. Serve with the baked eggs.

**✱ CALORIE SAVER**

Omit the mozzarella cheese and save **85** calories per serving (you will still have the Parm cheese for flavor), or omit the bread and save **71** calories per serving.

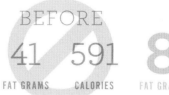

BEFORE
41 591
FAT GRAMS   CALORIES

AFTER
8 ☺ 251
FAT GRAMS   CALORIES

FAT GRAMS

# 3
---
CALORIES

# 253
---
FOOD VALUE POINTS

# 7

## WITH YOGURT
**Fat Grams 3, Calories 253, Food Value Points 7
(with nonfat Greek yogurt, such as 0% Fage Total)**

## AS TRAIL MIX
**Fat Grams 3, Calories 179, Food Value Points 4
(alone, as a trail-mix-type snack)**

## AS CEREAL WITH MILK
**Fat Grams 3, Calories 220, Food Value Points 6
(with ½ cup of skim milk)**

# Apple and Cranberry Granola Cereal

SERVES 4

**HERE'S MY RENDITION** of granola but without the sugar and fat that plagues most granolas. Rather than oats, to save calories, I've used kamut. If you've never heard of it, let me introduce you. Kamut is an ancient grain with origins in Egypt. Its kernels are 2 to 3 times larger than those of its modern wheat relatives. Kamut is increasingly used as an alternative to regular wheat. It has 20 to 40 percent more protein and is higher in good fats, amino acids, vitamins, and minerals. Plus, it can be tolerated by some with sensitivities to regular wheat. To cut the sugar but not the sweetness, I've used apple juice concentrate. It's a great way to lend a fruity sweetness to the kamut.

Make up a big batch of this. Eat it on its own as your very own healthy trail mix. Or mix it with yogurt for a fast, nutritious breakfast or dessert. If you prefer, serve it with skim milk for a filling breakfast.

## INGREDIENTS

| | |
|---|---|
| | Butter-flavored nonstick cooking spray |
| ¼ | cup apple juice concentrate |
| 2 | tablespoons agave nectar |
| ¼ | teaspoon vanilla extract |
| ¼ | teaspoon ground cinnamon |
| | Pinch of salt |
| 4 | cups puffed kamut, such as Arrowhead Mills |
| ¼ | cup unsweetened dried apples, cut into small dice |
| ¼ | cup dried cranberries, chopped into small pieces |
| ¼ | cup sliced almonds, toasted |
| 20 | ounces nonfat Greek yogurt, such as 0% Fage Total |

## METHOD

1 Preheat the oven to 250°F. Lightly spray 2 baking sheets with cooking spray and set aside.

2 In a medium bowl, add the apple juice concentrate, agave, vanilla, cinnamon, and salt if desired. Stir the mixture until well combined. Add the kamut and stir until well coated.

3 Spread the kamut in a thin layer on the baking sheets. Transfer to the oven and bake until the cereal is browned and slightly crisp, about 30 to 40 minutes, stirring once. Allow to completely cool.

4 Stir in the apples, cranberries, and almonds. Serve on top of the Greek yogurt.

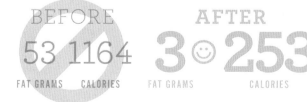

BEFORE 53 1164 AFTER 3 ☺ 253
FAT GRAMS CALORIES FAT GRAMS CALORIES

PER SERVING (with yogurt):
**253**calories **3g**fat ( **0g**sat / **1.8g**mono / **0.8g**poly )
**0mg**cholesterol **116mg**sodium
**42g**carbohydrate **4g**fiber **17g**protein

PER SERVING (with ½ cup skim milk):
**220**calories **3g**fat ( **0g**sat / **1.8g**mono / **0.8g**poly )
**2.5mg**cholesterol **116mg**sodium
**42g**carbohydrate **4g**fiber **8g**protein

PER SERVING (alone, as a trail-mix-type snack):
**179**calories **3g**fat ( **0g**sat / **1.8g**mono / **0.8g**poly )
**0mg**cholesterol **38mg**sodium
**26g**carbohydrate **4g**fiber **5g**protein

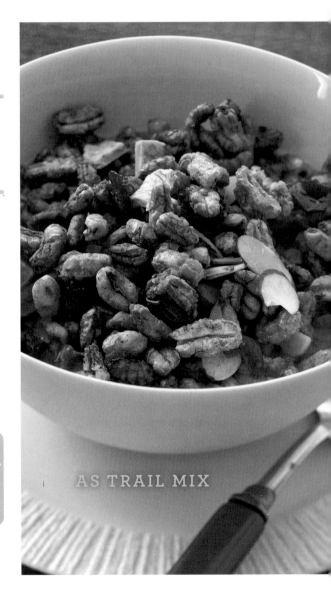

AS TRAIL MIX

**✱ CALORIE SAVER**

Omit the almonds and save **33** calories per serving.

WITH YOGURT

# Sunrise Sandwich

SERVES 4

**WHO IN THEIR WEAKEST** moment hasn't fallen prey to the allure of the delicious bacon and egg sandwich in the drive-through window? So rather than tempt myself, I created this delicious low-fat version of that famous breakfast sandwich. It is also low in calories and served on a whole wheat English muffin. Enjoy!

## INGREDIENTS

Nonstick cooking spray

1 vine-ripened tomato, sliced into ¼-inch slices

4 pieces (about 2½ ounces) Canadian bacon

1 garlic clove, minced

2 cups liquid egg substitute

Salt

Freshly ground black pepper

1 tablespoon chopped fresh flat-leaf parsley

4 slices 2% reduced-fat cheese, such as Borden's 2% Milk Reduced-Fat Sharp Singles

4 whole wheat English muffins

PER SERVING
**279** calories **6g** fat ( **3g** sat / **1g** mono / **0.7g** poly )
**19mg** cholesterol **1116mg** sodium
**33g** carbohydrate **5g** fiber **25g** protein

## METHOD

1 Heat a grill pan over high heat. When hot, remove it from the stove just while you coat it with cooking spray. Grill the tomato slices and the Canadian bacon until warmed through, about 5 minutes. Remove from the pan and set aside on a plate.

2 Heat a large nonstick sauté pan over medium-high heat. When hot, remove it from the stove while you coat it with cooking spray. Add the garlic. Sauté the garlic until it is browned, about 2 minutes. Add the egg substitute and with a heat-resistant rubber spatula, stir until the eggs begin to solidify and large curds form. Season with salt and pepper to taste. Scatter the parsley on top of the eggs, and then place the cheese on top of the eggs.

3 Meanwhile, toast the English muffins in the toaster oven.

4 To assemble the sandwiches, lay the bottom halves of the toasted English muffins on a cutting board. Divide the eggs into four equal portions and place on top of each muffin half. Top the eggs with the grilled bacon and tomato slices; then cover with the muffin tops. Serve immediately.

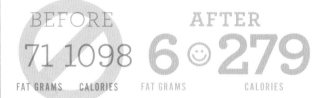

BEFORE
**71 1098**
FAT GRAMS   CALORIES

AFTER
**6** ☺ **279**
FAT GRAMS   CALORIES

**✳ CALORIE SAVER**

Omit the cheese and save **50** calories per serving.

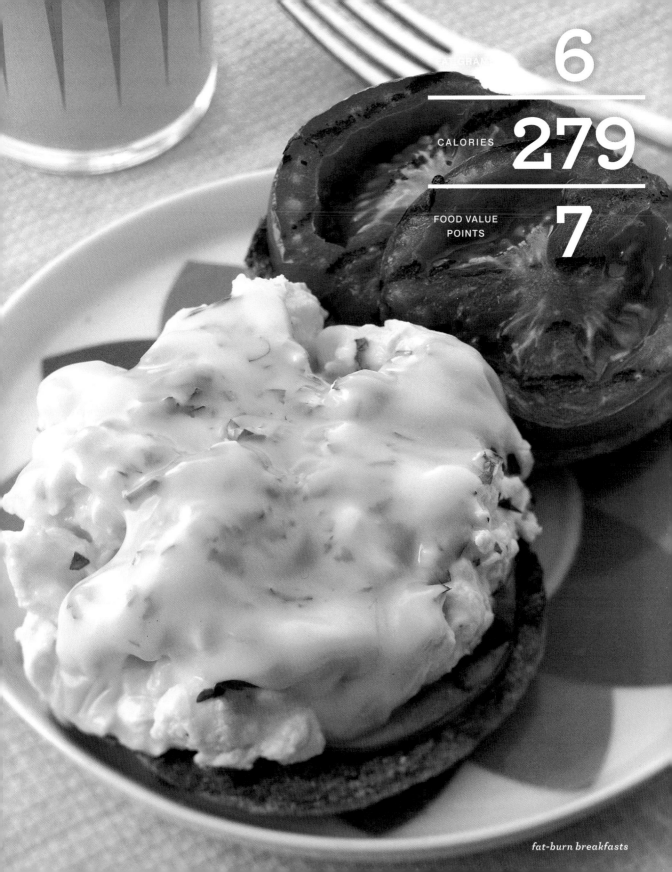

**6**
———
FAT GRAMS

CALORIES **279**
———
FOOD VALUE **7**
POINTS

*fat-burn breakfasts*

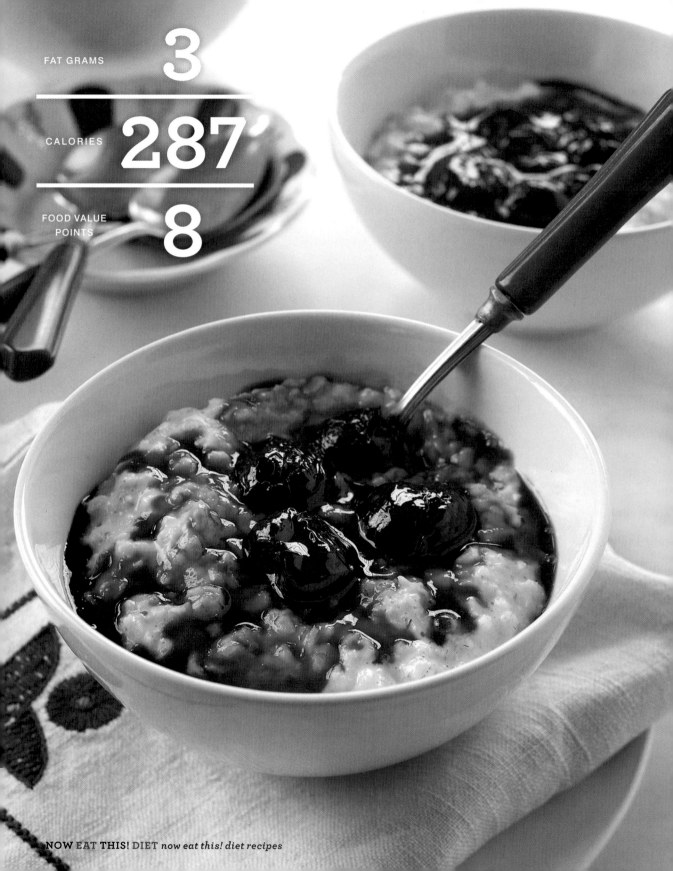

FAT GRAMS **3**

CALORIES **287**

FOOD VALUE POINTS **8**

# Cherry Red Oatmeal SERVES 4

**THERE'S A REASON WHY** things like Cherry Vanilla Coke and Cherry Vanilla Dr Pepper exist: because cherry and vanilla flavors are classic partners. So here's a quick and easy way to spruce up your morning oatmeal. Toss in frozen sweet cherries with some vanilla. Cherries are available year-round, unlike fresh sweet cherries, which come around only during the summer months. Also, like frozen grapes, they make for tasty bite-size treats. Cherries are loaded with antioxidants, too.

## INGREDIENTS

| | |
|---|---|
| 1 | cup frozen sweet cherries |
| ¼ | cup agave nectar |
| 1 | teaspoon vanilla extract |
| ¼ | cup water |
| ½ | teaspoon cornstarch |
| 2½ | cups skim milk |
| | Pinch of salt |
| 2 | cups quick-cooking oatmeal |

PER SERVING
287calories 3gfat ( 0.5gsat / 0.8gmono / 0.9gpoly )
3mgcholesterol 66mgsodium
57gcarbohydrate 4.5gfiber 11gprotein

## METHOD

1 In a small saucepan over medium heat, add the cherries, agave, vanilla, and 2 tablespoons water. In a small bowl, add the cornstarch and stir in the remaining water until smooth. Pour the mixture into the saucepan. Raise the heat, and bring the sauce to a boil, stirring occasionally. Turn down the heat and cook until the sauce has thickened and has a syrupy consistency, about 5 minutes.

2 Meanwhile, heat a medium saucepan over medium-high heat. When hot, add the milk and a pinch of salt, if desired, and bring to a boil. Add the oatmeal and cook until the oatmeal has thickened, about 1 minute, stirring occasionally.

3 Serve the oatmeal in bowls with the cherries and syrup drizzled over the top.

## ✱ CALORIE SAVER
Use water instead of milk and save 52 calories per serving.

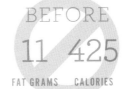
BEFORE
11 425
FAT GRAMS  CALORIES

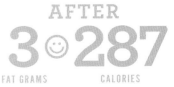
AFTER
3 ☺ 287
FAT GRAMS  CALORIES

*fat-burn breakfasts*

# Blue on Blueberry Silver Dollar Pancakes

**SOME PEOPLE LIKE** them any day of the week, and any time of the day. But pancakes make the perfect weekend breakfast or brunch meal. My quick blueberry "syrup" is a terrific complement to these pancakes, and it adds a nutritious fruit to your breakfast. Blueberries are a virtual powerhouse of great nutrition—and great for brain health. ✳ TIP: If you're using frozen blueberries, make sure they are frozen when you add them to the batter to ensure that they don't break or bleed. These pancakes are light and fluffy because I use whole wheat pastry flour and egg substitute. Anywhere else, blueberry pancakes would run up more than 1,000 calories a serving. Now you can eat blueberry pancakes without guilt, and your body will thank you for it.

## INGREDIENTS

- ¾ cup calorie-free pancake syrup, such as Walden Farms
- 1½ cups fresh or frozen blueberries
- 1½ cups whole wheat pastry flour
- 3½ teaspoons baking powder
- 4 packets (4 grams) powdered stevia, such as SweetLeaf
- ½ teaspoon salt
- 1¼ cups skim milk
- ½ cup liquid egg substitute
- 3 tablespoons canola oil
- Butter-flavored nonstick cooking spray

PER SERVING
**292** calories **12g** fat ( **1g** sat / **7g** mono / **3g** poly )
**1.5mg** cholesterol **830mg** sodium
**39g** carbohydrate **5g** fiber **10g** protein

## METHOD

1 In a small saucepan over low heat, add the pancake syrup and ½ cup blueberries. Stir until combined, and warm for 5 minutes. With the back of a spoon, crush some of the blueberries so they release their juices and give the syrup a purple hue. Turn off the heat and set aside.

2 In a large bowl, add the flour, baking powder, stevia, and salt. Whisk together until well combined.

3 Create a well in the center of the bowl and whisk in the milk, egg substitute, and oil. Be careful not to overmix. Once the mixture is blended, fold in the remaining blueberries with a spatula.

4 Heat a nonstick griddle or skillet over medium heat. When hot, remove it from the stove just while you coat it with cooking spray. Using a tablespoon measure, drop dollops of batter onto the griddle about an inch apart. Once bubbles form on the surface of the pancakes and the edges look dry, flip over. Continue with the remaining batter.

5 Serve pancakes with the blueberry syrup.

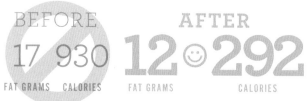

BEFORE 17 930
FAT GRAMS CALORIES

AFTER 12 ☺ 292
FAT GRAMS CALORIES

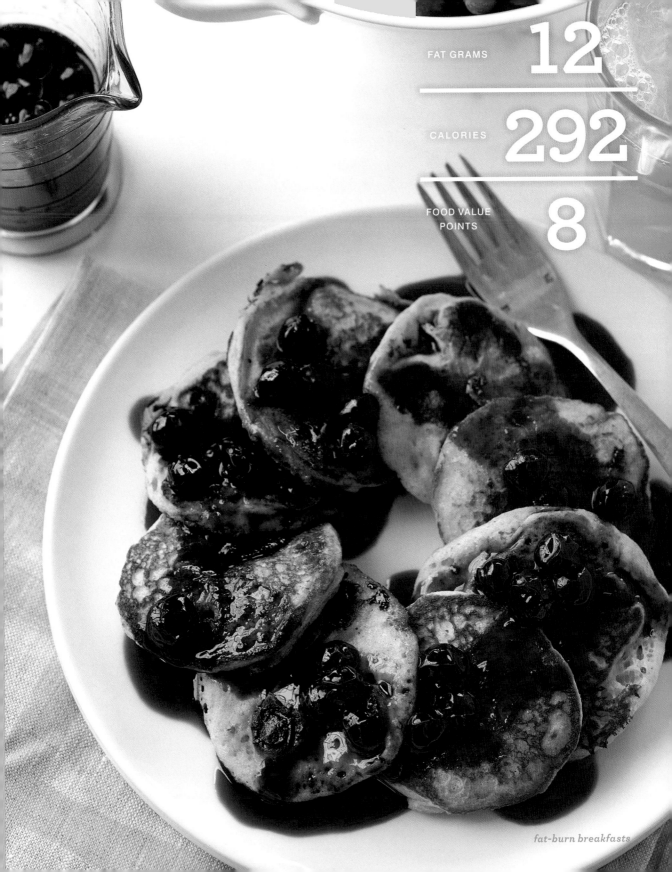

FAT GRAMS 12

CALORIES 292

FOOD VALUE POINTS 8

*fat-burn breakfasts*

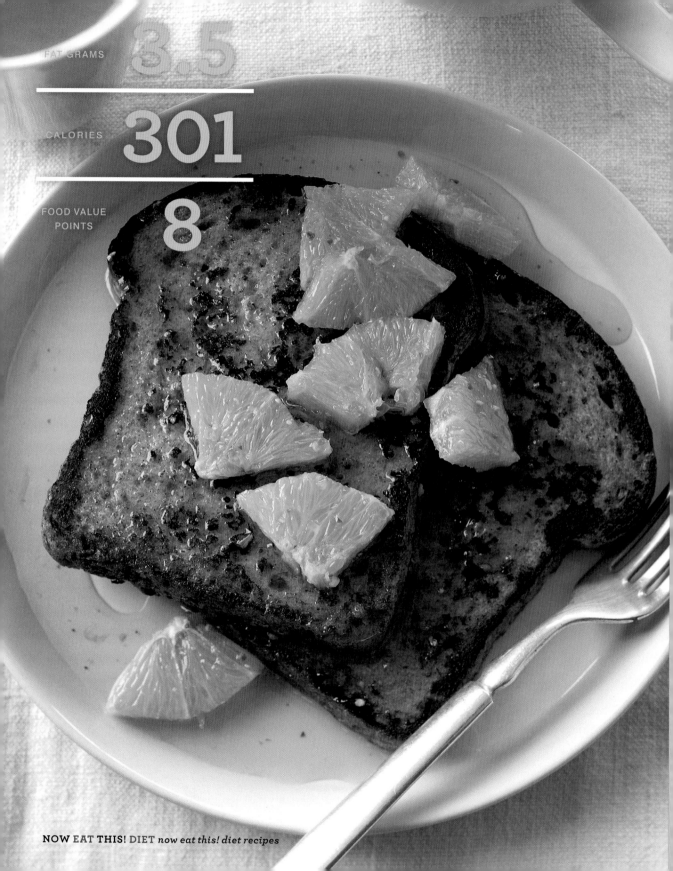

# French Toast à L'Orange

SERVES 4

**NO ONE REALLY** knows the exact origin of French toast, but most sources agree that the dish doesn't stem from classical French cuisine. One version of the story is that French toast was invented in 1724 at a roadside tavern near Albany, New York, by the tavern owner Joseph French. Whatever its background and whoever its inventor, French toast started as a thrifty breakfast food. When a loaf of bread got too stale to eat as sliced bread, a frugal cook sliced the stale loaf, soaked the slices in a little egg and milk, and fried them in oil. Mine aren't fried in oil, of course, but I use a just-as-delicious substitute: butter-flavored vegetable spray and a nonstick pan. I've tanged-up this classic dish with vitamin C–rich oranges for a nutritionally complete breakfast.

## INGREDIENTS

| | |
|---|---|
| 1 | medium navel orange |
| ½ | cup calorie-free pancake syrup, such as Walden Farms |
| 1 | cup liquid egg substitute |
| 1 | (12-ounce) can evaporated skim milk |
| 2 | teaspoons vanilla extract |
| ¾ | teaspoon ground cinnamon |
| 8 | pieces stale thin-sliced European whole-grain bread, such as Rubschlager |
| | Butter-flavored nonstick cooking spray |

PER SERVING
**301**calories **3.5g**fat ( **0g**sat / **0g**mono / **0g**poly )
**3mg**cholesterol **625mg**sodium
**50g**carbohydrate **5g**fiber **19g**protein

## METHOD

1 Using a rasp or grater, remove 1 teaspoon of the zest from the orange and set aside for the bread. Cut off the top and bottom of the orange. Position the orange so that the flat bottom end is resting on the cutting board. Using a sharp paring knife, cut the skin and white pith off in a downward curving motion. Continue cutting around the orange so that it is no longer surrounded by the skin and pith. Cut the orange crosswise into ¼-inch slices, and then cut the slices into quarters.

2 Transfer the orange quarters to a small saucepan over low heat. Add the pancake syrup, and stir to combine. Simmer for 5 minutes, and then turn off the heat and set aside.

3 In a large, shallow pan, add the egg substitute, evaporated milk, vanilla, cinnamon, and orange zest. Stir with a whisk or fork until well combined. Dip the bread slices into the egg mixture; turn to coat both sides.

4 Heat a griddle or large nonstick sauté pan over medium heat. When hot, remove it from the stove just while you coat it with cooking spray. Add the bread slices and cook, about 2 minutes each side. Repeat with remaining slices.

5 Serve with the orange syrup.

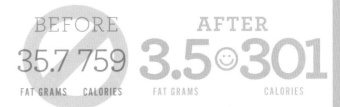

BEFORE 35.7 759 FAT GRAMS CALORIES    AFTER 3.5 ☺ 301 FAT GRAMS CALORIES

# Rocky Road Oatmeal

**WHEN IT COMES TO BREAKFAST,** it pays to think outside the box—the sugary cereal box, that is. I love rocky road ice cream, which inspired this recipe. The chocolate in rocky road ice cream can have a positive impact on your heart health due to the flavonoids, a health-building antioxidant in cocoa powder. Dark and bittersweet chocolate contain more cocoa powder, so choose those over milk or white chocolate. Chocolate still contains a fair amount of fat and sugar, so don't go overboard. Your kids will love this version of oatmeal, too. For nutrition and taste, it beats sugar-laced cocoa cereal in a box any day.

## INGREDIENTS

- 2½   **cups skim milk**
- **Pinch of salt**
- 2   **cups quick-cooking oatmeal**
- 1   **teaspoon vanilla extract**
- 2   **tablespoons agave nectar**
- 1   **ounce bittersweet (60%–70%) chocolate**
- ¼   **cup chopped walnuts, toasted**
- ¼   **cup minimarshmallows**

## METHOD

1  Heat a medium saucepan over medium-high heat. When hot, add the milk and salt, if desired, and bring to a boil.

2  Add the oatmeal, vanilla, and agave. Stir until combined. Cook until the oatmeal has thickened, about 5 minutes. Add the chocolate and stir until it has melted. Remove from heat.

3  Serve the oatmeal in bowls, and top with the toasted walnuts and minimarshmallows.

PER SERVING
**327**calories **10g**fat ( **2.8g**sat / **1.5g**mono / **4.4g**poly )
**3mg**cholesterol **76mg**sodium
**51g**carbohydrate **4g**fiber **12g**protein

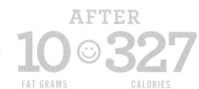

BEFORE
15  627
FAT GRAMS  CALORIES

AFTER
10 ☺ 327
FAT GRAMS   CALORIES

**✱ CALORIE SAVER**

Omit the walnuts  and save **48** calories per serving.

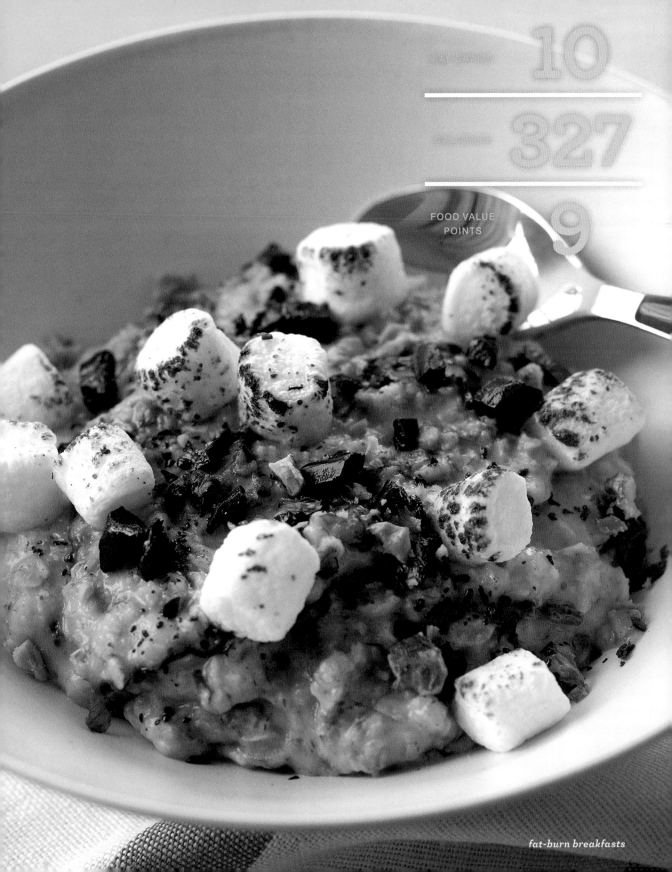

*fat-burn breakfasts*

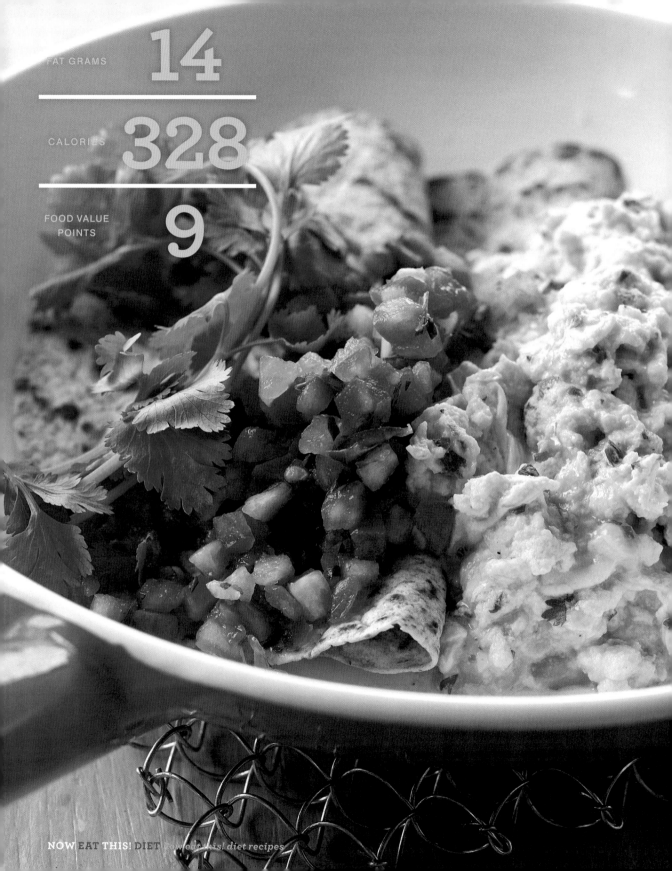

FAT GRAMS **14**

CALORIES **328**

FOOD VALUE POINTS **9**

# South of the Border Scramble with Chorizo and Salsa

SERVES 4

**THIS DISH IS MY TAKE** on huevos rancheros, a very popular breakfast item in the Southwest. Heck, they even eat them for lunch and dinner. As the story goes, this savory meal was cooked up on ranches and made from leftover taco fixin's. There are many different recipes for huevos rancheros, but for the most part, they all involve eggs (I use egg substitute to cut the fat and cholesterol), tortillas, reduced-fat chorizo (a sausage commonly used in Mexican cuisine), and some sort of sauce. I recommend freshly made, no-fat, store-bought salsa for the sauce here.

## INGREDIENTS

2    cups liquid egg substitute

     Salt

     Freshly ground black pepper

     Nonstick cooking spray

2    ounces reduced-fat chorizo sausage, such as Wellshire Farms, cut into ¼-inch slices

2    tablespoons chopped fresh cilantro

1    cup (about 4 ounces) shredded 50% reduced-fat cheddar, such as Cabot

8    (6-inch) low-carb tortillas, such as La Tortilla Factory

1    cup fresh salsa

½    cup reduced-fat sour cream, such as Breakstone's

## METHOD

1   Heat a large nonstick sauté pan over medium heat.

2   In a small bowl, add the egg substitute. Season with salt and pepper to taste. Mix well.

3   Remove the sauté pan from the stove just while you coat it with cooking spray. Add the chorizo and cook till slightly brown, about 3 minutes. Pour the egg mixture into pan. Using a heatproof rubber spatula, stir the eggs occasionally until large curds form. While the eggs are still wet, fold in the cilantro and cheese.

4   Meanwhile, using flameproof tongs, char the tortillas over an open flame until each side is slightly blackened (or toast them under a preheated broiler). Keep the tortillas warm by covering them with a kitchen towel as you go.

5   Serve the scrambled eggs with the charred tortillas and salsa. Add a dollop of reduced-fat sour cream to each serving.

### PER SERVING

**328** calories **14g** fat ( **6g** sat / **2g** mono / **1g** poly )
**43mg** cholesterol **1216mg** sodium
**30g** carbohydrate **14g** fiber **36g** protein

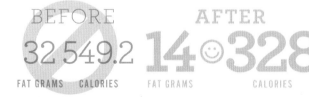

BEFORE
**32** FAT GRAMS  **549.2** CALORIES

AFTER
**14** FAT GRAMS  ☺  **328** CALORIES

**✱ CALORIE SAVER:** Use only 4 tortillas and save **50** calories per serving, or omit the sour cream and save **47** calories per serving. (Do both for a savings of **97** calories per serving.)

# Blueberry Graham Cheesecake Oatmeal

SERVES 4

**SINCE IT'S A GIVEN** by now that breakfast is the most important meal of the day, one that gives you the best start, the next subject to consider is the tasty one: what to have for breakfast. Oatmeal is one option that fulfills the job of a good breakfast: to fuel you with energy your body can use for activity and your brain can use for concentration and problem solving. But it doesn't always have to be the classic oatmeal in a bowl. So how about Blueberry Cheesecake Oatmeal? I know it sounds bizarre, but it works. This bowl of goodness has most of the elements of a cheesecake, but without all the hip-hugging fat and calories—including graham crackers, which were invented in the early 1800s and originally marketed as a health food. Add in blueberries, and you're definitely eating a superhealthy breakfast.

## INGREDIENTS

| | |
|---|---|
| 2½ | cups skim milk |
| | Pinch of salt |
| 2 | cups quick-cooking oatmeal |
| ½ | teaspoon vanilla extract |
| ¼ | cup agave nectar |
| ½ | teaspoon lemon zest |
| 1 | cup fresh or frozen blueberries |
| ¼ | cup reduced-fat cream cheese |
| ¼ | cup nonfat Greek yogurt, such as 0% Fage Total |
| 2 | squares (or 1 rectangle) graham crackers, crushed |

## METHOD

1 Heat a medium saucepan over medium-high heat. When hot, add the milk and salt, if desired, and bring to a boil.

2 Add the oatmeal, vanilla, agave, lemon zest, blueberries, and cream cheese. Stir until combined. Cook until the oatmeal has thickened, about 1 minute. Remove from heat and stir in the yogurt.

3 Serve the oatmeal in bowls, and sprinkle the crushed graham crackers on top.

PER SERVING
**339** calories **6g** fat ( **2g** sat / **1g** mono / **1g** poly )
**13mg** cholesterol **162mg** sodium
**60g** carbohydrate **5g** fiber **13g** protein

BEFORE
15 440
FAT GRAMS CALORIES

AFTER
6 ☺ 339
FAT GRAMS CALORIES

**\* CALORIE SAVER**
Use water instead of milk and save **52** calories per serving.

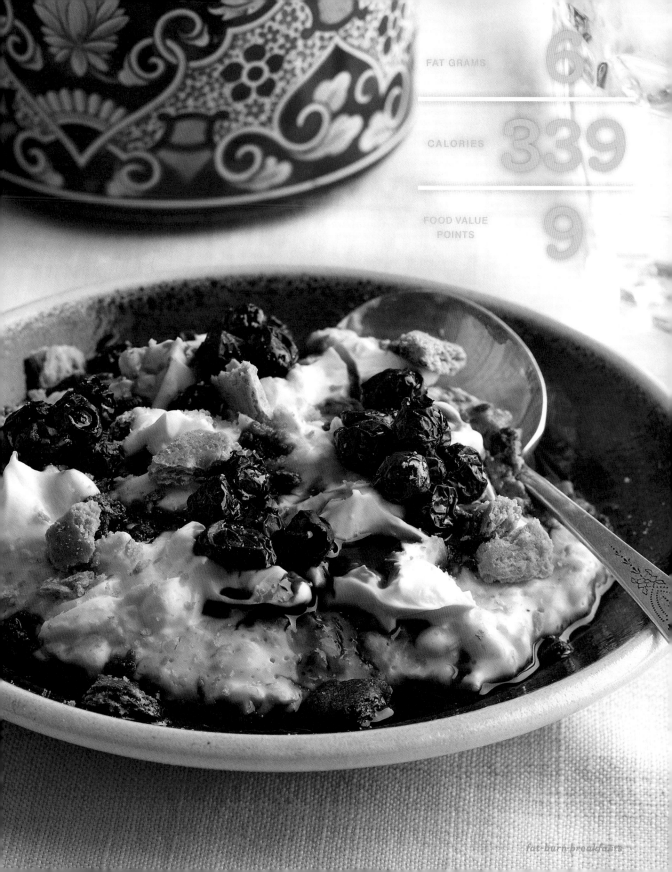

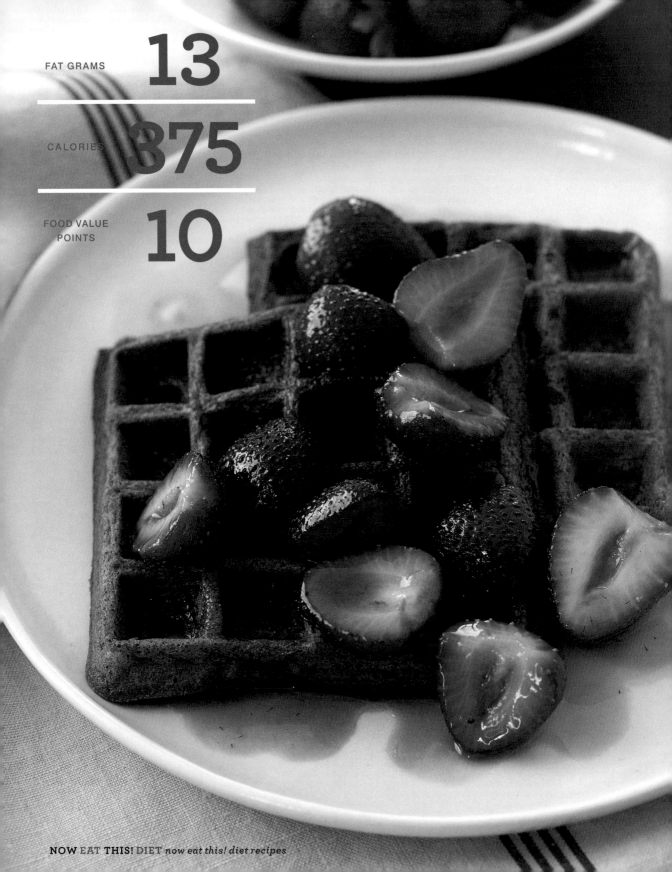

FAT GRAMS **13**

CALORIES **375**

FOOD VALUE POINTS **10**

# Strawberry Malted Belgian Waffles

SERVES 4

**THE "SECRET INGREDIENT"** here is malt powder, an intriguing and tasty ingredient originally invented as food for infants and invalids. The malty flavor of these waffles pairs beautifully with strawberries, cooked into a delicious syrup. It's a marriage made in heaven—well, in a kitchen, at least. ✳TIP: To keep the waffles warm while cooking the remaining batter, transfer the waffles to a baking sheet and pop them in an oven warmed to 200°F. The waffles will stay warm and take on a slightly crispy texture. Use butter-flavored nonstick cooking spray here; it helps add a nice buttery flavor to the waffles.

## INGREDIENTS

| | |
|---|---|
| 1 | cup calorie-free pancake syrup, such as Walden Farms |
| 2 | cups fresh strawberries, hulled and quartered |
| ¼ | teaspoon salt plus an additional pinch for the syrup |
| 1¾ | cups whole wheat pastry flour |
| ½ | cup malted milk powder, such as Carnation |
| 2 | teaspoons baking soda |
| 4 | packets (about 4 grams) powdered stevia, such as SweetLeaf |
| 1¾ | cups skim milk |
| 3 | tablespoons canola oil |
| 1 | teaspoon vanilla extract |
| 3 | large egg whites |
| | Butter-flavored nonstick cooking spray |

PER SERVING
375 calories 13g fat ( 1.5g sat / 7g mono / 3g poly )
5.5mg cholesterol 1023mg sodium
52g carbohydrate 5g fiber 13g protein

## METHOD

1 In a medium saucepan over low heat, add the pancake syrup, 1 cup strawberries, and a pinch of salt, if desired. Cook until the strawberries begin to soften and release juices, about 5 minutes. Mash the strawberries with the back of a spoon. Add the remaining strawberries, and stir to combine. Simmer for 2 minutes, and then turn off the heat and set aside.

2 Preheat the waffle iron to the highest temperature. Preheat the oven to 200°F.

3 In a medium bowl, whisk together the flour, malted milk powder, baking soda, ¼ teaspoon salt, and stevia. In a large bowl, whisk together the milk, oil, and vanilla. In two stages, mix the dry ingredients into the wet, making sure not to overmix. Set aside.

4 In a medium bowl, whip the egg whites with an electric mixer until soft peaks form.

5 Using a spatula, take a third of the egg whites and fold them into the batter. Once incorporated, fold in the remaining whites.

6 Coat the waffle iron with cooking spray. Pour batter into the iron and cook until golden. Transfer the waffle to a baking tray and keep warm in the oven while repeating the procedure with the remaining batter.

7 Serve immediately with the strawberry syrup.

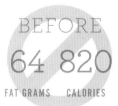

BEFORE
64 820
FAT GRAMS    CALORIES

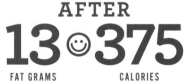

AFTER
13 ☺ 375
FAT GRAMS    CALORIES

*fat-burn breakfasts*

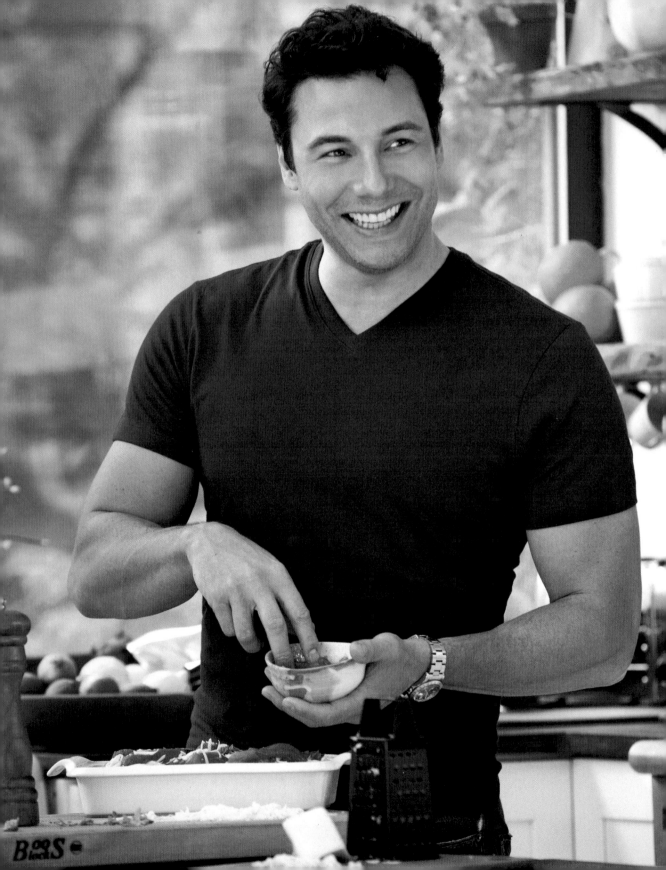

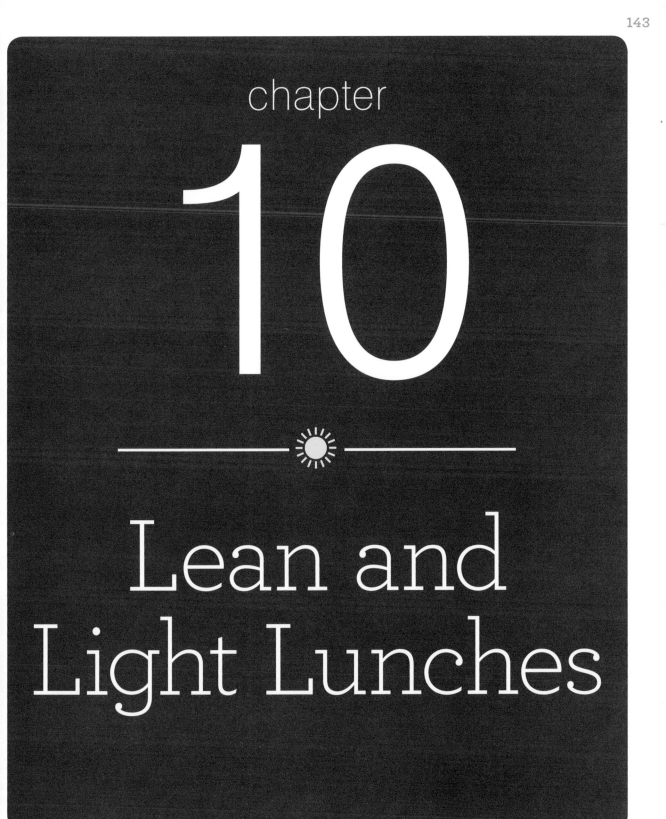

chapter

# 10

# Lean and Light Lunches

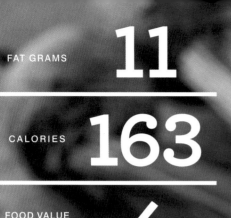

FAT GRAMS

# 11

CALORIES

# 163

FOOD VALUE
POINTS

# 4

# Red Beet, Goat Cheese, and Walnut Salad

SERVES 4

**MAYBE YOU'VE HEARD** that detox diets, in which you have to fast or otherwise go without much nourishment, are the "in" thing. Well, fasting sucks. It makes your body feel like it's going through shock therapy, and you can get pretty sick. Let beets be your detox. They contain phytochemicals and antioxidants that support detoxification. One of the best ways to enjoy beets is on a bed of arugula, a type of green that's healthier than nutritionally wimpy iceberg. ✳TIP: When buying beets, look for beets that are firm and have smooth skin. Avoid ones that are soft or show signs of damage. If they have the leaves intact, look for non-wilted leaves. And, when toasting nuts, keep a close eye on them. They can easily burn because of their high oil content. Enjoy this tasty version of a gourmet favorite—you just can't beet it. (I SWEAR, THEY MADE ME SAY THAT!)

## INGREDIENTS

| | |
|---|---|
| 4 | medium red beets |
| 6 | ounces (about 4 cups) baby arugula |
| ¼ | cup reduced-fat balsamic vinaigrette, such as Ken's Light Options |
| ¼ | cup chopped fresh flat-leaf parsley |
| 1 | tablespoon chopped fresh chives |
| | Salt |
| | Freshly ground black pepper |
| 2 | ounces (about ½ cup) crumbled goat cheese |
| ¼ | cup chopped walnuts, toasted |

## METHOD

1 Prick the skin of the beets with a fork. Place the beets on a microwave-safe plate, and microwave on high until tender, about 12 minutes (alternatively, wrap the beets in foil and roast them in the oven for 1 hour at 375°F). When they are cool enough to handle, peel the beets and cut them into bite-size wedges.

2 In a large bowl, combine the beets, arugula, vinaigrette, parsley, and chives. Toss thoroughly to combine. Season with salt and pepper to taste.

3 Divide the salad among 4 plates. Top each salad with crumbled goat cheese and toasted walnuts, and serve.

PER SERVING
**163**calories **11g**fat ( **3g**sat / **1.4g**mono / **3.7g**poly )
**7mg**cholesterol **235mg**sodium
**13g**carbohydrate **4g**fiber **6g**protein

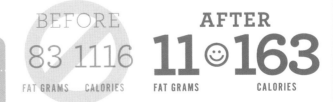

✳ CALORIE SAVER
Omit the cheese and save **38** calories a serving.

BEFORE
83 1116
FAT GRAMS   CALORIES

AFTER
11 ☺ 163
FAT GRAMS   CALORIES

*lean and light lunches*

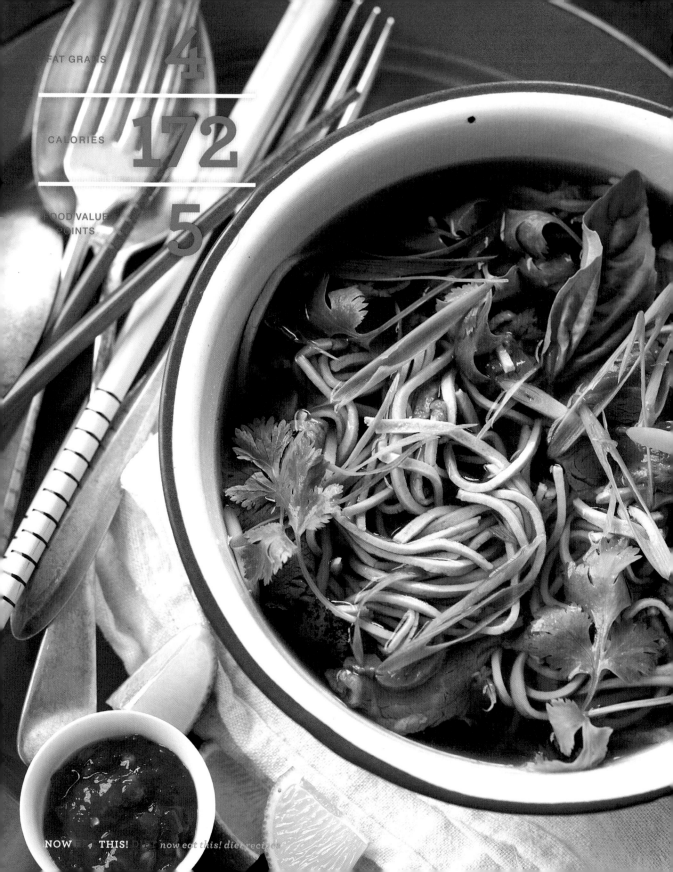

FAT GRAMS 4

CALORIES 172

FOOD VALUE
POINTS 5

# Rich Beef and Noodle Pho with Lime and Bean Sprouts

SERVES 4

**NO, I DIDN'T** misspell *hop*. This is a traditional Vietnamese comfort food (pronounced fuh) that originated in Hanoi after the turn of the nineteenth century, a culinary creation borne of French and Chinese influence. It's a simple soup filled with rice noodles swimming in a transparent, flavorful broth. My version uses low-carb, low-calorie shirataki noodles. Traditional pho soup takes about eight hours of simmering a cauldron of beef or chicken bones to create the broth, but I've cut that cooking time to less than 30 minutes, along with the calories.

> Eat Noodles to Your Heart's Content  Shiritaki noodles are becoming wildly popular. The reason is that they're virtually calorie-free. Not only that, but they're also gluten-free. This means you can have your "pasta" and eat a lot of it, too. What's the secret behind these guilt-free noodles? They're made mainly of soluble fiber. Soluble fiber acts to slow digestion. By doing this, it allows for the slower absorption of glucose and prolongs the sensation of fullness—great benefits for weight loss. Check out the website www.miraclenoodle.com for more information.

## INGREDIENTS

| | |
|---|---|
| 16 | ounces shirataki noodles, or tofu shirataki |
| 40 | ounces (5 cups) low-fat, low-sodium chicken broth |
| 4 | teaspoons agave nectar |
| ½ | cup chopped fresh basil |
| ¼ | cup chopped fresh cilantro |
| ¼ | cup chopped scallions (white and green parts) |
| 2 | limes |
| | Salt |
| | Freshly ground black pepper |
| 8 | ounces lean beef tenderloin, trimmed of all visible fat |
| 2 | teaspoons garlic-chili sauce, such as Huy Fong |
| 2 | cups bean sprouts |

## METHOD

1  To prepare the shirataki noodles, drain and rinse under hot water. Drain any remaining liquid.

2  In a large pot over medium-high heat, bring the chicken broth to a boil. Add the noodles and cook, about 2 minutes. Turn the heat to low and add the agave, basil, cilantro, and scallions. Cut one of the limes in half and squeeze the juice into the pot. Stir to combine. Season with salt and pepper to taste.

3  Slice the beef into very thin slices.

4  Divide the beef among 4 bowls. Ladle the hot soup into the bowls over the beef.

5  Cut the remaining lime into 4 wedges. Serve the soup with garlic-chili sauce, bean sprouts, and lime wedges.

PER SERVING
172 calories  **4g** fat ( **1.3g** sat / **1.5g** mono / **0g** poly )
**30mg** cholesterol  **182g** sodium
**18g** carbohydrate  **3g** fiber  **20g** protein

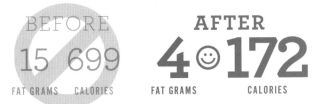

BEFORE
15 699
FAT GRAMS  CALORIES

**AFTER**
4 ☺ **172**
FAT GRAMS  CALORIES

*lean and light lunches*

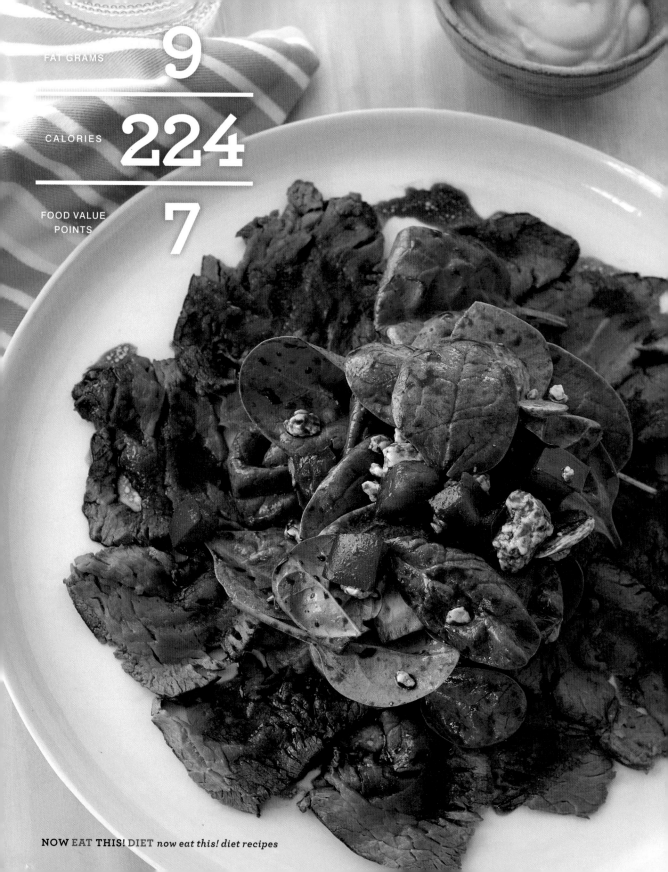

FAT GRAMS **9**

CALORIES **224**

FOOD VALUE POINTS **7**

# Sliced Steak with Tomato and Spinach Salad

SERVES 4

**THE TYPICAL RESTAURANT** nutritional information on this dish is just plain scary: The original recipe comes in at nearly 640 calories and 34 grams of fat. (Better warn your circulatory system it's coming.) I've knocked off a couple hundred calories, and it tastes just like any of the originals. If you don't like your beef medium-rare, feel free to adjust the cooking time of the meat in the oven.

## INGREDIENTS

| | |
|---|---|
| 1 | (1-pound) piece lean beef tenderloin, trimmed of all visible fat |
| | Salt |
| | Freshly ground black pepper |
| | Nonstick cooking spray |
| ¼ | cup balsamic vinegar |
| 2 | teaspoons Dijon mustard |
| 1 | tablespoon extra-virgin olive oil |
| 6 | ounces (about 8 cups) baby spinach |
| 2 | cups sliced white button mushrooms |
| 1 | cup diced vine-ripened tomatoes |
| ¼ | cup (about 1 ounce) crumbled reduced-fat blue cheese, such as Treasure Cave |

PER SERVING
**224** calories **9g** fat ( **3g** sat / **4g** mono / **0.5g** poly )
**60mg** cholesterol **287g** sodium
**15g** carbohydrate **3g** fiber **27g** protein

## METHOD

1 Preheat the oven to 450°F. Place a wire rack on a baking sheet lined with foil, and set it aside.

2 Heat a large cast-iron pan over high heat. Season the meat with salt and pepper to taste. When the pan is hot, remove it from the stove just while you coat it with cooking spray. Add the meat and sear, turning it occasionally until the meat is a deep golden brown all over, about 2 minutes per side. Transfer the meat to the wire rack on the baking sheet and continue to cook in the oven for 8 to 10 minutes or until the internal temperature reaches 125°F for medium-rare. Remove the baking sheet from the oven, and tent the meat with foil to keep it warm. Let the meat rest for at least 10 minutes before slicing.

3 In a medium bowl, whisk together the vinegar and mustard. Drizzle in the olive oil while continuing to whisk. Season with salt and pepper to taste. Add the spinach, mushrooms, tomatoes, and blue cheese to the bowl, and toss until well combined.

4 Slice the meat into very thin pieces and serve with the salad.

**✱ CALORIE SAVER**
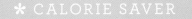
Cut the beef to 8 ounces and save **60** calories per serving.

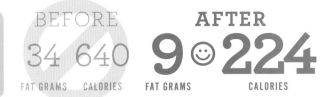

BEFORE
34 640
FAT GRAMS  CALORIES

**AFTER**
**9** ☺ **224**
FAT GRAMS  CALORIES

*lean and light lunches*

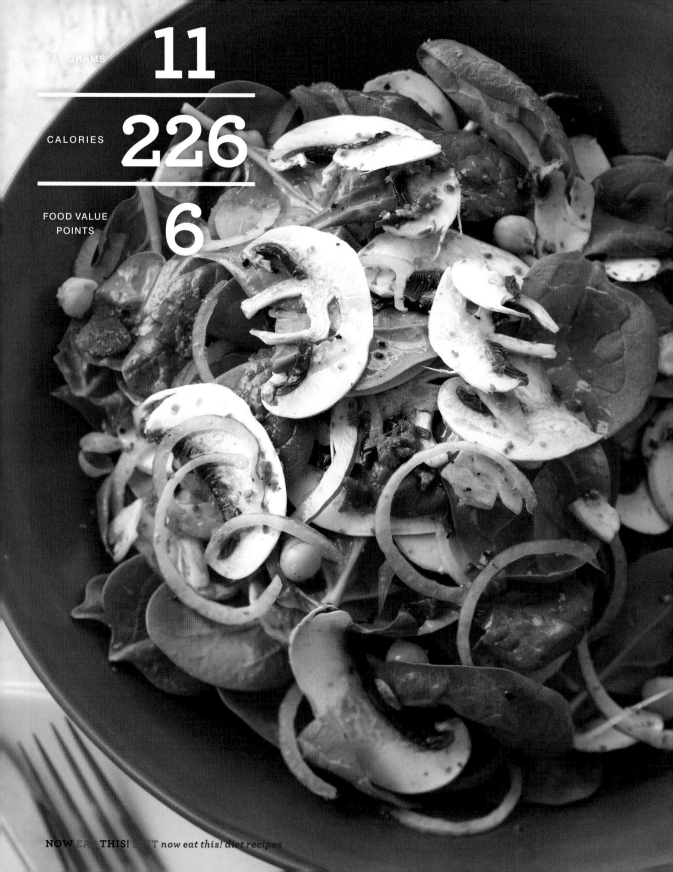

# Spinach and Bacon Salad

SERVES 4

**IF ANY SALAD** can claim the throne of "comfort food," it's the classic spinach salad, with its warm bacon-fat dressing. I've made this traditional salad a bit more waistline-friendly without sacrificing the taste (bring on the bacon) and texture (thanks to the high-fiber garbanzo beans). Of course, I lust for bacon. If someone said I could eat only one food for the rest of my life, it would be bacon. But my bacon is smart bacon. At one-third the fat and calories, we can keep this player in the game.

## INGREDIENTS

| | |
|---|---|
| ¼ | cup red wine vinegar |
| 1½ | teaspoons agave nectar |
| 1 | teaspoon Dijon mustard |
| 2 | tablespoons extra-virgin olive oil |
| | Salt |
| | Freshly ground black pepper |
| 6 | ounces (about 8 cups) baby spinach |
| ½ | medium red onion, thinly sliced |
| 2 | cups (about 6 ounces) sliced white button mushrooms |
| 1 | cup canned garbanzo beans, drained and rinsed |
| ½ | cup (about 2 ounces) real bacon bits, such as Hormel |

## METHOD

1 Heat a small saucepan over medium-low heat. Add the vinegar, agave, mustard, and olive oil, and whisk together. Season with salt and pepper to taste. When the dressing is warm, turn off the heat.

2 In a large bowl, add the spinach, onions, mushrooms, garbanzo beans, and bacon. Pour the dressing over the salad and toss thoroughly to combine. Season with salt and pepper to taste. Serve immediately.

PER SERVING
**226** calories **11g** fat ( **2g** sat / **5g** mono / **1g** poly )
**20mg** cholesterol **666mg** sodium
**23g** carbohydrate **5g** fiber **12g** protein

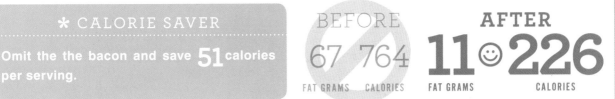

✱ CALORIE SAVER
Omit the the bacon and save **51** calories per serving.

BEFORE
67 764
FAT GRAMS   CALORIES

AFTER
11 ☺ 226
FAT GRAMS   CALORIES

# White Bean and Kale Soup with Rosemary and Parmigiano-Reggiano

SERVES 4

**SEVERAL YEARS AGO,** when bagged spinach was yanked from supermarkets after reports of contamination, we mourned its loss. But another green veggie stepped into its hallowed spot: kale. Yes, I know it looks like a pile of weeds sitting in the produce department, but kale is a miracle green. This veggie is loaded with calcium, fiber, and cancer-fighting antioxidants and abounds with beta-carotene and the compound sulforaphane, which research shows can help protect against certain cancers. Kale comes in green, purple, and dinosaur (so called because of its bumpy leaves) varieties. All work well with this soup.

I use canned white beans in this recipe. Compared to dry beans, the canned variety is already cooked, so you don't have to factor in the soaking time. When using canned beans, drain and rinse off the liquid, which can make the beans somewhat gooey. Use no-salt-added canned beans if you're watching your sodium intake.

By the way, bagged spinach seems to be okay now, despite having gone through some nasty times.

## INGREDIENTS

| | |
|---|---|
| 1 | tablespoon extra-virgin olive oil |
| ½ | medium yellow onion, cut into medium dice |
| 4 | cloves garlic, roughly chopped |
| 1 | (15.5-ounce) can white beans such as cannellini, great northern, or navy beans, drained and rinsed |
| ½ | teaspoon roughly chopped fresh rosemary |
| 1 | bay leaf |
| 4 | cups low-fat, low-sodium chicken broth |
| 5 | cups roughly chopped kale |
| | Salt |
| | Freshly ground black pepper |
| ¼ | cup grated Parmigiano-Reggiano |

## METHOD

1 Heat the olive oil in a medium pot over medium-high heat. When hot, add the onion and sauté for 3 minutes. Add the garlic and continue to cook for another 2 minutes or until the onions are soft and the garlic is browned.

2 Add the beans, rosemary, bay leaf, and chicken broth. Cover and bring to a boil. Turn down the heat and allow the soup to simmer for 5 minutes.

3 Add the kale to the pot. Cover and cook for about 2 minutes.

4 Remove the bay leaf from the soup. Season with salt and freshly ground black pepper to taste.

5 Serve the soup with a sprinkle of cheese over each bowl.

PER SERVING
**234**calories **7g**fat ( **1.8g**sat / **3.6g**mono / **1g**poly )
**4mg**cholesterol **473mg**sodium
**31g**carbohydrate **7g**fiber **17g**protein

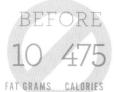

BEFORE
10 475
FAT GRAMS  CALORIES

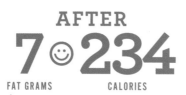

**AFTER**
**7** ☺ **234**
FAT GRAMS       CALORIES

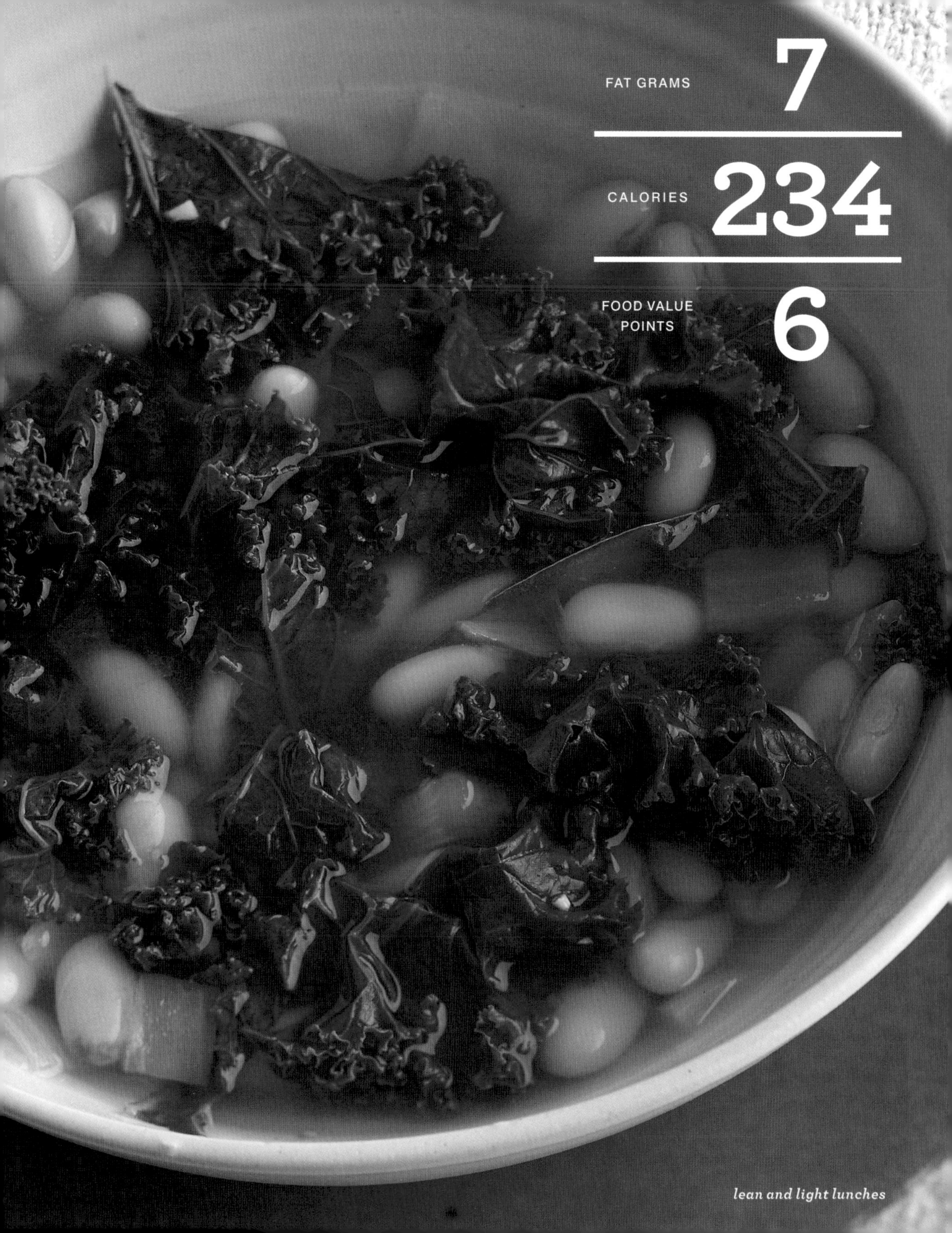

FAT GRAMS

**7**

CALORIES

**234**

FOOD VALUE
POINTS

**6**

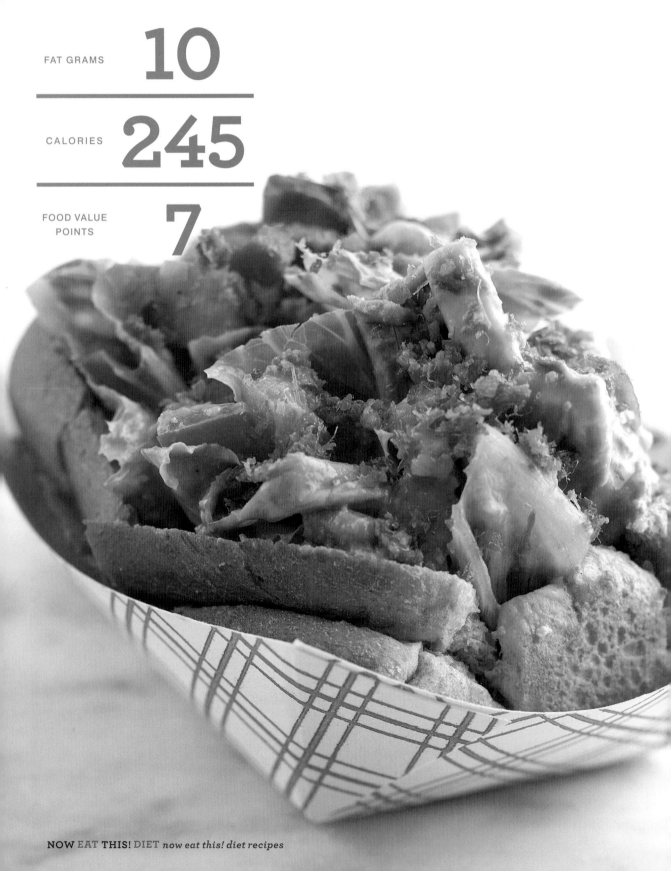

FAT GRAMS **10**

CALORIES **245**

FOOD VALUE
POINTS **7**

# Bacon Lettuce Tomato Roll

SERVES 4

**MOST PEOPLE LOVE BACON,** lettuce, and tomato sandwiches, but they aren't on many low-fat diets. I found that if I put the lettuce and tomato on the bread and then sprinkle it with some crumbled bacon bits and low-fat mayo, I get to have my favorite sandwich but not the fat! In my version I chop up all the ingredients to get the flavors to mingle, and then serve it on an open-face roll. My BLT also has avocado for added richness. Avocado is technically a fruit. It contains heart-healthy monounsaturated fats, which can lower cholesterol levels. Although I've never heard of anyone bingeing on avocados, don't try it. They still contain a hefty amount of calories. Oh, and did I mention I love bacon? I might live a shorter life, but give me bacon any day.

## INGREDIENTS

| | |
|---|---|
| 4 | whole wheat split-top hot dog buns, such as Matthew's Salad Rolls |
| ¼ | cup fat-free mayonnaise |
| 2 | teaspoons red wine vinegar |
| 4 | large romaine lettuce leaves, washed and chopped |
| 2 | medium red heirloom tomatoes, cut into small dice |
| 1 | Hass avocado, cut into small dice |
| ½ | cup (about 2 ounces) crumbled bacon, such as Hormel Real Bacon Bits |
| | Salt |
| | Freshly ground black pepper |

## METHOD

1 Toast both sides of the buns in a toaster oven.

2 In a large bowl, combine the mayonnaise and red wine vinegar with a whisk. Fold in the lettuce, tomatoes, avocado, and bacon. Season with salt and pepper to taste.

3 Divide the mixture among the 4 rolls, and serve immediately.

PER SERVING
245 calories **10g** fat ( **1.8g** sat / **3.6g** mono / **1.6g** poly )
**22mg** cholesterol **734mg** sodium
**29g** carbohydrate **5g** fiber **13g** protein

✱ CALORIE SAVER
Omit the avocado and save **57** calories per serving.

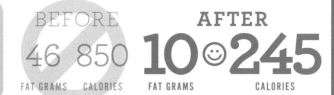

BEFORE
46 850
FAT GRAMS   CALORIES

AFTER
10 ☺ 245
FAT GRAMS   CALORIES

*lean and light lunches*

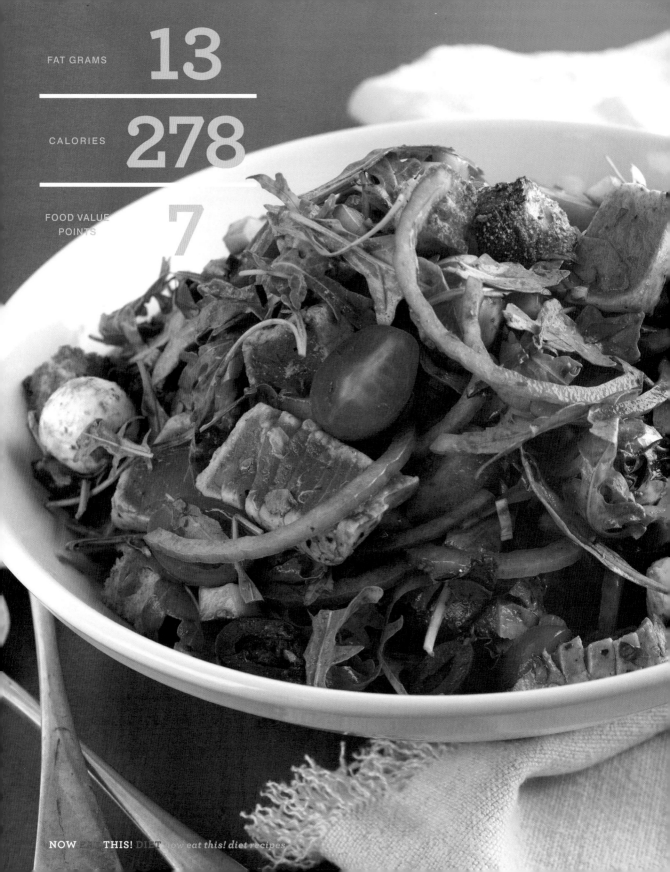

FAT GRAMS **13**

CALORIES **278**

FOOD VALUE
POINTS **7**

# Mediterranean Tuna, Bread, and Cheese Salad

SERVES 4

**HERE'S HOW MUCH** Italians love carbs: We can make a salad out of bread, otherwise known as panzanella. I wonder what the carb patrol would think of that—you know, those folks who randomly drive through your neighborhood hoping to catch you unawares with a slice of bread between your teeth. Okay, bread's not the only ingredient in this amazing, colorful salad. How do sushi-grade tuna, kalamata olives, and a special kind of fresh mozzarella cheese called bocconcini sound? The final ingredients needed to make this salad truly Italian are some tomatoes and passion. Being enthusiastic about making great food and then eating with even more enthusiasm is what we Italians thrive on.

## INGREDIENTS

| | |
|---|---|
| 2 | sushi-grade tuna steaks (6 ounces each) |
| | Salt |
| | Freshly ground black pepper |
| | Nonstick cooking spray |
| 1 | (1-inch-thick) slice whole wheat bread |
| 1 | cup grape tomatoes, halved |
| ¼ | English cucumber, cut into small dice |
| ½ | medium red onion, cut in half lengthwise and sliced into half moons |
| 1 | small head radicchio, sliced thin |
| 4 | ounces (about 3 cups) baby arugula |
| ½ | cup pitted kalamata olives, halved |
| 8 | ounces bocconcini |
| ¼ | cup reduced-fat vinaigrette, such as Ken's Light Options Olive Oil and Vinegar |

## METHOD

1 Season the tuna steaks with salt and pepper to taste. Heat a nonstick sauté pan over medium-high heat. When the pan is hot, remove it from the stove just while you coat it with cooking spray. Place the tuna steaks on the pan, and sear each side for about 1 to 2 minutes for medium-rare. Transfer the tuna to a platter and allow it to rest, uncovered, for 5 minutes.

2 Heat a grill pan over high heat. When hot, add the bread and grill on both sides until it is golden and toasted. Remove from pan and cut into ½-inch cubes.

3 Slice the tuna into ¼-inch strips.

4 In a large bowl, combine the tuna, bread, tomatoes, cucumber, red onion, radicchio, arugula, olives, and bocconcini. Toss the salad with the dressing. Season with salt and pepper to taste, and serve.

PER SERVING
**278** calories **13g** fat ( **4.5g** sat / **0g** mono / **0g** poly )
**61mg** cholesterol **537g** sodium
**13g** carbohydrate **2g** fiber **27g** protein

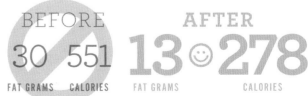

BEFORE
30 551
FAT GRAMS  CALORIES

AFTER
13 ☺ 278
FAT GRAMS  CALORIES

*lean and light lunches*

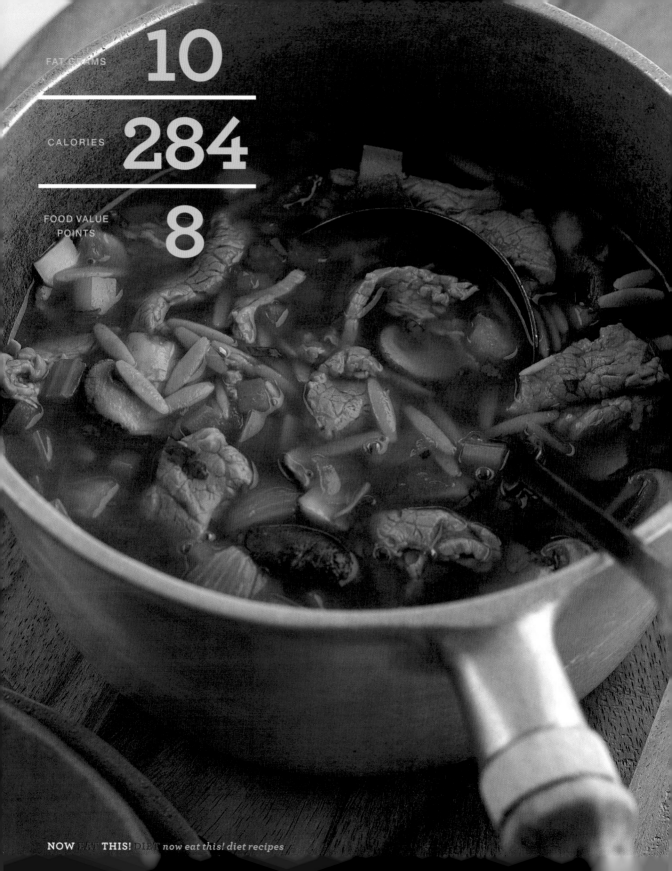

FAT GRAMS

# 10

CALORIES

# 284

FOOD VALUE
POINTS

# 8

# Beef and Orzo Soup

SERVES 4

**EVEN IF YOU WERE BORN** without veggie-craving taste buds, you'll love this meaty vegetable soup. Instead of using traditional barley in this soup, I used whole wheat orzo, which takes a fraction of the cooking time. Orzo is a rice-shaped pasta that can be used in soups and pasta salads. The beef tenderloin is so thinly sliced that it will cook rapidly once it's added to the hot soup. Chicken soup might be good for your soul, but this soup's good for your body and your soul.

## INGREDIENTS

| | |
|---|---|
| 2 | ounces 100% whole wheat orzo, such as RiceSelect |
| 1 | tablespoon extra-virgin olive oil |
| ½ | medium red onion, cut into small dice |
| 2 | celery stalks, cut into small dice |
| 2 | medium carrots, peeled and cut into small dice |
| ½ | pound (about 2 cups) sliced cremini mushrooms |
| | Salt |
| | Freshly ground black pepper |
| 2 | cloves garlic, chopped |
| 5 | cups low-fat, low-sodium chicken broth |
| 1 | (1-pound) piece lean beef tenderloin, trimmed of all visible fat |
| ¼ | chopped fresh flat-leaf parsley |

## METHOD

1 Bring a medium pot of salted water to a boil. Add the orzo and cook according to the package directions; drain.

2 Meanwhile, heat a large pot over medium heat. When hot, add the oil, and then the onion, celery, carrots, and mushrooms. Sauté until softened, about 5 to 7 minutes. Season with salt and pepper to taste. Add the garlic and cook until the garlic begins to brown, about 2 minutes.

3 Add the broth and orzo. Bring to a boil, and then reduce the heat so the soup is simmering. Season with salt and pepper to taste.

4 Slice the meat into very thin slices. (The meat will shred.) Add the meat to the soup. Sprinkle parsley on top, and serve immediately.

PER SERVING
**284** calories **10g** fat ( **2.5g** sat / **5g** mono / **0.8g** poly )
**60mg** cholesterol **201g** sodium
**22g** carbohydrate **4g** fiber **32g** protein

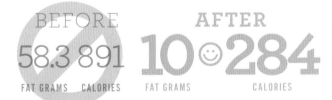

BEFORE 58.3 891
FAT GRAMS CALORIES

AFTER 10 ☺ 284
FAT GRAMS CALORIES

# Boston Blue Chicken and Apple Salad

SERVES 4

**WHEN I WAS A KID,** there was no way I was going to willingly put a piece of cheese that had mold in it into my mouth. You'd have to tie me down first. My taste for blue cheese changed, and now I adore it. In fact, it is one of my favorite cheeses. So, what makes a blue cheese "blue"? It's inoculated with a "good" mold to give the cheese its characteristics. But don't eat blue cheese on green bread. Green is a sign of a bad mold.

The pairing of blue cheese with the tartness of Granny Smith apples and the sweet char of sliced grilled chicken is an amazing combination of flavors, so brace your taste buds. ✱TIP: Once cut, apples have a tendency to turn brown because of oxidation. To help prevent this from happening, slice the apples right into the mixing bowl on a sharp-bladed mandoline at the very last minute. You can make your own vinaigrette for this salad, but there are some terrific brands you can buy at the store that are good and can save you some time.

## INGREDIENTS

| | |
|---|---|
| 4 | skinless, boneless chicken breasts (4 ounces each) |
| | Nonstick cooking spray |
| | Salt |
| | Freshly ground black pepper |
| 2 | heads Boston lettuce, leaves separated |
| 2 | medium Granny Smith apples, peeled, cored, and cut into ¼-inch-thick slices |
| ½ | cup (about 2 ounces) crumbled reduced-fat blue cheese, such as Treasure Cave |
| ¼ | cup reduced-fat vinaigrette, such as Ken's Light Options Olive Oil and Vinegar |
| ¼ | cup chopped walnuts, toasted |
| 2 | tablespoons chopped chives |

## METHOD

1 Heat a grill pan over high heat.

2 Spray the chicken breasts lightly with cooking spray, and season them with salt and pepper to taste. Grill the chicken until it is just cooked through, about 3 minutes per side. Transfer the chicken to a platter, and cover it with foil to keep it warm.

3 In large bowl, combine the lettuce, apples, blue cheese, and vinaigrette. Toss until the apples and lettuce are coated with dressing. Transfer to a serving bowl.

4 Slice the chicken into ½-inch-thick slices. Arrange the chicken with the salad, and scatter walnuts and chives on top.

PER SERVING
**294**calories **13g**fat ( **3g**sat / **1.7g**mono / **4g**poly )
**73mg**cholesterol **448g**sodium
**22g**carbohydrate **3g**fiber **30g**protein

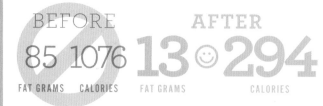

BEFORE
85 1076
FAT GRAMS  CALORIES

AFTER
13 ☺ 294
FAT GRAMS  CALORIES

### ✱ CALORIE SAVER

Omit the walnuts and save **48** calories per serving. Or omit the cheese and save **41** calories per serving; omit both and save **89** calories per serving.

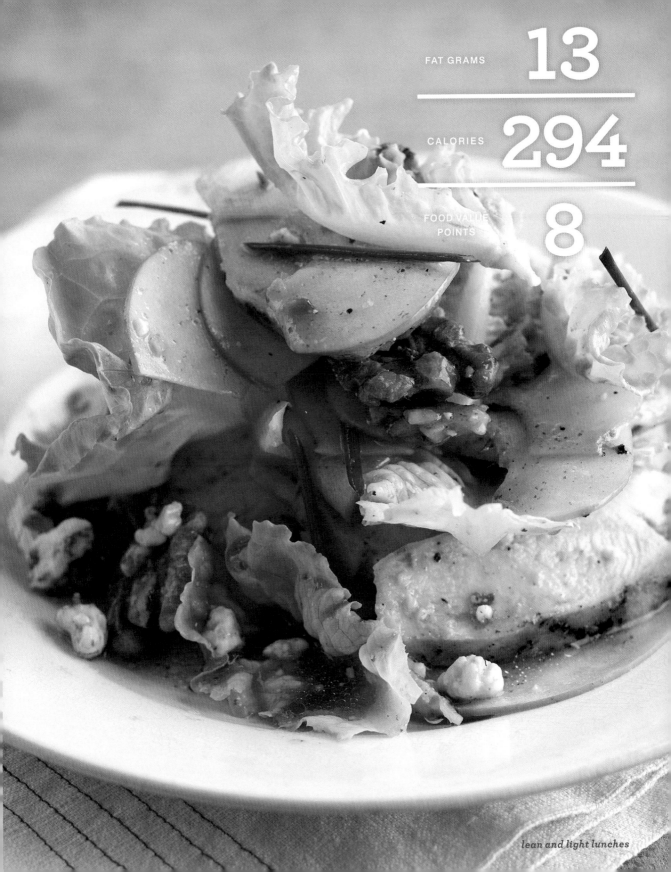

# Yellow Curry Shrimp and Green Pea Soup

SERVES 4

**IF YOU THOUGHT** you'd have to lose weight the old-fashioned way—tummy tuck—think again. Eating soups helps you lose weight. That's because, even though it's mostly water, soup satisfies you like a full meal. With this soup, your taste buds will abandon all things sweet and have a fling with all things spicy and savory. There's a lot of tangy stuff in this soup, but it takes only minutes to prepare. You can find yellow curry paste in the international section of your supermarket. The red variety is also readily available. Raw peeled and deveined shrimp are also available frozen if you can't find fresh. Make sure they are thawed before you use them. And don't you dare leave the tails on; that's just plain rude!

## INGREDIENTS

| | |
|---|---|
| 2 | tablespoons yellow curry paste, such as Karee Curry Paste |
| 1 | Vidalia onion, cut into small dice |
| 3 | cups low-fat, low-sodium chicken broth |
| 1 | cup canned peeled plum tomatoes, roughly chopped |
| 3 | tablespoons lime juice |
| 2 | tablespoons agave nectar |
| 1 | pound large shrimp, peeled and deveined, tails removed |
| 1 | cup frozen peas |
| 1 | cup 2% Greek yogurt, such as Fage Total |
| | Salt |
| | Freshly ground black pepper |
| ½ | cup chopped fresh cilantro |

## METHOD

1 Heat a large saucepan over medium heat. When the pan is hot, add the curry paste. Add the onions and sauté until softened, about 3 minutes.

2 Add the chicken broth, tomatoes, lime juice, and agave, and cover. Reduce the heat to medium-low and simmer for 5 minutes. Add the shrimp and cook till they are no longer translucent, about 1 minute. Add the peas and cook for another minute. Remove the pan from the heat and stir in the yogurt. Season with salt and pepper to taste. Sprinkle the cilantro over the soup.

PER SERVING
**302** calories **5g** fat ( **1.5g** sat / **0.8g** mono / **1g** poly )
**176mg** cholesterol **687g** sodium
**30g** carbohydrate **4g** fiber **35g** protein

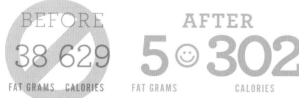

BEFORE
38 629
FAT GRAMS   CALORIES

AFTER
5 ☺ 302
FAT GRAMS        CALORIES

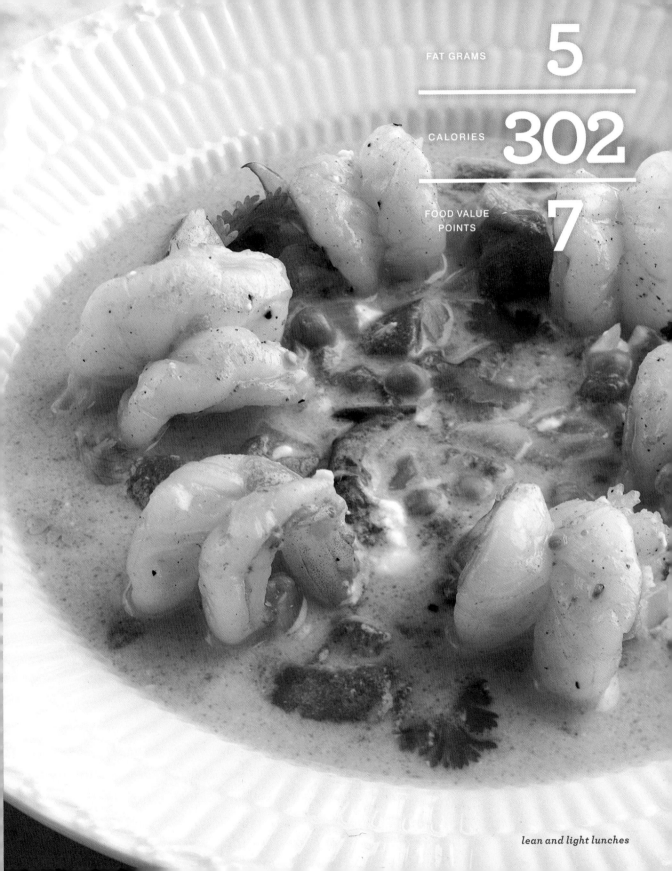

*lean and light lunches*

# Faux-Fried Filet o' Fish Sandwich

SERVES 4

**DID YOU KNOW** that just one fast-food fish sandwich might furnish all the calories an adult needs in a single day? I suppose you could eat one fish sandwich and nothing else each day, and drop some pounds. But that would get pretty boring. I have a better idea: Try my version. It has two-thirds fewer calories and practically none of the fat.

## INGREDIENTS

½    cup whole wheat flour

1½   cups whole wheat panko bread crumbs, such as Ian's All-Natural

2    large egg whites

8    ounces cod fillet, cut on the bias into 4 equal pieces

     Salt

     Freshly ground black pepper

     Nonstick cooking spray

½    cup fat-free mayonnaise

1    tablespoon no-sugar-added sweet relish, such as Mt. Olive

4    whole wheat hamburger buns

4    leaves romaine lettuce, shredded

4    slices (about ½ ounce each) cheddar cheese

4    slices vine-ripened tomato

## METHOD

1 Preheat the oven to 450°F. Place a wire rack on a foil-lined baking sheet, and set it aside.

2 Put the flour in a shallow dish. Put the panko in another shallow dish. In a medium bowl, whip the egg whites with a whisk until they are extremely foamy but not quite holding peaks.

3 Season the fish with salt and pepper to taste. Working in batches, dredge the fish in the flour, shaking off any excess. Add the fish to the egg whites and toss to coat completely. Add the fish, a few pieces at a time, to the bowl of panko, and coat completely.

4 Spread the fish out on the wire rack, and spray it lightly with cooking spray. Bake the fish until the breading is golden and crispy and the fish is cooked through, about 10 to 14 minutes.

5 Meanwhile, in a small bowl, add the mayonnaise and relish. Stir till combined.

6 Toast the hamburger buns in the toaster oven.

7 To assemble the sandwiches, spread the tartar sauce on the bottom buns. Layer shredded lettuce on top of the sauce and then top with the fish. Continue to layer with the cheese and tomato slices. Finally, complete the sandwich with the top bun. Serve immediately.

PER SERVING

**313** calories **8g** fat ( **3.6g** sat / **2.5g** mono / **1.3g** poly )
**39mg** cholesterol **628g** sodium
**42g** carbohydrate **6g** fiber **20g** protein

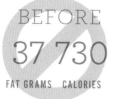

BEFORE
37 730
FAT GRAMS   CALORIES

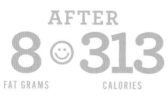

AFTER
8 ☺ 313
FAT GRAMS   CALORIES

**✱ CALORIE SAVER**

Omit the cheese and save **70** calories per serving.

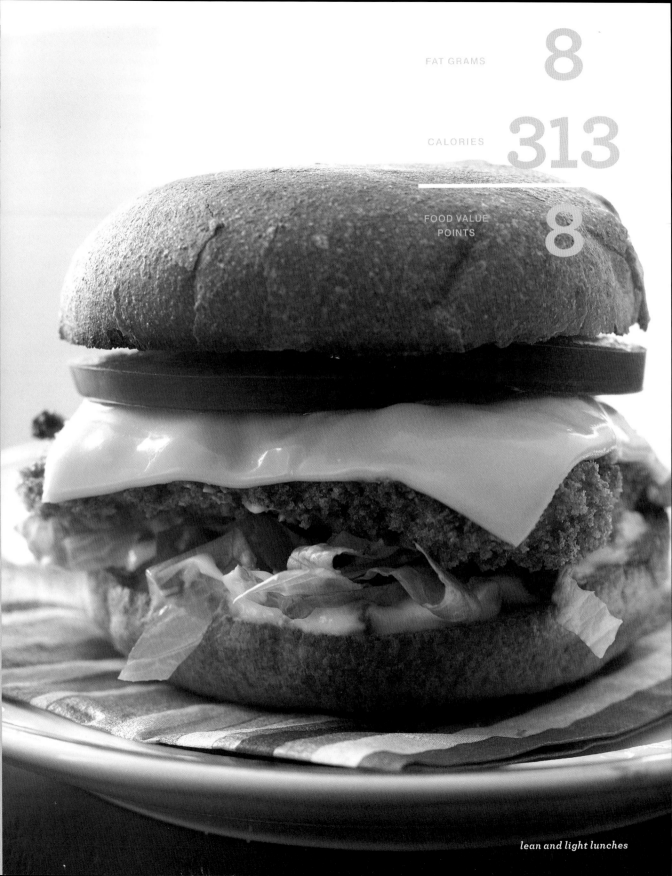

FAT GRAMS **8**

CALORIES **313**

FOOD VALUE
POINTS **8**

*lean and light lunches*

# Individual Crispy "Loaded" Pizza

SERVES 6

**PIZZA IS A UNIVERSAL** crowd-pleaser, and part of its charm is the doughy bed it rests on, along with gooey, wonderful cheese. You'll get no argument from me. I love pizza. But not all pizzas are created equally. This pizza is loaded with cheese, mushrooms, sausage, and peperoncini, but not calories. So for watching your weight, this pizza is a delicious solution. It's meaty, yet amazingly low in fat. You'll love the crust's wholesome taste.

## INGREDIENTS

¾ cup warm (110°F) water

½ teaspoon molasses

1½ teaspoons active dry yeast

½ teaspoon salt

1¾ cups whole wheat flour, plus additional for rolling and kneading

Nonstick olive oil spray

1 tablespoon cornmeal

¾ cup low-fat store-bought marinara sauce, such as Trader Joe's

½ cup torn fresh basil leaves

6 medium (about 4 ounces) cremini mushrooms, thinly sliced (about 2 cups)

8 ounces low-fat turkey sausage, such as Butterball, crumbled and cooked (about 1⅓ cups)

6 whole bottled peperoncini, such as BandG, stems removed and cut into ¼-inch slices

1½ cups shredded reduced-fat mozzarella cheese, such as Weight Watchers

2 tablespoons grated Parmigiano-Reggiano

## METHOD

1 Stir the water and molasses together in a large bowl until the molasses is dissolved. Sprinkle the yeast over the water, and let stand in a warm place until foamy, about 10 minutes.

2 Stir the salt into the yeast mixture; then stir in the 1¾ cups flour until the dough starts to come together. Scrape this rough dough out onto a work surface that has been sprinkled lightly with flour. Knead the dough until it becomes smooth and pulls back when you stretch it, about 5 minutes. If necessary, add just enough flour as you knead to keep the dough from sticking to your hands and the work surface. Make a neat round out of the dough and place it in a large bowl that has been sprayed with the olive oil spray. Cover the bowl loosely with a clean kitchen towel. Let the dough sit in a warm place until it has doubled in size, about 1 hour.

3 Turn the dough out onto a lightly floured surface. Divide it into 6 equal wedges. Form each wedge into a tight ball by rolling it in the palm of your hand until the edges have rounded. Spray a baking sheet with olive oil spray. Arrange the dough balls a few inches apart on the prepared baking sheet. Cover them with plastic wrap and let rise in a warm place until doubled, about 45 minutes.

4 With a rack in the center position, preheat the oven to 500°F or its highest setting. (Remove any other racks or position them below the center rack. This will make it easier to slide the pizzas onto the stone and remove them once they're cooked.) Place a pizza stone on the rack and let it heat for 20 minutes.

BEFORE
42 610
FAT GRAMS CALORIES

AFTER
10 ☺ 316
FAT GRAMS CALORIES

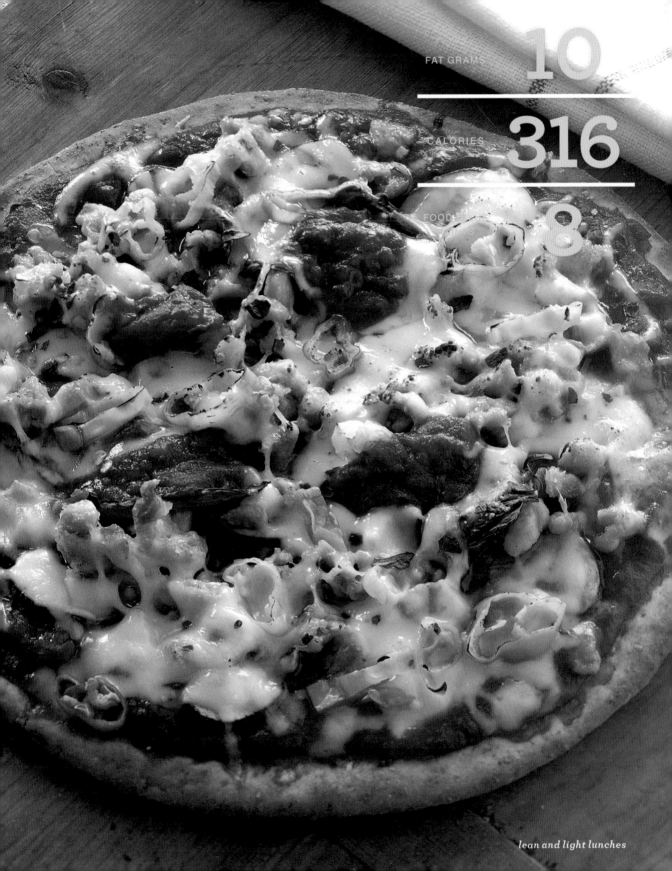

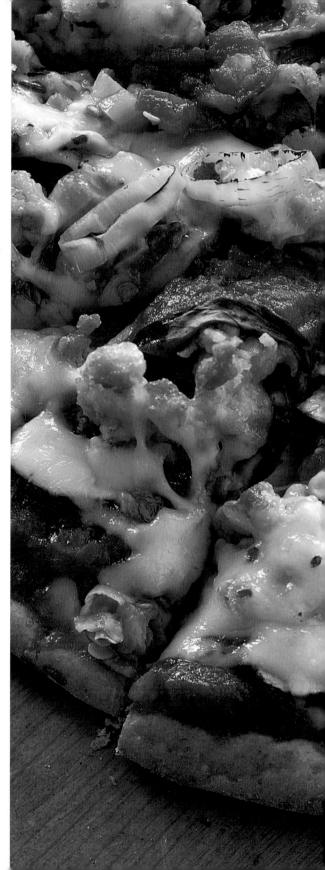

## METHOD

5   Dust a wooden pizza peel with the cornmeal. If you don't have a pizza peel, dust a cookie sheet (flat—no rims) with cornmeal. Lightly flour the work surface and roll one ball of the dough out with a rolling pin until it will not stretch any further. Drape the circle of dough over both of your fists so the edges of the dough barely overhang your knuckles, and gently pull the edges outward while rotating the crust. Keep stretching and rotating the dough gently until the dough is about 9 inches in diameter. Don't worry about a few small tears; they can be repaired once the dough is on the peel. Place the dough on the prepared peel. Prick the dough in about 8 places with a fork. Pinch together any little tears.

6   Slide the dough onto the hot pizza stone in the oven, and bake until the dough is puffed and the underside is lightly browned, 2 to 3 minutes. Remove the dough and flip it bottom (browned) side up on your work surface. Repeat with the remaining balls of dough. When you've had some practice, you should be able to roll out and stretch one piece of dough while another is baking on the stone.

7   Spread about 2 tablespoons of the marinara sauce onto each crust, leaving a ½-inch border. Scatter the basil over the sauce. Scatter the mushrooms, cooked sausage, and peperoncini evenly over the sauce. Mix the cheeses together in a bowl, and sprinkle ¼ cup of the mixture over each pizza. One at a time, slide the pizzas back onto the pizza stone. Bake until the cheese is golden brown and bubbling and the crust is brown and crispy, 3 to 4 minutes. If your pizza stone is large enough, you may be able to bake the topped pizzas two at a time.

8   Cut the pizzas into wedges, if desired, and serve.

PER SERVING
**316**calories **10g**fat ( **3g**sat / **0g**mono / **0g**poly )
**35mg**cholesterol **1013g**sodium
**36g**carbohydrate **6g**fiber **21g**protein

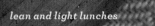
lean and light lunches

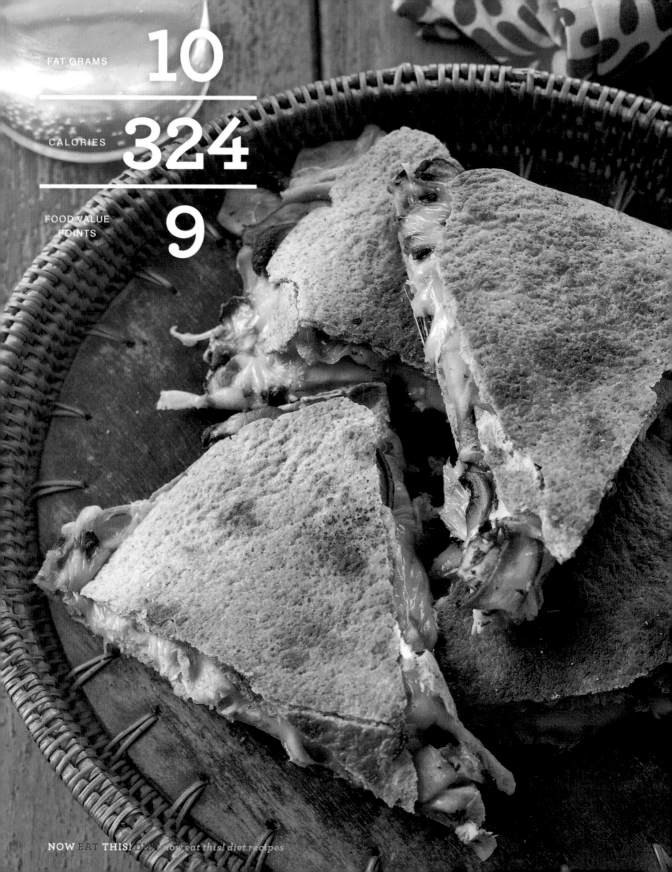

FAT GRAMS

**10**

CALORIES

**324**

FOOD VALUE
POINTS

**9**

# Chicken and Mushroom Quesadilla

**QUESADILLAS** are the grilled cheese sandwich's Mexican cousin. Made with tortillas, they're thin and crispy on the outside, with smooth melted cheese on the inside, and can be adapted to a variety of fillings and flavors. Mine uses chicken, but feel free to try whatever meats or fillings you like. The glory of quesadillas is that anything can go in them. No need to dip these wedges into salsa, because it's already in the quesadilla! Not only does it add flavor, but it makes the filling juicy. Serve them as appetizers for parties, and you'll hit a home run. No one knows who invented quesadillas—maybe cartoon hero Slowpoke Rodriguez; he seemed to know how to enjoy life.

## INGREDIENTS

Nonstick cooking spray

1 pound sliced white button mushrooms

Salt

Freshly ground black pepper

2 tablespoons finely chopped shallots

2 tablespoons chopped fresh flat-leaf parsley

4 (9-inch) low-carb tortillas, such as La Tortilla Factory

6 ounces (about 1½ cups) shredded 75% reduced-fat cheddar, such as Cabot

7 ounces (about 2 cups) shredded skinless breast meat from a rotisserie or roast chicken

1 cup jarred tomatillo salsa

PER SERVING
**324** calories **10g** fat ( **3.5g** sat / **3.3g** mono / **1.5g** poly )
**64mg** cholesterol **1237g** sodium
**29g** carbohydrate **13g** fiber **44g** protein

## METHOD

1 Heat a large nonstick sauté pan over medium heat. When hot, remove it from the stove just while you coat it with cooking spray. Add mushrooms and season with salt and pepper to taste. (You might have to cook in batches.) Cook the mushrooms until they are tender, about 6 to 8 minutes. If they appear too dry, add 1 or 2 tablespoons of water. Add the shallots and cook for 1 minute. When they are just about done, stir in the parsley. Set aside.

2 Heat 2 large nonstick sauté pans over medium heat.

3 Lay 2 tortillas on a work surface. Divide the cheddar cheese between the 2 tortillas. Scatter the chicken over the cheese and spoon the salsa over both tortillas. Divide the mushrooms between the tortillas. Season the toppings with salt and pepper to taste. Top each with another tortilla.

4 When the pans are hot, hold them away from the stove and spray them generously with cooking spray. Carefully place 1 quesadilla in each of the pans. Cook until the tortillas are golden and crispy, about 4 minutes.

5 Carefully flip the quesadillas, using a plate if necessary, and continue to cook until the bottom tortillas are golden brown and crispy and the filling is hot throughout, about 4 minutes.

6 Transfer the quesadillas to a cutting board. Cut into wedges and serve immediately.

BEFORE
70 1089
FAT GRAMS   CALORIES

AFTER
10 ☺ 324
FAT GRAMS   CALORIES

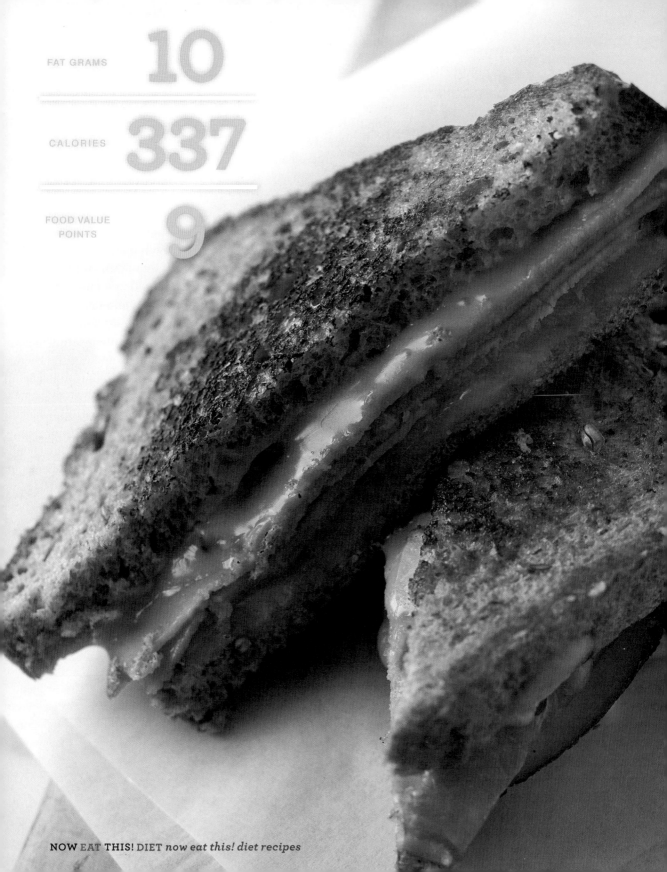

FAT GRAMS **10**

CALORIES **337**

FOOD VALUE
POINTS **9**

# Grilled Cheese and Ham

**EVER WANT TO CRAWL** into a dark corner with some comfort food? Sure, something like a gooey grilled cheese seems like the perfect antidote to a bad funk. But this fat-laden favorite can do serious diet damage. Here's a way to get the comfort you need, without padding your thighs. My Grilled Cheese and Ham is distinguished by its perfect, buttery crispness and the yummy cheese melting inside. ✱TIP: Another way to brown each side of the sandwiches is to just toast in a toaster oven. And, when buying whole wheat bread, check the ingredient list on the bag before selecting to make sure it's 100 percent whole wheat.

## INGREDIENTS

8    pieces thin-sliced European whole-grain bread, such as Rubschlager

4    ounces shredded 75% reduced-fat cheddar, such as Cabot

8    slices (about 6 ounces) high-quality deli ham

4    slices 2% reduced-fat-milk cheese, such as Borden's 2% Milk Reduced-Fat Sharp Singles

2    tablespoons Dijon mustard

    Butter-flavored nonstick cooking spray

PER SERVING
**337**calories **10g**fat ( **3.9g**sat / **0.6g**mono / **0g**poly )
**47mg**cholesterol **1415mg**sodium
**39g**carbohydrate **4g**fiber **26g**protein

## METHOD

1  Preheat the oven to 350°F. Heat 2 nonstick sauté pans over medium-low heat.

2  Meanwhile, assemble the sandwiches: Lay 4 slices of bread on a work surface. Divide the shredded cheddar among the 4 pieces of bread. Lay 2 slices of ham on top of the cheese. Place the cheese slices on top of the ham. Spread the mustard on each of the remaining 4 slices of bread. Place the bread slices, mustard side down, on top of the cheese.

3  Away from the stove, spray the sauté pans with cooking spray. Spray both sides of the sandwiches with cooking spray, and place 2 sandwiches in each pan. Brown each side of the sandwiches, about 3 minutes per side. Transfer the sandwiches to a baking sheet, and bake until they are warmed through, about 5 minutes. Cut each sandwich in half, and serve.

✱ CALORIE SAVER
Omit the shredded cheese (keep the slices) and and save **60** calories per serving.

BEFORE
30 680
FAT GRAMS   CALORIES

AFTER
10 ☺ 337
FAT GRAMS   CALORIES

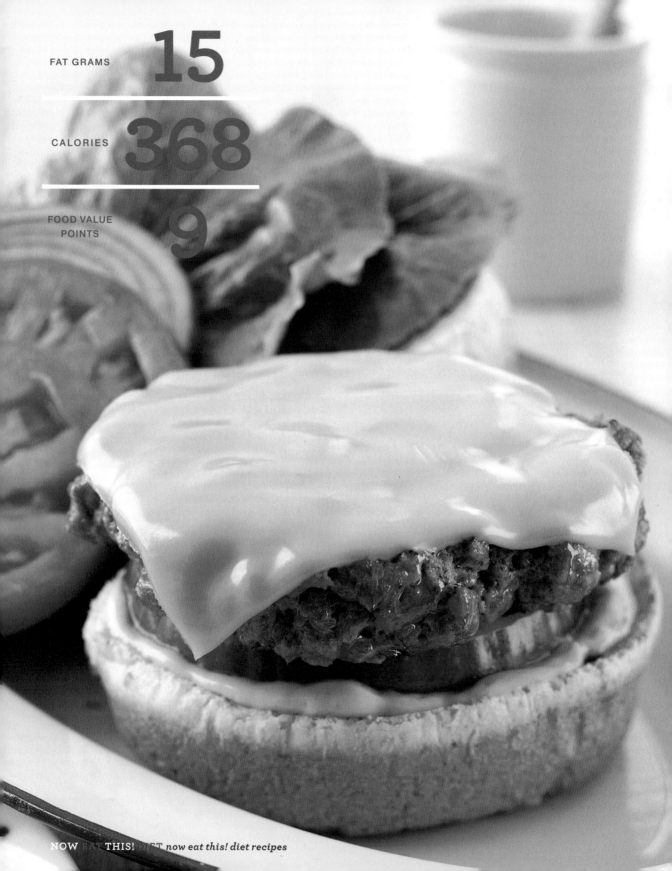

FAT GRAMS **15**

CALORIES **368**

FOOD VALUE
POINTS **9**

# Yes, a Cheeseburger!

SERVES 4

**WHILE WORKING ON THIS BOOK,** the thought kept running through my mind: "A cheeseburger sure sounds good right about now." Thankfully, for my health's sake, that wasn't the only thing rattling around my brain. I had to think about how to create a healthy cheeseburger. I know that sounds like the ultimate contradiction—"healthy" and "cheeseburger"—but I think I got it: This one is fewer than half the calories of a typical one you'd get at a restaurant. I even made my own "special" sauce to go with the burgers by blending fat-free mayonnaise, sugar-free relish, and reduced-sugar ketchup.

## INGREDIENTS

4   whole wheat hamburger buns

    Nonstick cooking spray

16  ounces 90% lean ground beef, formed into 4 patties

    Salt

    Freshly ground black pepper

4   slices 2% reduced-fat-milk cheese, such as Borden's 2% Milk Reduced-Fat Sharp Singles

⅓   cup fat-free mayonnaise

2   tablespoons no-sugar-added sweet relish, such as Mt. Olive

1   tablespoon reduced-sugar ketchup, such as Heinz

4   leaves romaine lettuce, broken in half

4   slices tomato

4   slices red onion

## METHOD

1   Preheat a grill pan over high heat.

2   Split the buns in half, and spray the split surfaces lightly with cooking spray. Place the buns, cut side down, on the grill. Allow the buns to char slightly, and then transfer them to a platter.

3   Hold the grill pan away from the stove while you coat the surface with cooking spray. Season the burger patties with salt and pepper to taste. Place the burger patties on the grill, and cook for about 2½ minutes per side for rare. During the last minute, put 1 slice of cheese on each burger.

4   In small bowl, mix together the mayonnaise, sweet relish, and ketchup. Set aside.

5   To assemble the burgers, place the burgers on top of the bottom buns. Pile lettuce, tomato, red onion, and Russian dressing on top of each burger, and set the bun tops in place. Serve.

PER SERVING
**368** calories **15g** fat ( **6g** sat / **4.8g** mono / **1.3g** poly )
**81mg** cholesterol **795mg** sodium
**30g** carbohydrate **4g** fiber **29g** protein

## ✱ CALORIE SAVER

Omit the cheese and save **50** calories per serving, or omit the Russian dressing and save **28** calories per serving.

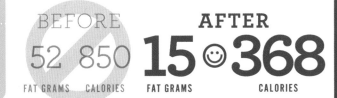

BEFORE
52 850
FAT GRAMS   CALORIES

AFTER
15 ☺ 368
FAT GRAMS   CALORIES

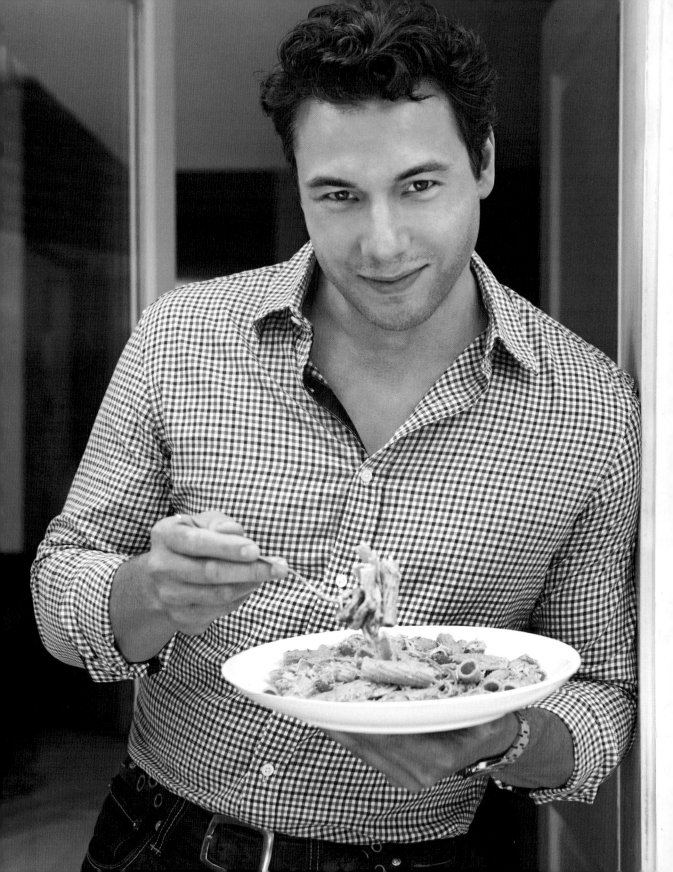

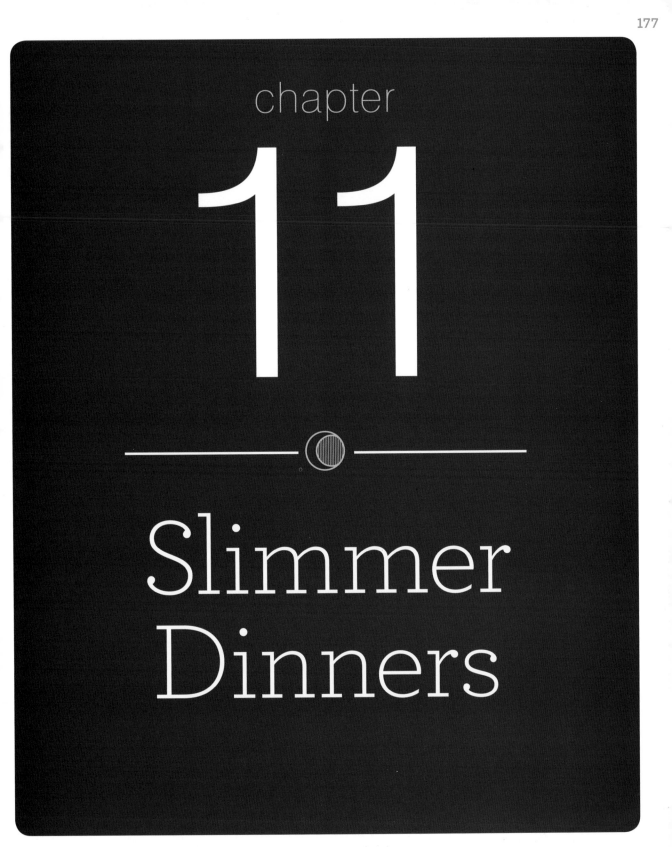

chapter

# 11

# Slimmer
# Dinners

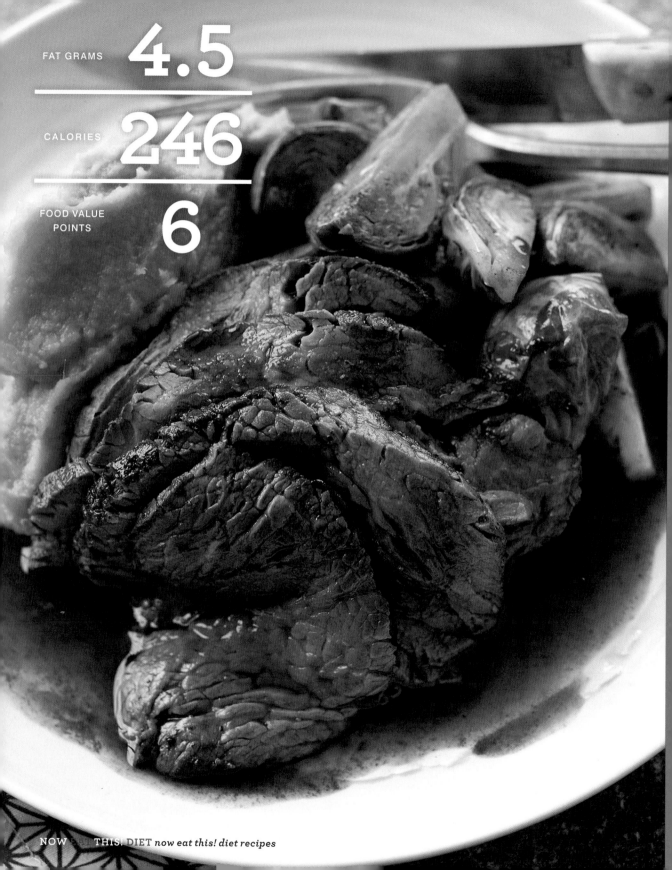

FAT GRAMS **4.5**

CALORIES **246**

FOOD VALUE
POINTS **6**

# Roast Beef with Brussels Sprouts and Balsamic Jus

SERVES 4

**HERE'S A WONDERFUL WAY TO ENJOY ROAST BEEF**—with Brussels sprouts. For some reason, many people think they hate Brussels sprouts. That's a shame, but I think I know why. Most people parboil them. This makes them smell like rotten cabbage, and they disintegrate in the mouth like a soggy mess. Try my way of preparing them: roasting. It brings out their sweetness and crunch. Balsamic vinegar is a great go-to sauce starter. At about 10 calories per tablespoon, it's the perfect sweet and sour addition to most dishes.

## INGREDIENTS

| | |
|---|---|
| 1 | (1-pound) piece lean beef tenderloin, trimmed of all visible fat |
| | Salt |
| | Freshly ground black pepper |
| | Nonstick cooking spray |
| 2 | medium sweet potatoes |
| ½ | cup evaporated skim milk |
| 1 | tablespoon agave nectar |
| 2 | cups Brussels sprouts, trimmed and sliced into quarters |
| ¼ | cup balsamic vinegar |

PER SERVING
**246**calories **4.5g**fat ( **1.6g**sat / **1.6g**mono / **0g**poly )
**61mg**cholesterol **127mg**sodium
**26g**carbohydrate **3.5g**fiber **27g**protein

## METHOD

1. Preheat the oven to 450°F. Place a wire rack on a baking sheet lined with foil, and set it aside.

2. Heat a large cast-iron pan over high heat. Season the meat with salt and pepper to taste. When the pan is hot, remove it from the stove while you coat it with the cooking spray. Add the meat to the pan and sear all the sides, about 2 minutes per side. Transfer the tenderloin to the wire rack on the baking sheet and continue to cook in the oven for 8 to 10 minutes or until the internal temperature reaches 125°F for medium-rare. Remove the baking sheet from the oven, and tent the meat with foil to keep it warm. Let the meat rest for at least 10 minutes before slicing.

3. Microwave the sweet potatoes covered with plastic wrap on high for 7 to 8 minutes, until tender, turning them halfway through. Remove the skin of the potatoes and then mash the flesh with a potato masher in a medium bowl. Combine the mash with the evaporated milk and agave nectar. Season with salt and pepper to taste. Cover with foil to keep warm. Set aside.

4. Heat the same cast-iron pan over medium-high heat. When hot, remove it from the stove just while you coat it with the cooking spray. Add the Brussels sprouts and cook till just browned, about 8 minutes, stirring occasionally. Deglaze the pan with the balsamic vinegar, making sure to scrape the flavorful bits off the bottom of the pan. Cover and continue to cook the Brussels sprouts till they are tender, adding a few tablespoons of water if they begin to look dry.

5. Cut the meat into thin slices, and serve with the sweet potatoes and Brussels sprouts. Spoon the balsamic jus over the meat.

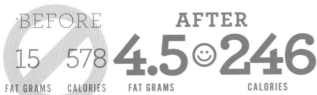

BEFORE
15 578
FAT GRAMS   CALORIES

AFTER
4.5 ☺ 246
FAT GRAMS   CALORIES

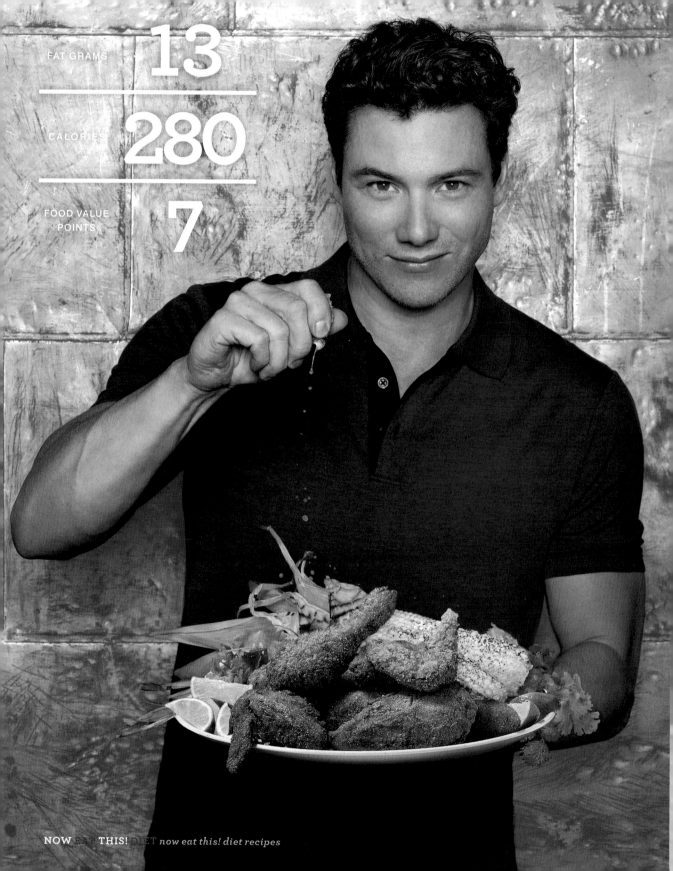

# Flash-Fried Chicken "Carnitas"

**CARNITAS ARE CHUNKS OF PORK** that are first simmered in a flavorful broth and then fried in their own rendered fat until crispy. Needless to say, they are loaded with fat and calories. To keep the flavor level high and the calorie and fat count low, I used chicken simmered in broth, a well-seasoned cornmeal coating, and a method for flash frying that I developed. The buttermilk stands in for Mexican crema and has about 10 percent of the fat and calories of its Mexican counterpart.

Simmering is a slow cooking method that works best at 160°F—use a thermometer.

## INGREDIENTS

For the *carnitas:*

3 cups low-fat, low-sodium chicken broth

4 pieces of chicken (skinless, boneless chicken breasts with wings attached, thighs, and drumsticks; about 1 pound total)

2 quarts grapeseed oil or corn oil

¾ cup fine-ground yellow cornmeal

¾ cup whole wheat flour

3 tablespoons adobo powder, Goya or similar

Salt

Freshly ground black pepper

2 cups low-fat buttermilk

## INGREDIENTS

For the salad:

½ medium Hass avocado, peeled and sliced paper thin

4 cups shredded iceberg lettuce

2 ripe roma tomatoes, halved and thinly sliced

1 small red onion, halved lengthwise and thinly sliced

Salt

Freshly ground black pepper

2 tablespoons lime juice

1 bunch cilantro

8 lime wedges

PER SERVING
**280**calories **13g**fat ( **2g**sat / **4g**mono / **6g**poly )
**75mg**cholesterol **747mg**sodium
**13g**carbohydrate **3g**fiber **27g**protein

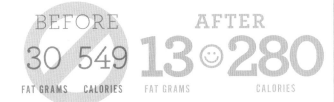

BEFORE
30 549
FAT GRAMS CALORIES

AFTER
13 ☺ 280
FAT GRAMS CALORIES

## Oil is flammable.

Follow these tips to be safe when deep-fat frying:

1. Have a fire extinguisher handy.
2. Never cover the pot while heating oil.
3. Always use a thermometer, 400°F is the max temp needed.
4. Water + hot oil = IED (improvised explosive device); keep water away from hot oil.
5. Use longs tongs or a fry basket; do not put fingers inside the pot for any reason.

## METHOD

1 Heat the chicken broth to simmering (160°F) in a large saucepan over high heat, seasoning it generously with salt. Add the chicken to the pan, and return the broth to a simmer (160°F). Cover the pan and reduce the heat to low. Cook until the chicken is tender when you poke it with a fork and no longer pink, about 30 minutes. Remove the chicken from the broth, pat it dry, and set it aside on a platter. Cover the platter with foil to keep the chicken warm. Reserve the stock for another use.

2 Pour the grapeseed oil into a large pot with high sides. (There should be at least 2 inches of oil in the pot.) Clip a deep-frying thermometer to the side of the pot and be sure the point of the thermometer is not touching the bottom of the pot. Heat the oil to 400°F over medium heat.

3 Set a wire rack in a rimmed baking sheet or over several layers of paper towels (for draining the chicken). In a shallow dish, whisk together the cornmeal, flour, adobo, 2 teaspoons salt, and black pepper until thoroughly combined.

4 Prepare the salad: In a medium bowl, toss the avocado, lettuce, tomato, and red onion and season with salt and pepper and lime juice. Divide the salad among 4 serving plates.

5 Pour the buttermilk into a bowl. Cut the chicken into 1½-inch pieces and add them to the buttermilk. Turn the chicken pieces gently in the buttermilk, coating them completely. Lift the chicken pieces from the buttermilk one at a time with a fork, and let any excess buttermilk drip back into the bowl. Add a few pieces of coated chicken to the cornmeal mix and coat them completely in the mix. Bounce the coated chicken gently in your palm to shake off any excess flour. Put the coated chicken on the baking sheet, and repeat this step with the remaining chicken. Sift any remaining coating mix to remove bits of chicken or buttermilk and store it covered in a cool place for up to a few weeks.

6 Fry the chicken, 6 to 8 pieces at a time, in the hot oil until deep golden brown, 30 seconds to 1 minute. Drain on the wire rack, and serve immediately on top of or alongside the salad. Serve with cilantro and lime wedges. (Let the oil cool completely, and then strain it through a very fine sieve. It will keep in the refrigerator for a few weeks and can be used 2 to 3 more times before discarding.)

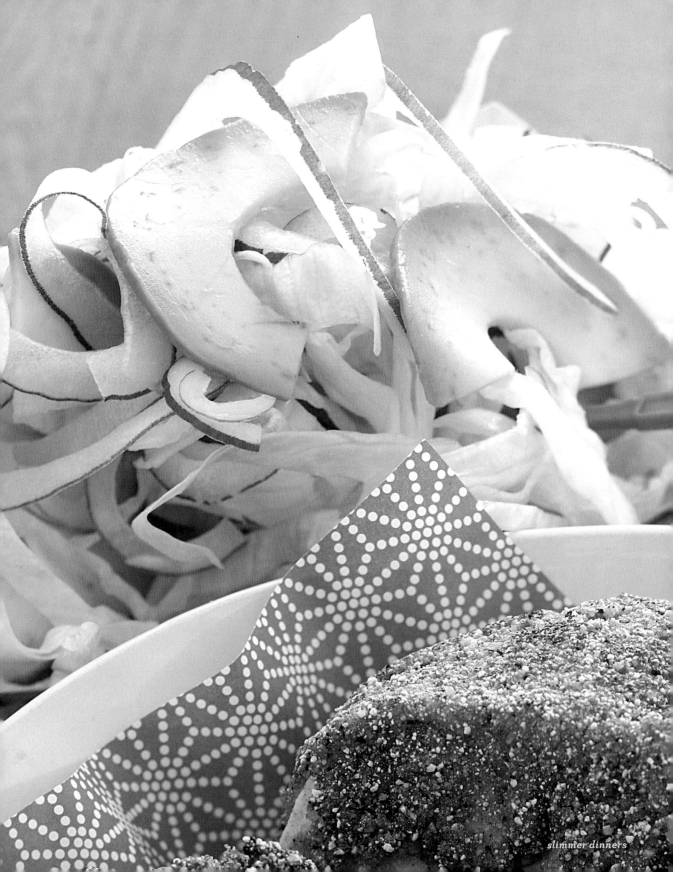

*slimmer dinners*

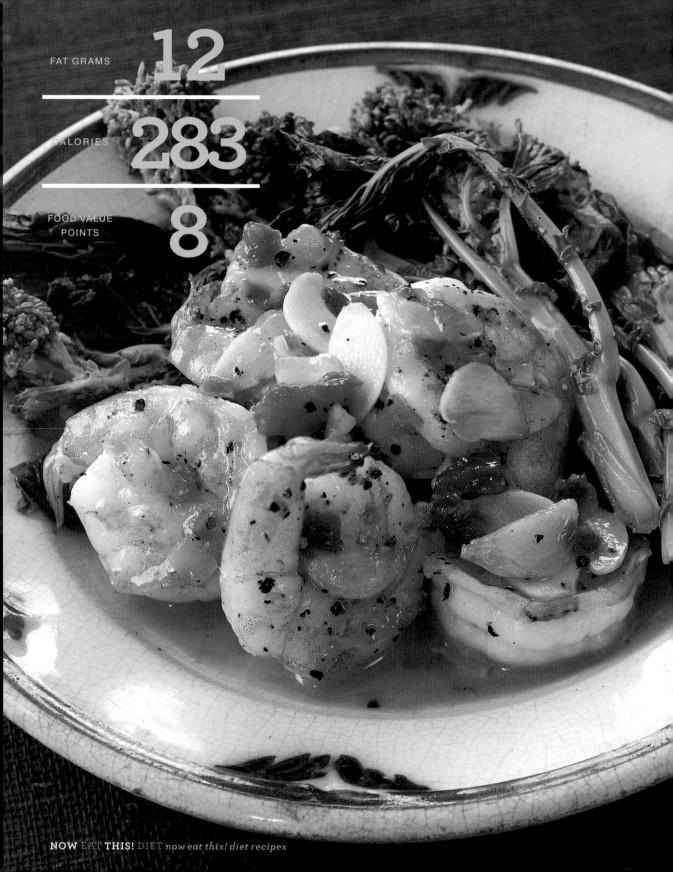

FAT GRAMS

# 12

CALORIES

# 283

FOOD VALUE
POINTS

# 8

# Lemon Pepper Shrimp

SERVES 4

**THIS AMAZING SHRIMP DISH FEATURES BROCCOLI RABE.** First question: What is broccoli rabe and why should you care? Broccoli rabe does everything for you but your laundry. It's inexpensive, quick and easy to prepare, and very delicious. As a matter of fact, it's so surprisingly useful it should be appointed to a cabinet position in the White House. It's loaded with protein, calcium, potassium, iron, and vitamins A, C, and K. So if you ever get stranded on a desert island, I hope broccoli rabe grows there. This veggie isn't broccoli, even though it looks like tiny clusters of broccoli florets. It's a closer relative to turnips. It can be bitter, so we need to serve it with sweetened foods and brown it to make it as sweetly balanced as possible.

Next question: Who played Chandler's father on *Friends*? Just kidding; you'll love this light, scrumptious, low-carb meal.

## INGREDIENTS

1    pound large shrimp, peeled and deveined, tails removed

     Salt

2    teaspoons coarsely ground black pepper

2    tablespoons extra-virgin olive oil

¼    cup fresh lemon juice

¼    cup hot pepper jelly, such as Stonewall Kitchen

1    tablespoon unsalted butter

2    cloves garlic, thinly sliced

1    bunch broccoli rabe

## PER SERVING

**283** calories **12g** fat ( **3g** sat / **6g** mono / **1.6g** poly )
**180mg** cholesterol **207g** sodium
**18g** carbohydrate **0g** fiber **27g** protein

## METHOD

1   Heat a large nonstick sauté pan over medium-high heat.

2   Meanwhile, blot the shrimp with paper towels to ensure that they are dry. Season one side of the shrimp with salt to taste. Sprinkle 1 teaspoon of the pepper onto one side of the shrimp and lightly press so that the pepper adheres. Repeat on the other side with the remaining pepper. Add 1 tablespoon of the olive oil to the pan, and then add the shrimp, salted side down. After about 2 minutes season the other side with salt and turn the shrimp over. Cook the shrimp till done, about 2½ minutes each side. Transfer the shrimp to a plate and set aside.

3   Turn off the heat, and while the pan is still hot, add the lemon juice, pepper jelly, and butter. Stir until well mixed. Toss the shrimp back into the pan and coat in the sauce. Set aside.

4   Heat another large nonstick sauté pan over medium-high heat. Add the remaining oil and garlic. Sauté until the garlic begins to brown, about 2 minutes. Add the broccoli rabe and cook until tender, about 5 minutes. Season with salt and pepper to taste.

5   Serve the shrimp with the broccoli rabe.

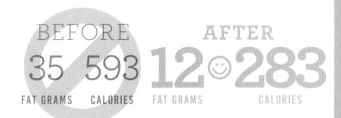

BEFORE
**35** FAT GRAMS   **593** CALORIES

AFTER
**12** FAT GRAMS ☺ **283** CALORIES

# Ginger Sweet Chicken and Broccoli Stir-Fry

SERVES 6

**THERE WAS A CHINESE TAKEOUT PLACE** in the Queens neighborhood where I grew up. The owner was a vision of beauty, and the food was delicious. My family and I went there all the time and feasted on heaps of food, pork-fried rice, wonton soup, shrimp with lobster sauce—all for about $10. To this day, I love Chinese food. Employees at my neighborhood Chinese restaurant know my first, last, and middle name. So in any interaction between myself and Chinese food, I have to exercise a bit of self-control. One way I do that is by cooking light stir-fry dishes at home, like this one. The chicken and broccoli are not coated in loads of sugar and sodium, and you can taste the subtle flavor of ginger in here. Here's some trivia you can impress your friends with: There are more than forty thousand Chinese restaurants in the United States alone, more than the number of McDonald's, Burger Kings, and KFCs combined.

## INGREDIENTS

4    cups fresh broccoli florets

¼    cup water

2    teaspoons canola oil

1    pound skinless, boneless chicken breast, cut into medium-size chunks

     Salt

     Freshly ground black pepper

     1-inch knob of fresh ginger, cut into disks and smashed with the side of a large chef's knife

¼    cup sugar-free apricot preserves, such as Smucker's

¼    cup low-sodium soy sauce

2    tablespoons chopped fresh cilantro

½    teaspoon garlic-chili sauce, such as Huy Fong

2    cups cooked brown rice

## METHOD

1   Place the broccoli in a microwave-safe dish. Add the water and cover with a microwave-safe plate or plastic wrap. Microwave on high for 3 to 4 minutes or until the florets are tender. Set aside.

2   Meanwhile, heat a large nonstick sauté pan over medium-high heat. When hot, add 1 teaspoon canola oil and the chicken. Season with salt and pepper to taste. Cook the chicken until both sides are browned, about 2 minutes for each side. Move the chicken to the perimeter of the pan, and then add the remaining oil to the center. Add the ginger to the oil and sauté until fragrant, about 1 minute. Add the apricot preserves and the soy sauce. Stir together and bring to a simmer.

3   Drain the broccoli and add to the pan. Toss together, and then add the cilantro and garlic-chili sauce.

4   Serve immediately with brown rice.

PER SERVING
**298** calories **6g** fat ( **1g** sat / **2.7g** mono / **1.6g** poly )
**73mg** cholesterol **702mg** sodium
**33g** carbohydrate **4g** fiber **30g** protein

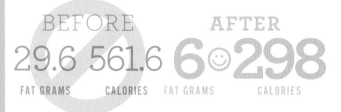

BEFORE
29.6  561.6
FAT GRAMS  CALORIES

AFTER
6 ☺ 298
FAT GRAMS  CALORIES

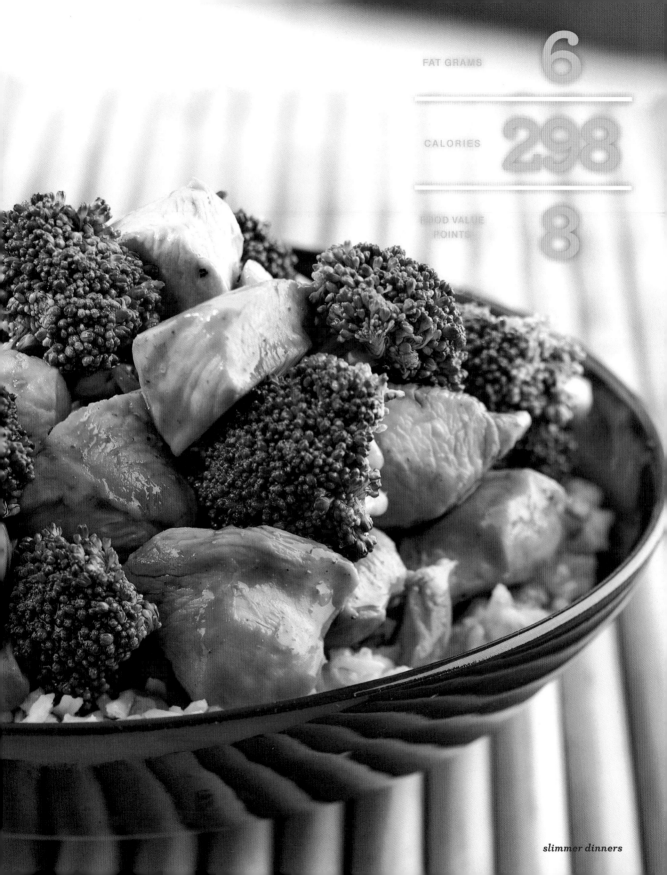

FAT GRAMS 6

CALORIES 298

FOOD VALUE POINTS 8

*slimmer dinners*

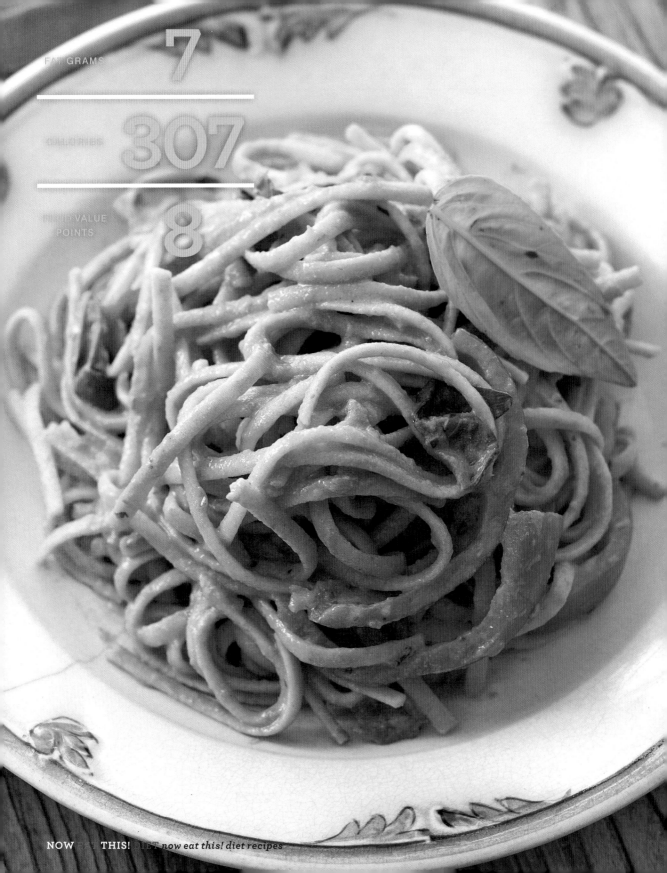

# Spicy-Sweet Linguine alla Vodka

SERVES 4

**THE SPICE COMES FROM PEPPER SAUCE,** the sweet from roasted red pepper, and the creaminess from yogurt and Parmigiano-Reggiano. Look for roasted peppers that say "fire-roasted" on the label. They will have a nicer flavor. You'll quickly notice that there is no vodka in this recipe, and that's intentional. It doesn't add much except for empty calories, and who wants to waste a great cocktail in a dish of pasta?

## INGREDIENTS

| | |
|---|---|
| 8 | ounces whole wheat linguine |
| 1½ | cups store-bought low-fat marinara sauce |
| 1 | large bottle fire-roasted red peppers (about 4 ounces) cut into thin strips (about ¾ cup) |
| ¼ | cup 2% Greek yogurt, such as Fage Total |
| 1 | cup chopped fresh basil |
| 1 to 1½ | teaspoons hot pepper sauce |
| | Salt |
| | Freshly ground black pepper |
| 6 | tablespoons grated Parmigiano-Reggiano cheese |

PER SERVING
**307** calories **7g** fat ( **2g** sat / **1g** mono / **0.5g** poly )
**8mg** cholesterol **772mg** sodium
**52g** carbohydrate **8g** fiber **14g** protein

## METHOD

1 Bring a large pot of lightly salted water to a boil. Add the pasta and cook according to the package directions, about 9 minutes.

2 Meanwhile, bring the marinara sauce and sliced peppers to a simmer in a large nonstick sauté pan over medium heat. Cook the sauce, stirring it occasionally with a heat-resistant rubber spatula, until it is slightly thickened, about 5 minutes. Remove the sauce from the heat.

3 Put the yogurt in a small bowl. Stir about ½ cup of the warmed sauce into the yogurt until smooth (this tempers it and prevents the yogurt from curdling). Then whisk the yogurt mixture into the marinara sauce. Keep the sauce off the heat, and cover the pan to keep the sauce warm.

4 Drain the linguine in a colander. Slide it into a large serving bowl, and add the sauce, basil, and 1 teaspoon of the hot pepper sauce. Toss gently until the linguine is evenly coated with sauce. Season with salt and pepper to taste and, if you like, the remaining ½ teaspoon hot pepper sauce. Sprinkle the cheese on top, and serve.

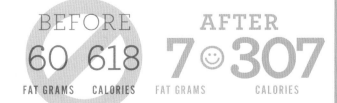

BEFORE
60 618
FAT GRAMS   CALORIES

AFTER
7 ☺ 307
FAT GRAMS   CALORIES

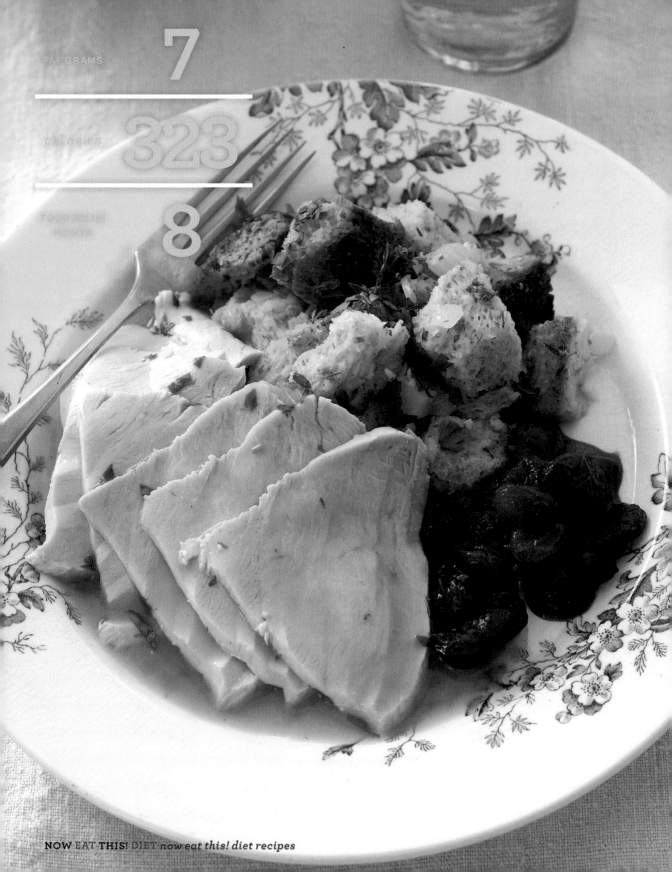

# Turkey Dinner with All the Trimmings

SERVES 4

**AT CHRISTMAS,** don't be one of those greedy people who asks for a 50-inch plasma TV or a 2-carat diamond. Instead, how about a holiday meal that doesn't make you gain a pound per forkful? Here it is: my version of roast turkey dinner. This meal takes less than an hour to make, a fraction less than typical turkey dinners. Poaching the turkey keeps the turkey moist without any added fat. Plus, the poaching liquid is used for the stuffing and to make the gravy.

One more thing: Let's remind ourselves that holidays aren't a celebration of the perfect turkey or the smoothest mashed potatoes. It's the time to think about family and togetherness. And football.

## INGREDIENTS

| | |
|---|---|
| 4 | cups low-fat, low-sodium chicken broth |
| 1 | pound fresh or completely thawed boneless, skinless turkey breast, trimmed of all visible fat |
| 1 | tablespoon extra-virgin olive oil |
| ¼ | cup chopped onions |
| ¼ | cup chopped celery |
| | Salt |
| | Freshly ground black pepper |
| 1½ | teaspoons poultry seasoning, such as Spice Hunter |
| 4 | ounces cubed stale 100% whole wheat bread |
| 1 | tablespoon chopped fresh flat-leaf parsley |
| 4½ | teaspoons cornstarch |
| ½ | cup no-sugar-added cranberry sauce, such as Steel's Gourmet Agave |

PER SERVING
**323** calories **7g** fat ( **1g** sat / **3.7g** mono / **1g** poly )
**45mg** cholesterol **345mg** sodium
**30g** carbohydrate **4g** fiber **38g** protein

## METHOD

1 In a medium pot with a candy or deep-fry thermometer attached, heat the broth. When the liquid reaches 165°F, with barely any bubbles reaching the surface, add the turkey. Adjust the heat, if necessary, to keep the temperature at 165°F. Using foil, cover the pot around the thermometer and poach the turkey until the internal temperature of the turkey reaches 150°F, about 30 to 40 minutes. Turn off the heat and let the turkey rest in the poaching liquid for an additional 15 to 20 minutes.

2 Meanwhile, heat a large nonstick pan over medium heat. When hot, add the olive oil. Add the onions and celery and cook until the vegetables are soft, about 5 minutes. Season with salt and pepper to taste. Add the poultry seasoning and bread. Stir to combine. Lower the heat to low and add the poaching liquid, ½ cup at a time (about 1 cup total), to the pan to moisten the bread. Stir well, and then cover. Cook until the bread is moist and hot, about 5 minutes. Stir in the parsley, and season with salt and pepper to taste. Set aside.

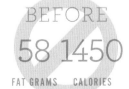

BEFORE
58 1450
FAT GRAMS    CALORIES

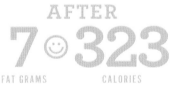

AFTER
7 ☺ 323
FAT GRAMS    CALORIES

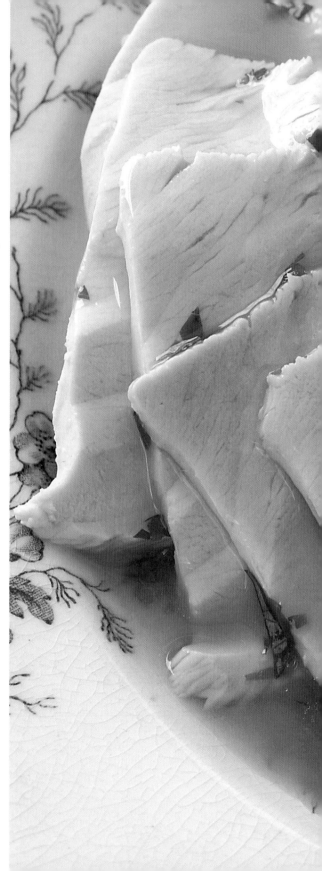

## METHOD

3 Remove the turkey from the poaching liquid, and tent with foil to keep warm.

4 Remove the thermometer from the pot and bring the poaching liquid up to a simmer. In a small bowl, add the cornstarch. Whisk in about ½ cup of the poaching liquid, and then pour the mixture back into the pot. Turn up the heat so that the liquid boils. Turn down the heat and simmer until the liquid thickens and reduces in volume by a third, about 10 minutes. If the liquid is too thin, mix more cornstarch with some liquid from the pot and stir it back into the simmering gravy. Season with salt and pepper to taste.

5 Slice the turkey breast as thinly as possible. Serve with the stuffing, gravy, and cranberry sauce.

**\* CALORIE SAVER**

Omit the cranberry sauce and save **30** calories per serving.

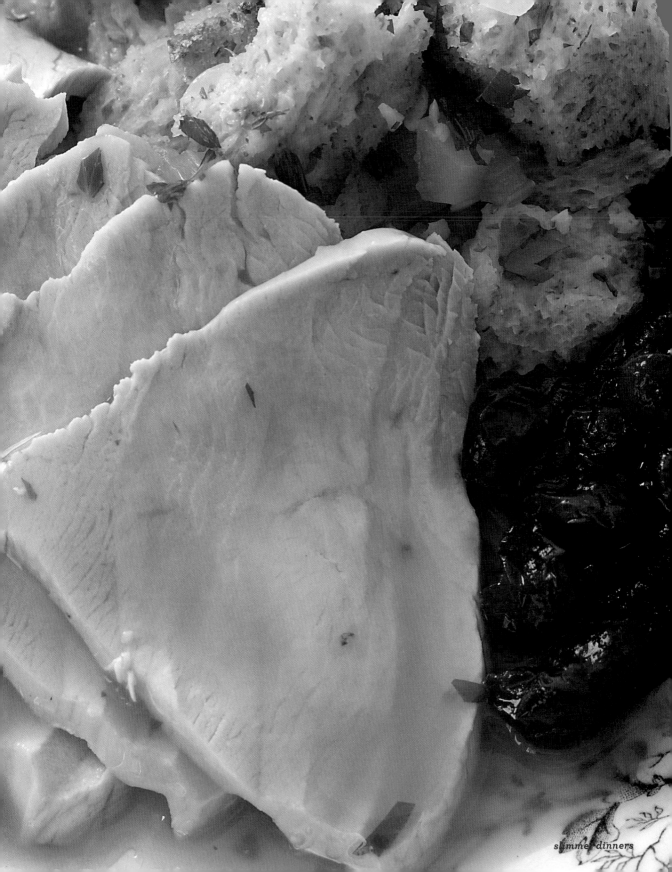

simmer dinners

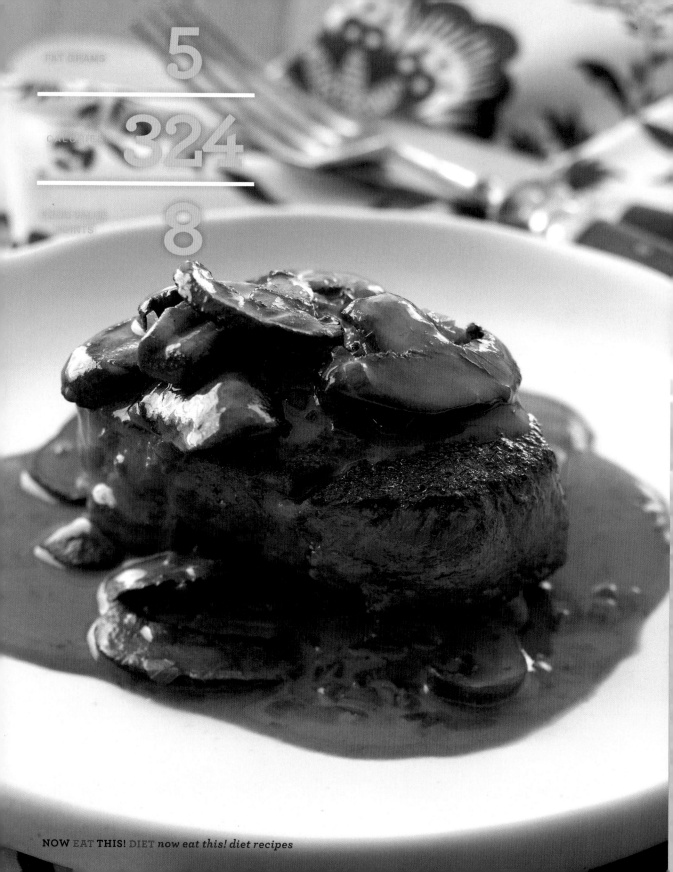

FAT GRAMS
5

CALORIES
324

WEIGHT WATCHERS
POINTS
8

# Sautéed Steak with Mushrooms

SERVES 4

**FOR MANY YEARS,** I worked as a restaurant chef. It was a great way to turn my appetite into a profit center to help me pay the tab for giant T-bones, cheeseburgers, and foie gras. But what it did was give me a cholesterol count well above the acceptable range of 200. My weight shot up, too, requiring an incremental series of bigger sizes. These days, I know better. To satisfy my appetite for beef, I now cook mostly with beef tenderloin, among the leanest of cuts, and match it up with nutritious veggies like sweet potatoes and cremini mushrooms (smaller versions of Portobello mushrooms). This dish turns off the fat and turns up the flavor.

## INGREDIENTS

2    **large sweet potatoes (about 1¾ pounds)**

     **Nonstick cooking spray**

4    **lean beef tenderloin steaks (4 ounces each), trimmed of all visible fat**

     **Salt**

     **Freshly ground black pepper**

4    **cups sliced cremini mushrooms**

¼    **cup chopped shallot**

6    **tablespoons balsamic vinegar**

2    **teaspoons cornstarch**

1    **cup low-fat, low-sodium chicken broth**

½    **cup fat-free evaporated milk**

¼    **cup chopped fresh flat-leaf parsley**

PER SERVING
**324**calories **5g**fat ( **2g**sat / **2g**mono / **0g**poly )
**61mg**cholesterol **165mg**sodium
**42g**carbohydrate **4g**fiber **30g**protein

## METHOD

1  Prick the skin of the sweet potatoes with a fork, and microwave them covered with plastic on high for 7 to 8 minutes, until they are completely cooked, turning once halfway through. Set aside and cover with foil to keep warm.

2  Heat a large cast-iron skillet over medium-high heat. When the skillet is hot, remove it from the stove just while you spray it with cooking spray. Season the steaks with salt and pepper. Add the steaks to the skillet and sauté until golden brown, about 4 minutes per side. Transfer the steaks to a platter, and cover with foil to keep them warm.

3  Spray the skillet with more cooking spray, again away from the stove, and add the mushrooms. Sauté until the mushrooms start to become tender, about 5 minutes. Add the shallots and sauté for 1 minute. Add the vinegar, scraping up any flavorful bits with a wooden spoon.

4  In a small bowl, add the cornstarch and chicken broth. Whisk until the cornstarch is dissolved. Add the mixture to the skillet, and bring the sauce to a boil. Stir in the evaporated milk and parsley and simmer until the sauce has slightly thickened. Season with salt and pepper to taste.

5  Split the sweet potatoes in half lengthwise. Serve the steaks with the pan sauce and the sweet potato halves.

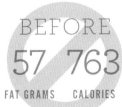

BEFORE
**57** / **763**
FAT GRAMS   CALORIES

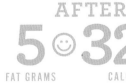

AFTER
**5** ☺ **324**
FAT GRAMS   CALORIES

**✱ CALORIE SAVER**

Omit the sweet potatoes and save **118** calories per serving.

*slimmer dinners*

# Chicken Amandine with Green Beans and Lemon Butter

SERVES 4

**I REMEMBER WHEN FRIED CHICKEN** was touted as a diet food during the carbophobia days. Colonel Sanders, who was no stranger to a greasy tide of fried meals, touted the low-carbohydrate content of KFC products on TV. C'mon now, could anyone really look at a bucket of fried chicken and honestly think it was "health food"?

If you like fried chicken that's a bona fide health food, try this dish. I use the faux-frying method to create a chicken breast that tastes fried. Mixing in the toasted almonds creates another dimension by lending a nutty, warm flavor, and the careful use of just enough but not too much butter certifies this recipe as pure good.

## INGREDIENTS

¼ cup whole wheat flour

½ cup whole wheat panko bread crumbs, such as Ian's All-Natural

½ cup toasted sliced almonds, broken into pieces

½ cup liquid egg substitute

4 skinless, boneless chicken breasts (4 ounces each)

Salt

Freshly ground black pepper

Nonstick cooking spray

1 tablespoon unsalted butter

1 pound haricots verts or slim green beans, trimmed

⅔ cup low-fat, low-sodium chicken broth

¼ cup chopped fresh flat-leaf parsley

¼ cup fresh lemon juice

PER SERVING
**327**calories **12g**fat ( **3g**sat / **5.4g**mono / **2g**poly )
**80mg**cholesterol **188mg**sodium
**22g**carbohydrate **6g**fiber **33g**protein

## METHOD

1 Preheat the oven to 400°F. Place a wire rack on a baking sheet lined with foil, and set it aside.

2 Put the flour in a shallow dish. Mix the panko and almonds in another shallow dish. In a shallow plate, put the egg substitute.

3 Season the chicken with salt and pepper to taste. Working in batches, dredge the chicken in the flour, shaking off any excess. Add the chicken to the egg substitute and coat completely. Add the chicken, a few pieces at a time, to the panko and almond mixture and coat completely.

4 Spread the chicken out on the wire rack. Spray lightly with cooking spray. Bake the chicken until the breading is golden and crispy and the chicken is cooked through, about 10 minutes. Remove the baking sheet from the oven, and tent the meat with foil to keep warm.

5 Heat a large nonstick sauté pan over medium-high heat. When hot, add the butter and green beans and cook, about 1 to 2 minutes. Add the chicken broth and bring to a boil. Reduce the heat to medium-low and simmer until the sauce has slightly thickened, about 2 minutes. Add the parsley and lemon juice and season with salt and pepper to taste.

6 Serve the chicken with the beans and the lemon-butter sauce.

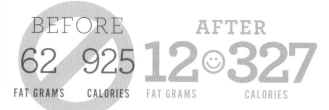

BEFORE
**62** **925**
FAT GRAMS  CALORIES

AFTER
**12** ☺ **327**
FAT GRAMS  CALORIES

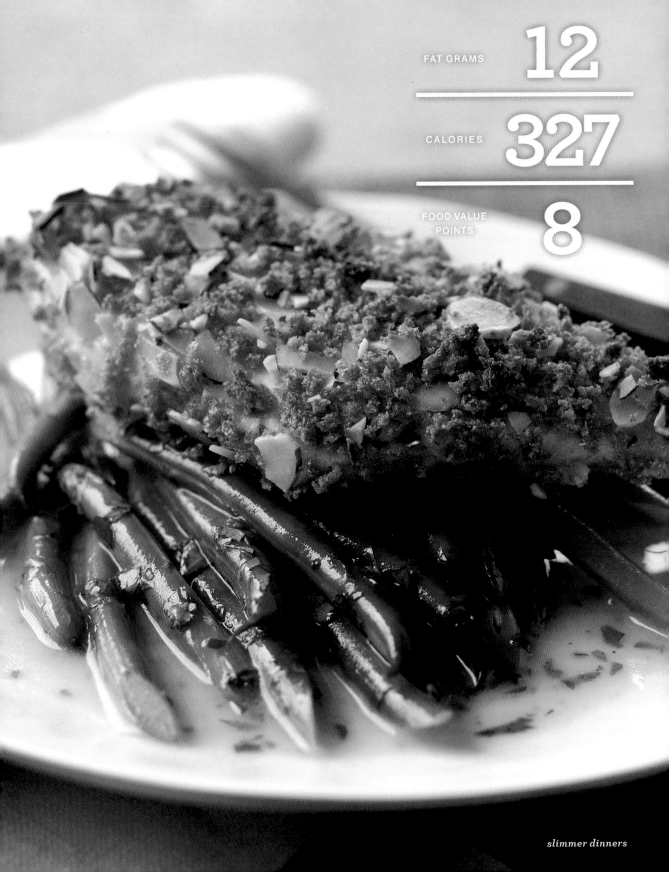

FAT GRAMS 12

CALORIES 327

FOOD VALUE POINTS 8

*slimmer dinners*

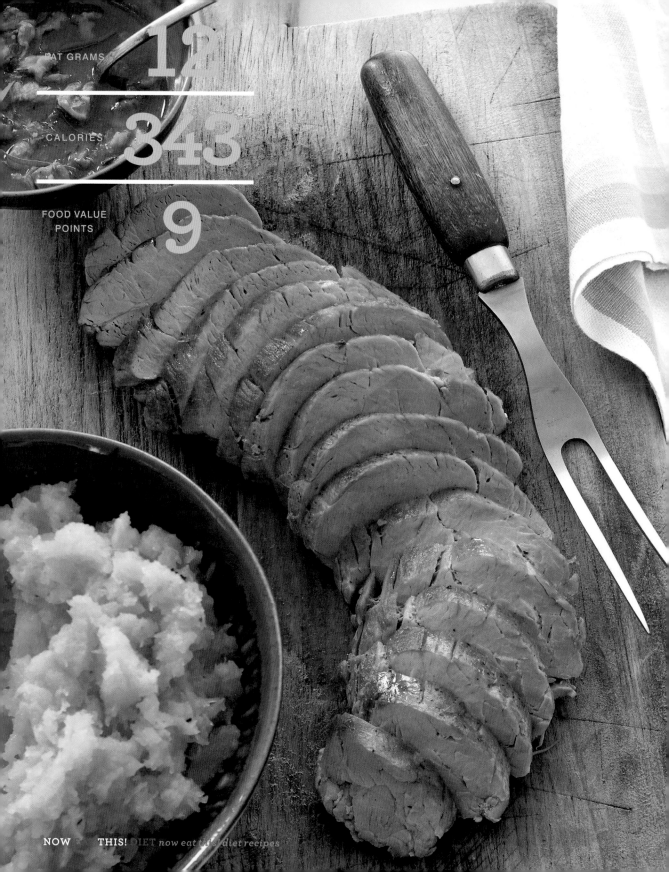

FAT GRAMS **12**

CALORIES **343**

FOOD VALUE
POINTS **9**

# Roasted Pork Tenderloin with Butternut Squash Mash and Tarragon Gravy

SERVES 4

**I JUST ATE A MEAL OF SOME MELTINGLY TENDER PORK,** butternut squash, and toasted walnuts. No, this isn't my food journal. I'm sharing this information with you because the above foods are supposed to reduce the incidence of many diseases that might come my way. Okay, maybe you're not interested in your arteries working at peak capacity; maybe what you want is to enjoy food to the maximum and not have to force it down your throat because it's good for you. That said, you'll love this dish, whether or not its health benefits ever cross your mind.

## INGREDIENTS

1   medium butternut squash, cut in half lengthwise, seeds removed

1   pound lean pork tenderloin, trimmed of all visible fat
    Salt
    Freshly ground black pepper
    Nonstick butter-flavored cooking spray

½   cup unsweetened applesauce

4   teaspoons Dijon mustard

½   cup apple cider or low-fat, low-sodium chicken broth

1   tablespoon plus 2 teaspoons agave nectar

2   teaspoons chopped fresh tarragon

2   grates of a nutmeg

½   cup toasted walnuts, broken into small pieces

## METHOD

1   Preheat the oven to 400°F.

2   Place the butternut squash, cut side down, on a microwave-safe plate. Microwave on high till the squash is tender, about 12 to 15 minutes.

3   Meanwhile, heat a large cast-iron skillet over high heat. Season the pork with salt and pepper to taste. When the pan is hot, remove it from the stove just while you coat it with the cooking spray. Add the pork to the pan and sear on all sides, about 3 minutes per side. Transfer the pork to a baking sheet and continue cooking in the oven till done, about 10 to 15 minutes, or until the internal temperature reaches 155°F. Remove the baking sheet from the oven, and tent the meat with foil to keep it warm. Let the meat rest for at least 10 minutes before slicing.

4   In the same pan over medium-low heat, add the applesauce, scraping up any flavorful bits with a wooden spoon. Add the mustard, apple cider, 2 teaspoons agave, and tarragon. Stir continuously until the sauce thickens. Season with salt and pepper to taste.

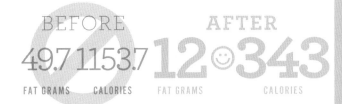

BEFORE 49.7 1153.7  AFTER 12 343

FAT GRAMS   CALORIES   FAT GRAMS   CALORIES

## PORK TENDERLOIN

What is quick-cooking, healthy, and as close to foolproof as you can get without hiring me to do the cooking? Answer (hint: it's not a low-cal frozen dinner):

It's pork tenderloin, a very lean cut of meat with just 147 calories and 4 grams of fat in 3½ ounces. It's also the most tender cut on the hog. You can stir-fry it, broil it, roast it, or grill it. Just about any way you prepare it, it's cooked to juicy perfection in 25 minutes or less. Throw in a couple of creative side dishes to round out the meal, and you're set.

I like pork tenderloin for its versatility, too. You can use thinly sliced pork tenderloin in any recipe calling for thin-sliced boneless chicken breast, veal, or beef tenderloin. It's a terrific dinner solution.

When shopping for pork tenderloin, please don't confuse it with "center loin," which is dry and definitely undesirable.

One more advantage: Pork tenderloin is sometimes sold in vacuum-packed bags, so it can be stored for weeks in your fridge.

### ✱ CALORIE SAVER

Omit the walnuts and save **96** calories per serving.

## METHOD

5 With a spoon, scoop the flesh of the squash into a medium bowl. Mash the squash with a fork, and add the nutmeg grates and remaining agave. Stir till combined. Season with salt and pepper to taste.

6 With a sharp knife, thinly slice the pork. Serve the pork with the reduced sauce and the butternut squash. Sprinkle the walnuts on top of the pork.

### PER SERVING
**343**calories **12g**fat ( **1.8g**sat / **2.3g**mono / **7.4g**poly )
**74mg**cholesterol **190mg**sodium
**33g**carbohydrate **4g**fiber **27g**protein

*slimmer dinners*

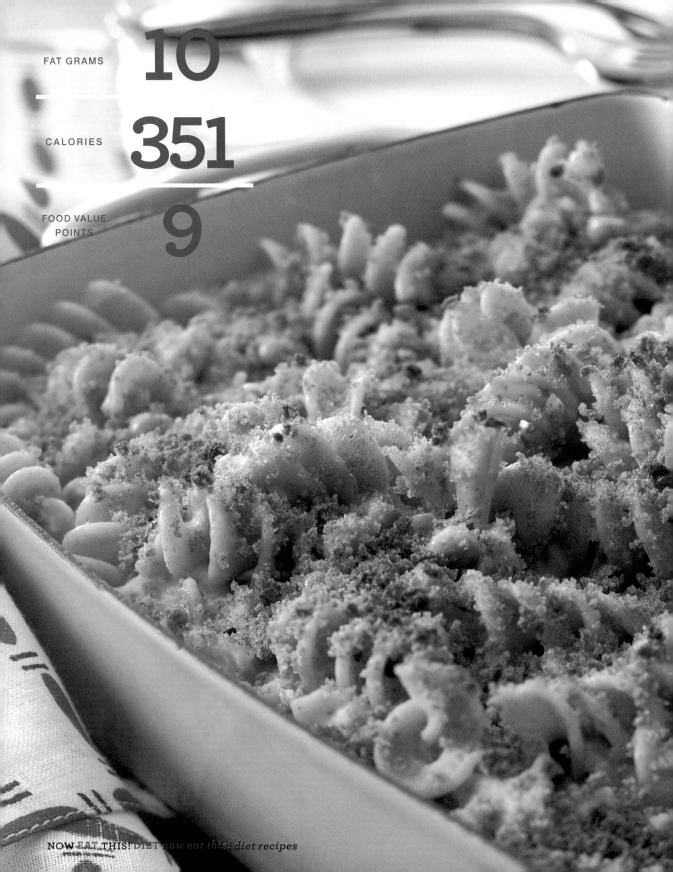

FAT GRAMS **10**

CALORIES **351**

FOOD VALUE POINTS **9**

# Crispy-on-the-Top Tuna and Green Pea Casserole

SERVES 6

**WHO GREW UP EATING TUNA CASSEROLE?** Raise your hands. That's just about everybody. Okay, this is not your mother's tuna casserole . . . nor does it use Tuna Helper. But it does taste just as wonderful—without losing any of its comfort-food flavor.

I've wowed it up a bit with Dijon mustard, and I used whole wheat panko bread crumbs for that traditional crunchy topping. If you can't find these particular bread crumbs, you can always toast leftover whole wheat bread and break it into crumbs with a rolling pin.

## INGREDIENTS

Nonstick cooking spray

6   ounces whole wheat rotini, such as Ronzoni Healthy Harvest

¾   cup reduced-fat sour cream, such as Breakstone's

¾   cup 2% Greek yogurt, such as Fage Total

3   tablespoons Dijon mustard

5   ounces (1¼ cups) shredded 50% reduced-fat cheddar cheese, such as Cabot

18   ounces canned albacore tuna, packed in water, drained

1½   cups frozen peas

Salt

Freshly ground  black pepper

¼   cup whole wheat panko bread crumbs, such as Ian's All-Natural

## METHOD

1 Preheat the oven to 425°F. Spray an 8 x 8 x 2-inch baking dish with cooking spray, and set aside.

2 Bring a large pot of salted water to a boil. Add the pasta and cook according to package directions; drain.

3 In a medium bowl, mix the sour cream, yogurt, mustard, and cheese together. Add the cooked noodles, tuna, and peas. Stir until the pasta is coated with the sauce. Season with salt and pepper to taste.

4 Pour the mixture into the prepared baking dish, and sprinkle the panko over the top.

5 Bake until the rotini is hot throughout, about 10 minutes. Serve immediately.

PER SERVING
**351** calories **10g** fat ( **5g** sat / **1g** mono / **0.5g** poly )
**64mg** cholesterol **589mg** sodium
**34g** carbohydrate **6g** fiber **36g** protein

**∗ CALORIE SAVER**
Omit the peas and save **31** calories per serving.

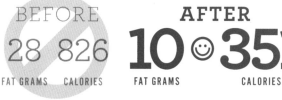

BEFORE
28 826
FAT GRAMS   CALORIES

AFTER
10 ☺ 351
FAT GRAMS   CALORIES

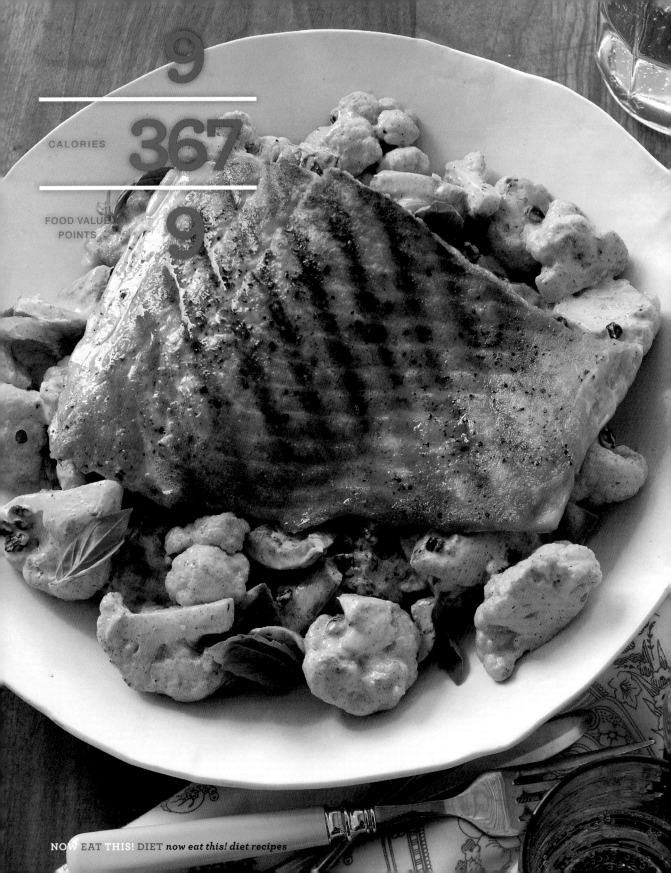

9

CALORIES

367

FOOD VALUE
POINTS

9

# Grilled Salmon with Curried Cauliflower

SERVES 4

**IF YOU'RE NOT EATING ENOUGH SALMON,** you'll be arrested by the food police and made to swim upstream until the end of your days. Salmon contains omega-3 fatty acids that are good for your heart and may protect against Alzheimer's disease. But you have to make sure that your salmon is not farm-raised or fished from rivers deemed toxic. Otherwise you'll get too much mercury and cut your life short. At least you'll be able to remember stuff up until then.

I've paired salmon with cauliflower here. Cauliflower is a "good catch," too. It's an excellent source of vitamin C and cancer-fighting phytochemicals. Although frozen cauliflower is very convenient and well-suited for some dishes, the texture can get a little chewy when defrosted. In this dish, I used fresh florets. The success of the dish also depends on the curry you are using. Since curry is a spice blend, it can vary tremendously from brand to brand. Use one that you like, or you can even try making your own.

## INGREDIENTS

| | |
|---|---|
| | Nonstick cooking spray |
| 4 | (4-ounce) salmon fillets |
| | Salt |
| | Freshly ground black pepper |
| 4 | cups fresh cauliflower florets |
| 2 | cloves garlic, chopped |
| 1 | green pepper, cut into large dice |
| ½ | medium red onion, cut into large dice |
| 4 | teaspoons mild curry powder |
| 1 | cup low-fat, low-sodium chicken broth |
| 2 | tablespoons currants |
| ½ | cup 2% Greek yogurt, such as Fage Total |
| 2 | cups cooked brown rice |

## METHOD

1 Heat a grill pan over medium-high heat. When pan is hot, remove it from the stove to coat it with cooking spray.

2 Season the salmon fillets on both sides with salt and freshly ground black pepper to taste. Lay the fillets on the hot grill pan and cook, about 2 to 3 minutes per side. Transfer the salmon to a serving platter, and tent it with foil to keep it warm.

3 Heat a large nonstick sauté pan over medium-high heat. When hot, coat with cooking spray, away from the stove. Add the cauliflower and sauté till browned, about 4 minutes. Add the garlic, green pepper, onion, curry powder, chicken broth, and currants. Stir to combine. Cover and simmer till the vegetables have softened, about 5 minutes, stirring occasionally. Season with salt and pepper to taste.

4 Remove the pan from heat and stir in the yogurt till well incorporated.

5 Serve the salmon with the curried cauliflower and brown rice.

PER SERVING
**367**calories **9g**fat ( **2g**sat / **3g**mono / **3g**poly )
**53mg**cholesterol **120mg**sodium
**38g**carbohydrate **6g**fiber **34g**protein

**✳ CALORIE SAVER**

Omit the rice and save **108** calories per serving.

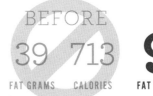

BEFORE
39 713
FAT GRAMS   CALORIES

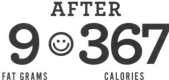

**AFTER**
9 ☺ **367**
FAT GRAMS   CALORIES

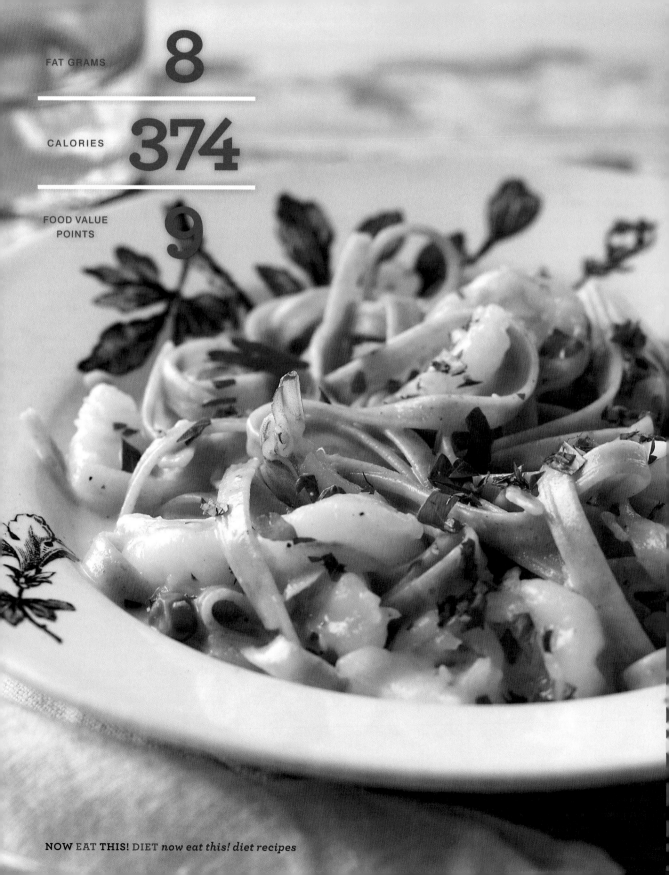

FAT GRAMS **8**

CALORIES **374**

FOOD VALUE POINTS **9**

# Fettuccine Alfredo with Shrimp

SERVES 4

**FETTUCCINE IS MOST CLOSELY ASSOCIATED WITH** the classic dish fettuccine Alfredo. There really was an Alfredo, by the way. Alfredo Di Lelio created this dish in 1914 to help his wife, who was pregnant, restore her appetite. His concern and creativity paid off, not only for his wife, but for people around the world who have enjoyed this dish.

Several years ago, fettuccine Alfredo was dubbed "a heart attack on a plate" because of its rich fattiness. You don't have to worry about that with my rendition. There's virtually no fat, except the scant amount in the yogurt and cheese. The nutmeg adds extra "oomph." I make this with whole wheat pasta, which punches up the nutrition and fiber. This dish will satisfy your craving for cheesy, carby comfort food while keeping your thighs and butt in check.

## INGREDIENTS

| | |
|---|---|
| 6 | ounces whole wheat fettuccine |
| ¾ | pound large shrimp, peeled and deveined, tails removed |
| 1 | cup frozen peas |
| 2 | teaspoons unsalted butter |
| 3 | garlic cloves, minced |
| 2 | teaspoons cornstarch |
| 2 | grates of a nutmeg |
| ¾ | cup low-fat, low-sodium chicken broth |
| ½ | cup grated Parmigiano-Reggiano |
| ¾ | cup 2% Greek yogurt, such as Fage Total |
| | Salt |
| | Freshly ground black pepper |

## METHOD

1. Bring a large pot of salted water to a boil. Add the fettuccine and cook according to the package directions. In the last few minutes of cooking, add the shrimp and peas and cook until the shrimp is pink and no longer translucent; drain.

2. While the pasta is cooking, melt the butter in a large nonstick sauté pan over medium heat. Add the garlic and cook until it is fragrant, about 2 minutes.

3. Meanwhile, combine the cornstarch and nutmeg grates in a small bowl. Whisk in the chicken broth until smooth. Pour the mixture into the sauté pan, raise the heat, and bring the sauce to a simmer, whisking occasionally. Whisk in ¼ cup of the cheese until it has melted. Remove the sauté pan from the heat and whisk in the yogurt until the sauce is smooth.

4. In a large bowl, toss the cooked fettuccine, shrimp, and peas with the sauce. Season with salt and pepper to taste, if desired. Top the pasta with the remaining ¼ cup cheese, and serve.

### PER SERVING

**374** calories **8g** fat ( **4g** sat / **1.8g** mono / **1.1g** poly )
**146mg** cholesterol **339mg** sodium
**43g** carbohydrate **6g** fiber **34g** protein

**\* CALORIE SAVER**

Omit the peas and save **31** calories per serving.

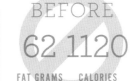

BEFORE
62 1120
FAT GRAMS  CALORIES

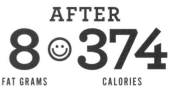

**AFTER**
**8** ☺ **374**
FAT GRAMS       CALORIES

# Chicken Pesto Pasta

SERVES 4

**IF YOU WANT TO FIND ROMANCE WITHOUT ONLINE SEARCHES,** dating services, singles bars, or speed dating, grow some basil and put it on your doorstep. In Italy, basil was (and is) renowned as a sign of love. As tradition goes, a pot of basil placed on her balcony signified that a woman was ready to receive a lover. Moreover, if the lover gifted her with a sprig of this herb upon his arrival, she would surely fall in love with him and never leave his side. Now, doesn't that sound a lot easier?

Italy, of course, is also the home of pesto, basil's signature dish, and now so ubiquitous that it adorns pizzas, burgers, even potato chips. But while this puree of basil, garlic, and pine nuts has a healthy, fresh image, it packs serious fat and calories because it's loaded with oil, sometimes even butter. So I've gone where no cook has gone before: I've created a no-oil pesto. Try it in this chicken pasta dish and let me know what you think. Oh—and let me know how the basil-on-the-doorstep thing works out for you, too.

## INGREDIENTS

8 ounces whole wheat rigatoni pasta, such as Bionaturae Organic

2 large garlic cloves, coarsely chopped

½ cup reduced-fat sour cream, such as Breakstone's

1 cup packed fresh basil leaves

2 tablespoons chopped fresh flat-leaf parsley

Pinch of crushed red pepper

½ cup grated Parmigiano-Reggiano cheese

1 tablespoon chopped toasted pine nuts

Salt

Freshly ground black pepper

6 ounces (about 2 cups) chopped skinless breast meat from a rotisserie or roast chicken

1 cup grape or cherry tomatoes, cut in half

## METHOD

1 Bring a large pot of salted water to a boil. Add the rigatoni and cook according to package directions; drain.

2 While the pasta is cooking, combine the garlic and sour cream in the bowl of a food processor, and pulse until the garlic is finely chopped. Add the basil, parsley, crushed red pepper, ¼ cup of the Parmigiano-Reggiano, and pine nuts. Puree until the sauce is smooth. Season with salt and pepper to taste. Set aside.

3 In a large bowl, toss the pasta, chicken, and tomatoes with the pesto. Season with salt and pepper to taste, if desired. Top the pasta with the remaining cheese, and serve.

PER SERVING
**385** calories **10g** fat ( **5g** sat / **3g** mono / **1.4g** poly )
**56mg** cholesterol **225mg** sodium
**47g** carbohydrate **6g** fiber **26g** protein

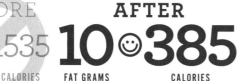

BEFORE
103 1535
FAT GRAMS   CALORIES

AFTER
10 ☺ 385
FAT GRAMS   CALORIES

**\* CALORIE SAVER**
Omit the Parm cheese and save **43** calories per serving.

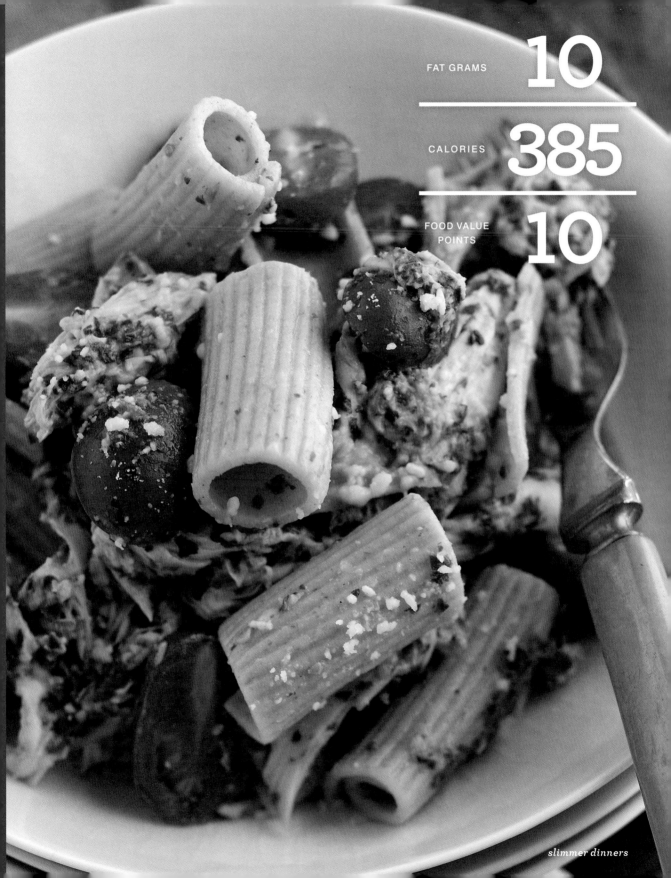

FAT GRAMS **10**

CALORIES **385**

FOOD VALUE POINTS **10**

*slimmer dinners*

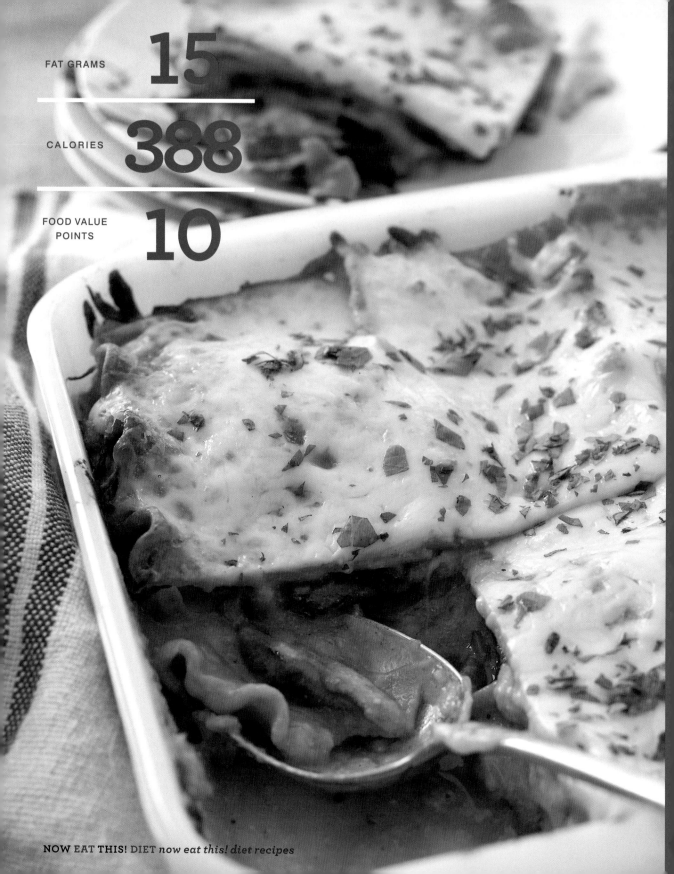

FAT GRAMS **15**

CALORIES **388**

FOOD VALUE
POINTS **10**

# No-Boil Mushroom Lasagna

SERVES 4

**YEARS AGO,** after she came to Hollywood and became an international film star, Sophia Loren gave the media her most sultry pose one day and reportedly said, "All you see, I owe to pasta." Americans now know what Italians and others have known for centuries: Pasta is cheap, chic, and healthy. I don't like diets that give you scheduled feedings of birdseed, so, my friends, thank you for coming back to the pasta fold. This recipe uses no-boil noodles. Mushrooms and no-boil lasagna noodles were made for each other. Because mushrooms release a lot of water during cooking, they essentially steam the noodles, thereby cooking them.

## INGREDIENTS

Nonstick cooking spray

2 cups reduced-fat ricotta cheese, such as Sargento

½ cup chopped fresh basil

2 tablespoons chopped fresh flat-leaf parsley

1 cup grated Parmigiano-Reggiano

Salt

Freshly ground black pepper

4 ounces (about 8 sheets) no-boil whole wheat lasagna noodles, such as Dalallo

10 ounces sliced cremini mushrooms

4 ounces white button mushrooms

½ cup shredded reduced-fat mozzarella cheese

PER SERVING
**388**calories **15g**fat ( **8g**sat / **2.6g**mono / **1.2g**poly )
**57mg**cholesterol **510mg**sodium
**34g**carbohydrate **3g**fiber **28g**protein

## METHOD

1 Preheat the oven to 350°F. Coat the inside of an 8 x 8 x 2-inch baking pan with cooking spray and set aside.

2 In a medium bowl, add the ricotta, basil, parsley, and ¾ cup Parmigiano-Reggiano. Mix with a spoon until blended. Season with salt and pepper to taste. Set aside.

3 Line the bottom of the prepared baking pan with two lasagna sheets. Top with ½ cup of the cheese mixture. Using the back of a spoon, spread the mixture so that the noodles are covered. Top with a layer of mushrooms. Repeat the procedure two more times. On the last layer, place two lasagna sheets on top of the mushrooms. Spread a layer of the remaining cheese mixture on top. Scatter the mozzarella and remaining Parmigiano-Reggiano on top.

4 Cover tightly with foil and bake in the oven for 30 minutes.

5 Raise the temperature of the oven to 425°F, and bake for another 15 minutes. Uncover the dish and continue to bake for another 15 minutes or until the top is golden brown.

**✳ CALORIE SAVER**

Cut the Parm cheese in half and save **43** calories per serving.

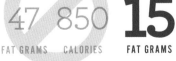
BEFORE
47 850
FAT GRAMS   CALORIES

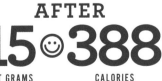
**AFTER**
**15** ☺ **388**
**FAT GRAMS**   CALORIES

*slimmer dinners*

# BBQ Pork Chops

SERVES 4

**I LOVE RIBS THAT HAVE BEEN SMOKED SO LONG,** they should be in rehab. But I don't love the fat or what it does to my heart. Here's my version: large, meaty pork chops you can pick up in your hands (if you want) and sink your teeth into—all covered with a tangy, peppery, sweet flavor that will definitely make you want to pork out. What's kale doing in there? For all its nutritional charms, kale isn't a vegetable I'd recommend serving plain, because the flavor is assertive. Instead, I suggest kale in a dish that has some meaty flavor to round out the taste. Pork is perfect.

## INGREDIENTS

¾   cup reduced-sugar ketchup, such as Heinz

½   cup plus 2 tablespoons apple cider vinegar

4   teaspoons molasses

¾   teaspoon garlic powder

¾   teaspoon onion powder

1   tablespoon agave nectar

    Nonstick cooking spray

8   (about 2 pounds) thinly cut pork chops, trimmed of all visible fat

1   teaspoon extra-virgin olive oil

4   cloves garlic, sliced

1   bunch kale, washed, ribs and stems removed, and roughly chopped

    Salt

    Freshly ground black pepper

## METHOD

1 In a large shallow dish, combine the ketchup, ¼ cup plus 2 tablespoons cider vinegar, molasses, garlic powder, onion powder, and agave. Stir together. Reserve ½ cup and set aside. Add the pork to the sauce and allow the pork to marinate for 10 minutes.

2 Heat a grill pan over high heat. When hot, remove it from the stove just while you coat it with cooking spray. Place the pork on the pan. Cook until the pork is charred and cooked through, about 3 minutes each side, continually brushing with the leftover barbecue sauce marinade. Transfer the pork to a serving platter, and tent it with foil to keep it warm.

3 Heat a large nonstick pan over medium-high heat. When hot, add the olive oil and garlic. Cook the garlic until it is browned and toasted. Add the kale and cook till just wilted. Add the remaining cider vinegar and cook for another minute. Season with salt and pepper.

PER SERVING
**398** calories **16g** fat ( **5g** sat / **7g** mono / **1.8g** poly )
**81mg** cholesterol **665mg** sodium
**36g** carbohydrate **4g** fiber **31g** protein

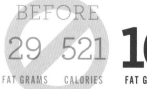
BEFORE 29 FAT GRAMS 521 CALORIES

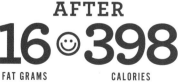
AFTER 16 ☺ 398 FAT GRAMS CALORIES

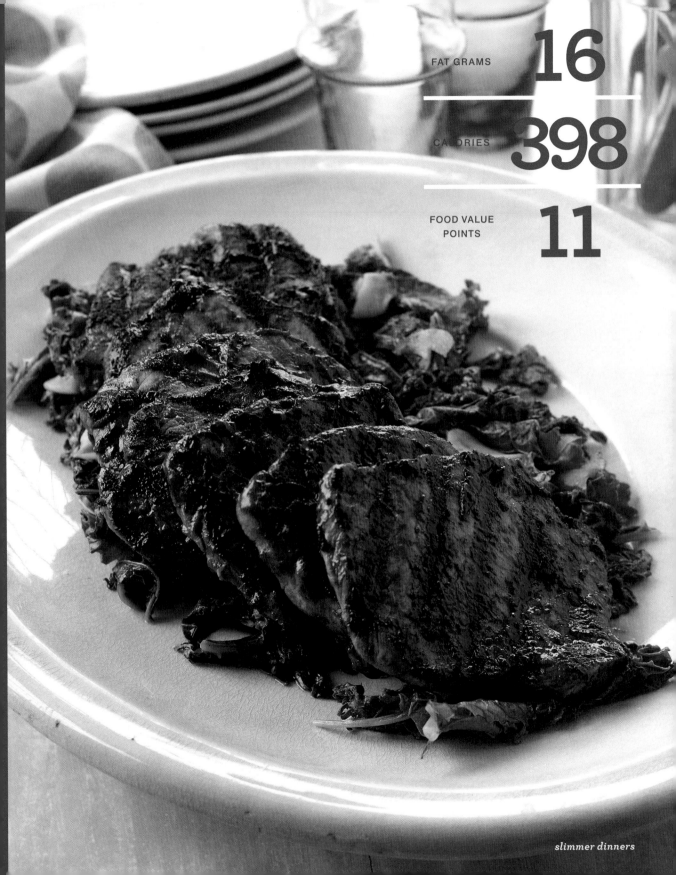

FAT GRAMS **16**

CALORIES **398**

FOOD VALUE
POINTS **11**

*slimmer dinners*

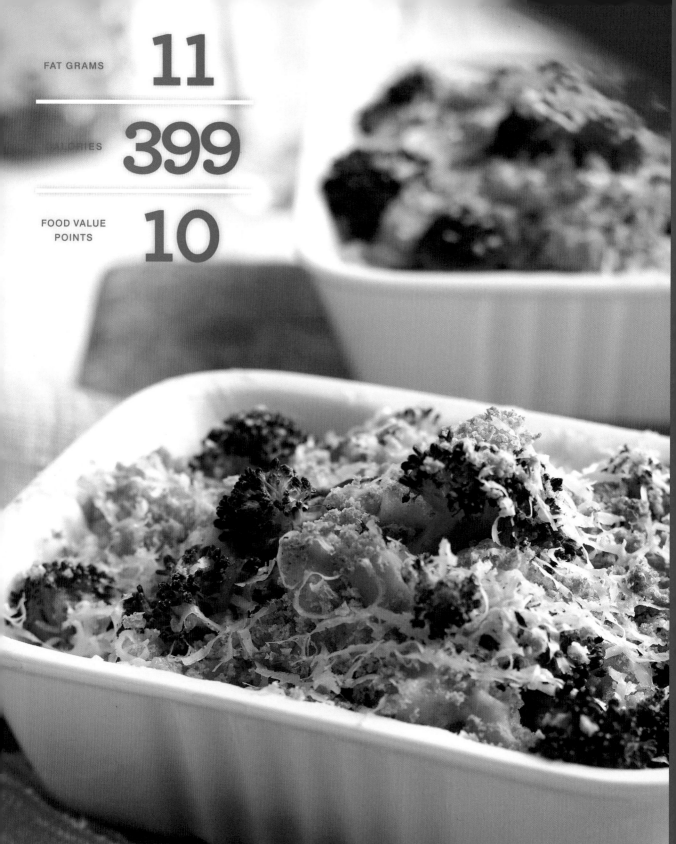

FAT GRAMS **11**

CALORIES **399**

FOOD VALUE
POINTS **10**

# Mac and Cheese with Ham and Broccoli

SERVES 4

**MACARONI AND CHEESE IS MY QUINTESSENTIAL COMFORT FOOD.** It always has been, from the time my mother made it when I was a kid. Although I like to think my mom created this homey dish, mac and cheese is thought to have been introduced to America by Thomas Jefferson, who was an acknowledged foodie. He even had his own pasta-making machine. The first U.S. macaroni factory was built in 1848 in Brooklyn, New York, not by an Italian, but by an enterprising French flour miller from Lyon named Antoine Zerega.

History lesson over. Now you can eat this big, bubbling dish to your heart's content (well, almost). I use pureed onions and garlic in the cheese sauce for added creaminess. Canadian bacon is actually quite lean. Unlike regular bacon, which comes from the pig belly, Canadian bacon is from the loin of the pig. An ounce of cooked bacon packs in 160 calories, whereas an ounce of cooked Canadian bacon contains only 50 calories.

## INGREDIENTS

Nonstick cooking spray

1 large Vidalia onion, roughly chopped

9 garlic cloves, roughly chopped

½ cup water

Salt

Freshly ground black pepper

6 ounces whole wheat elbow macaroni

2 cups broccoli florets

½ teaspoon dry mustard

Pinch of cayenne pepper

1¾ cups (about 7 ounces) shredded 50% reduced-fat cheddar, such as Cabot

⅓ cup nonfat Greek yogurt, such as Fage Total

½ cup (about 2 ounces) diced Canadian bacon

⅓ cup whole wheat panko bread crumbs, such as Ian's All-Natural

⅓ cup grated Parmigiano-Reggiano cheese

## METHOD

1 Preheat the oven to 425°F. Spray an 8 x 8 x 2-inch baking dish with cooking spray, and set aside.

2 Combine the onion, garlic, and water in a microwave-safe bowl. Season with salt and pepper to taste. Cover the bowl tightly with plastic wrap, and microwave on high for 10 minutes. Pour the mixture into a blender and blend it until it is completely smooth.

3 Bring a large pot of salted water to a boil. Add the macaroni and cook according to the package directions. In the last 2 minutes of cooking, add the broccoli florets; drain.

4 While the pasta is cooking, bring the pureed onion mixture, mustard, and cayenne to a simmer in a small saucepan over medium heat, stirring often. Whisk in the cheddar until it has melted. Remove the pan from the heat and whisk in the yogurt.

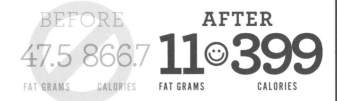

BEFORE 47.5 FAT GRAMS 866.7 CALORIES

AFTER 11 FAT GRAMS 399 CALORIES

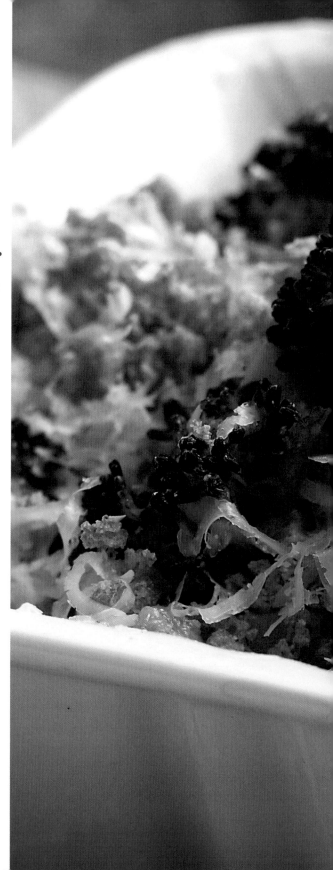

## METHOD

5 In a medium bowl, toss the cooked macaroni and the Canadian bacon with the cheese sauce to coat thoroughly. Season with salt to taste. Pour the macaroni into the prepared baking dish, and sprinkle the panko over the top. Top with the Parmigiano-Reggiano.

6 Bake until the cheese has melted and the macaroni is hot throughout, about 10 minutes. Serve immediately.

PER SERVING
**399** calories **11g** fat ( **7g** sat / **0.9g** mono / **0.4g** poly )
**40mg** cholesterol **880mg** sodium
**51g** carbohydrate **7g** fiber **29g** protein

### * CALORIE SAVER

Omit the panko and Parm and save **39** calories per serving.

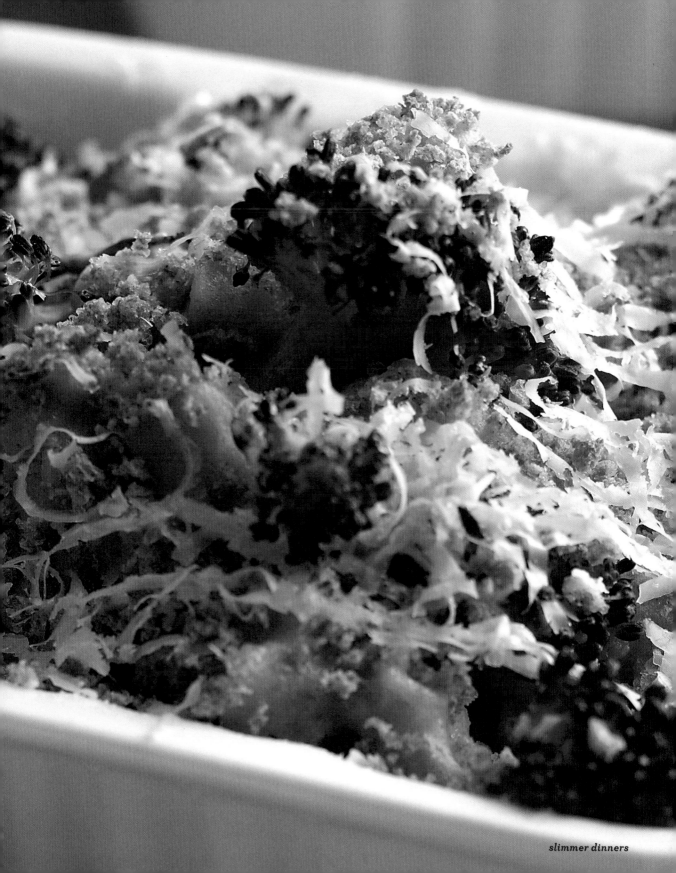

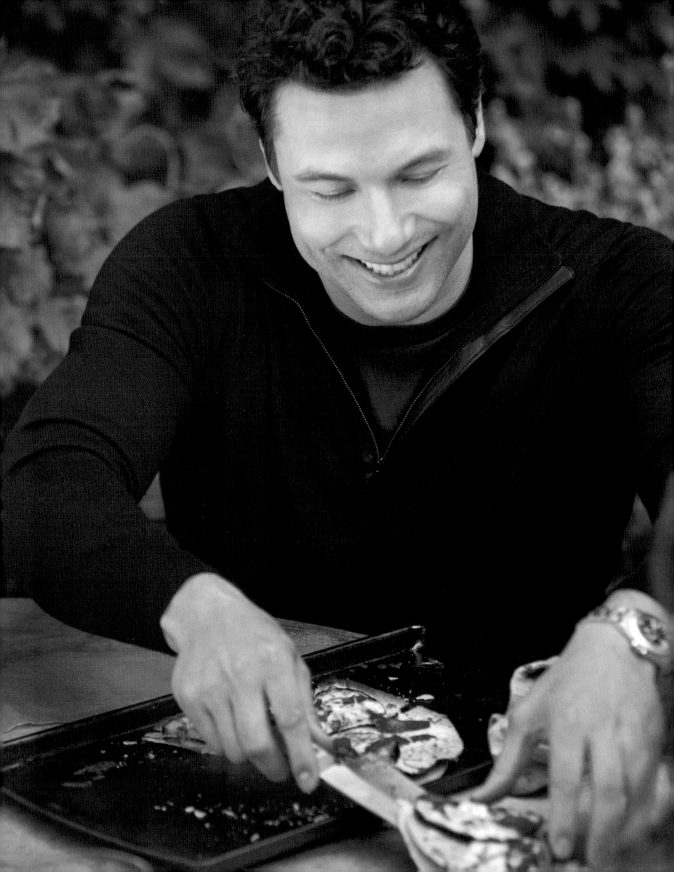

chapter

# 12

# Savory Snacks

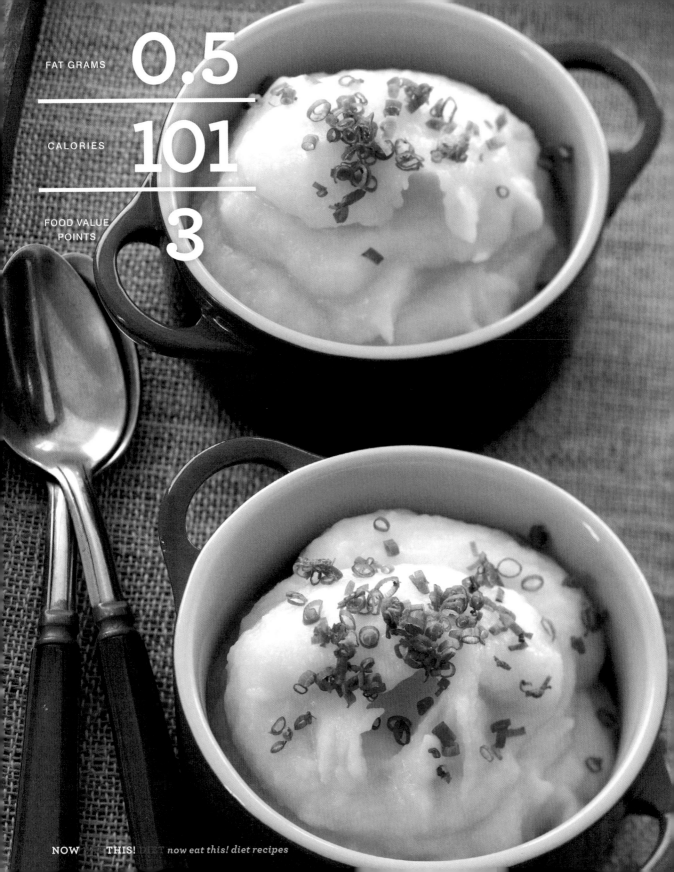

FAT GRAMS

0.5

CALORIES

101

FOOD VALUE
POINTS

3

# Garlic Mashed Potatoes

SERVES 4

**IF YOU'VE BEEN SUBSISTING** on bunless hamburgers for six months because you're cutting carbs, pick up your fork *now*. Have I got a bit of culinary heaven for you. These mashed potatoes are mostly mashed cauliflower, but you'd never know it. And your kids won't either. This is great way to sneak some veggies into your children's diets.

## INGREDIENTS

1   large russet potato, peeled and cut into ½-inch pieces

4   cups fresh cauliflower florets

6   garlic cloves

¼   cup low-fat buttermilk

    Salt

    Freshly ground black pepper

1   tablespoon chopped fresh chives

### PER SERVING
**101**calories **0.5g**fat ( **0g**sat / **0g**mono / **0g**poly )
**1mg**cholesterol **53mg**sodium
**22g**carbohydrate **3g**fiber **4g**protein

## METHOD

1   In a large saucepan, combine the potatoes, cauliflower, and garlic. Add water to cover and bring to a boil over high heat. Once the mixture boils, reduce the heat so that it simmers. Cook until the vegetables are tender, about 15 minutes; drain and return to the pan.

2   Add the buttermilk to the pan. With a hand-held blender, puree the mixture until it is smooth. (You can also use a food processor or a potato masher.) Season with salt and pepper to taste.

3   Transfer the mixture to a bowl and sprinkle the chives over the potatoes.

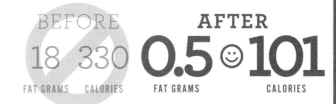

BEFORE
18   330
FAT GRAMS   CALORIES

AFTER
**0.5** ☺ **101**
FAT GRAMS   CALORIES

*savory snacks*

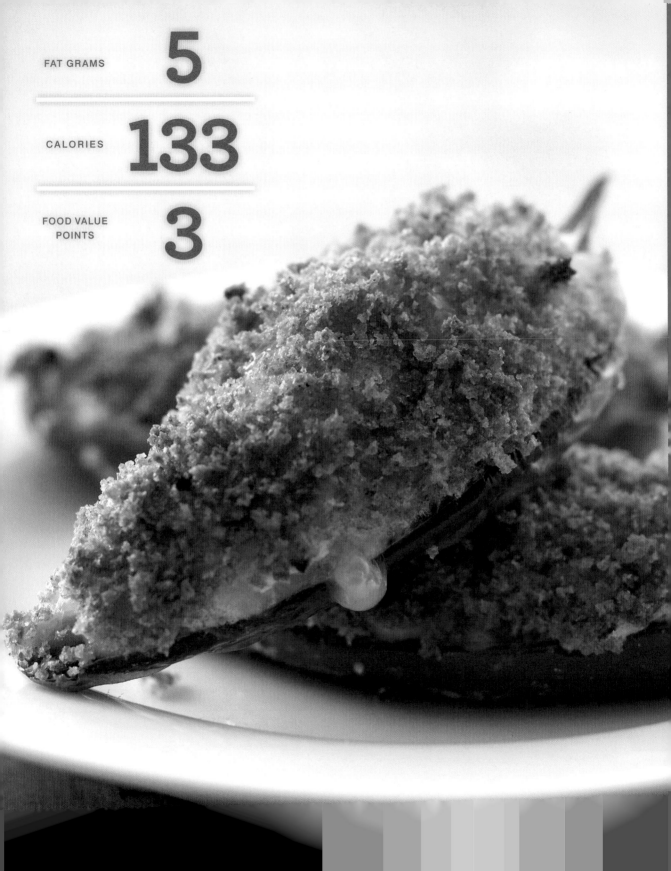

FAT GRAMS **5**

CALORIES **133**

FOOD VALUE
POINTS **3**

# Chicken and Cheese Poppers

**WHEN I'M NOT COOKING,** I'm thinking about food. In fact, I often make up little lists in my head involving food and food-related experiences to divert myself while I'm standing in checkout lines or waiting in airports. The other day, I was thinking about what's the best deep-fried thing ever. Jalapeño poppers was the answer. I had to figure out how to make them without deep-frying. Here's what I came up with. I don't think you'll ever go back to the oily version.

## INGREDIENTS

| | |
|---|---|
| 6 | jalapeño peppers |
| 1 | cup (about 3.5 ounces) shredded skinless breast meat from a rotisserie or roast chicken |
| ¼ | cup reduced-fat cream cheese |
| ¼ | cup reduced-fat sour cream, such as Breakstone's |
| ¼ | cup chopped scallions (white and green parts) |
| ½ | cup (about 2 ounces) shredded 75% reduced-fat cheddar, such as Cabot |
| | Salt |
| | Freshly ground black pepper |
| ½ | cup whole wheat flour |
| 1½ | cups whole wheat panko bread crumbs, such as Ian's All-Natural |
| 4 | large egg whites |
| | Nonstick cooking spray |

PER SERVING
**133**calories **5g**fat ( **2.5g**sat / **0.8g**mono / **0g**poly )
**29mg**cholesterol **205mg**sodium
**11g**carbohydrate **2g**fiber **12g**protein

## METHOD

1 Preheat the broiler on high. Place a wire baking rack on a foil-lined baking sheet.

2 Cut each jalapeño in half and scrape out the seeds and membrane. Place the jalapeños on the prepared baking sheet, and broil until they begin to char slightly and are partially cooked, about 2 minutes. Allow the jalapeños to cool completely.

3 Preheat the oven to 450°F.

4 In a small bowl, mix together the chicken, cream cheese, sour cream, scallions, and cheese. Season with salt and pepper to taste. Divide the filling into 12 equal parts and fill each jalapeño half with the chicken mixture, packing it in tightly.

5 Put the flour in a shallow dish. Put the panko in a small dish. In a medium bowl, whip the egg whites with a whisk until they are extremely foamy but not quite holding peaks.

6 Working in batches, dredge the jalapeños in the flour, shaking off any excess. Add the jalapeños to the egg whites and toss to coat completely, being careful not to let the filling come out. Add the jalapeños, a few pieces at a time, to the panko and coat completely.

7 Spread the jalapeños out on the wire rack and season them generously with salt and pepper. Spray the jalapeños lightly with cooking spray. Bake until the breading is golden brown and crispy and the cheese is melted throughout, about 20 minutes.

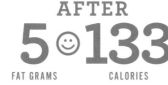

BEFORE
27.5 432
FAT GRAMS CALORIES

AFTER
5 ☺ 133
FAT GRAMS CALORIES

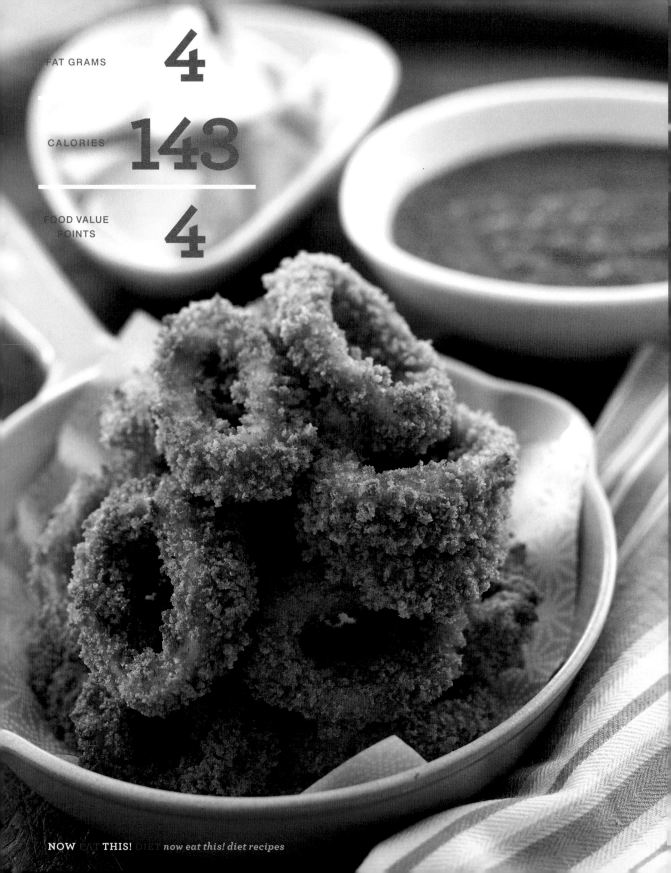

FAT GRAMS **4**

CALORIES **143**

FOOD VALUE POINTS **4**

# Spicy Fried Calamari with Cherry Tomato Dipping Sauce

SERVES 4

**THERE ARE A LOT OF AMAZING DISHES THAT START WITH THE LETTER C:** chocolate, cashews, calzones, cannelloni, chateaubriand, cheese—and calamari. Calamari is the Italian word for squid. The delicate circlets are usually served lightly breaded and fried, then dipped in a tomato-based sauce. It's a very popular appetizer, but it's loaded with fat and calories. I love calamari, so I had to find a way to lighten it. Here it is!

You can find decent cherry tomatoes even in the dead of winter, so keep this simple sauce in mind for spooning over omelets or underneath broiled fish fillets or as a dunk for other foods—like zucchini—that are "fried" using this method. ✱TIP: When doing the shopping for this recipe, buy larger calamari bodies. Rings cut from larger calamari are easier to coat than small rings.

## INGREDIENTS

**FOR THE SAUCE** (makes about ½ cup):

1   pint cherry or grape tomatoes

2   teaspoons olive oil

2   cloves garlic, smashed, peeled, and sliced thin

    Large pinch crushed red pepper flakes

    Salt

## INGREDIENTS

**FOR THE CALAMARI:**

¾   cup whole wheat flour

2½  cups whole wheat panko bread crumbs, such as Ian's All-Natural

4   large egg whites

8   ounces cleaned calamari bodies, cut into ¼-inch rings

    Garlic salt

    Freshly ground black pepper

    Nonstick cooking spray

4   lemon wedges

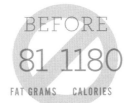

BEFORE
81 1180
FAT GRAMS   CALORIES

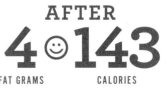

AFTER
4 ☺ 143
FAT GRAMS   CALORIES

*savory snacks*

## METHOD

1 To make the sauce, rinse the tomatoes and drain them. Choose a heavy pan that has a cover and will hold the tomatoes in an even layer. Pour in the oil and heat over medium heat. Add the garlic and cook, shaking the pan, until the edges just begin to brown. Toss in the red pepper, cook a second, and then add the tomatoes all at once. Cover the pan and cook, shaking the pan, for a minute or so. Lift the lid a little to see if the tomatoes have started to burst. If not, cover and shake for a little bit longer. When the tomatoes have started to burst, stir in 2 tablespoons water and lower the heat slightly. Stir and mash until all the tomatoes are a big mush. Cool the sauce slightly, and then pour it into a not-too-fine sieve over a bowl. Gently force the sauce through the sieve using the back of a ladle. Check and add salt as you like. Discard the solids in the sieve and pour the sauce into a small microwave-safe bowl.

2 Preheat the oven to 450°F. Place a wire rack on a foil-lined baking sheet, and set it aside.

3 To prepare the calamari, put the flour and panko in separate shallow dishes. In a medium bowl, whip the egg whites with a whisk until they are extremely foamy but not quite holding peaks.

4 Blot the calamari dry with paper towels. Working with a few calamari rings at a time, dredge the calamari in the flour, making sure the insides of the rings are coated. Bounce the calamari in your palm, a few pieces at a time, to shake off any excess flour. Add the calamari to the egg whites and toss to coat completely. Remove the calamari, letting excess egg white drip back into the bowl (a regular dinner fork works well for this). Drop the rings into the panko and coat them completely, opening the rings and pressing the panko lightly onto the calamari to help it stick. If necessary, rebeat the egg whites to keep them foamy while coating the calamari.

5 Spread the calamari out on the wire rack, and season generously with garlic salt and pepper. Spray the calamari lightly with nonstick cooking spray. Bake until the breading is cooked through, about 14 minutes.

6 Meanwhile, heat the sauce in the microwave until it is hot, about 2 minutes.

7 Serve the calamari with the lemon wedges and the sauce for dipping.

PER SERVING

**143** calories **4g** fat ( **0.5g** sat / **2g** mono / **0.6g** poly )
**132mg** cholesterol **158mg** sodium
**16g** carbohydrate **3g** fiber **13g** protein

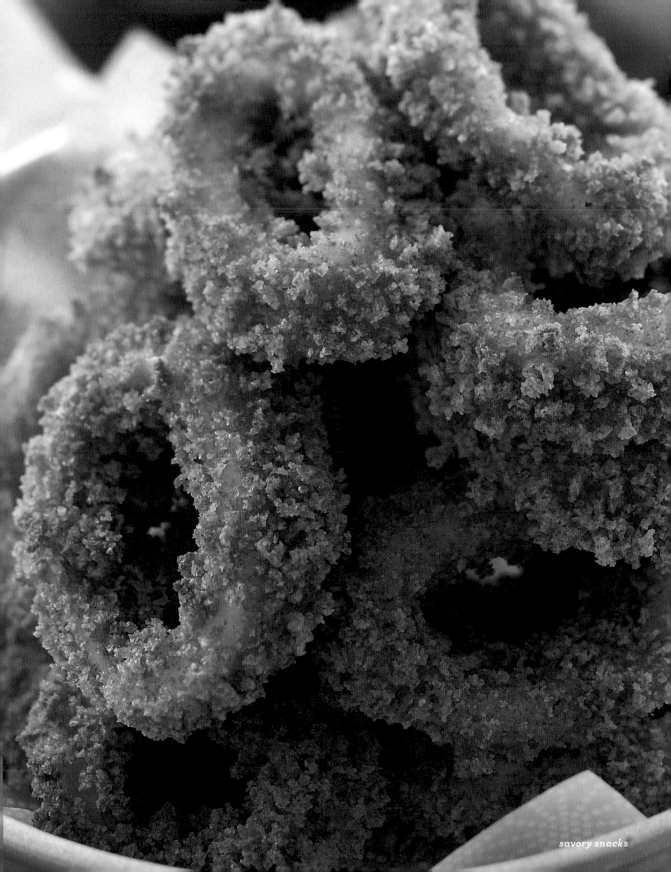

savory snacks

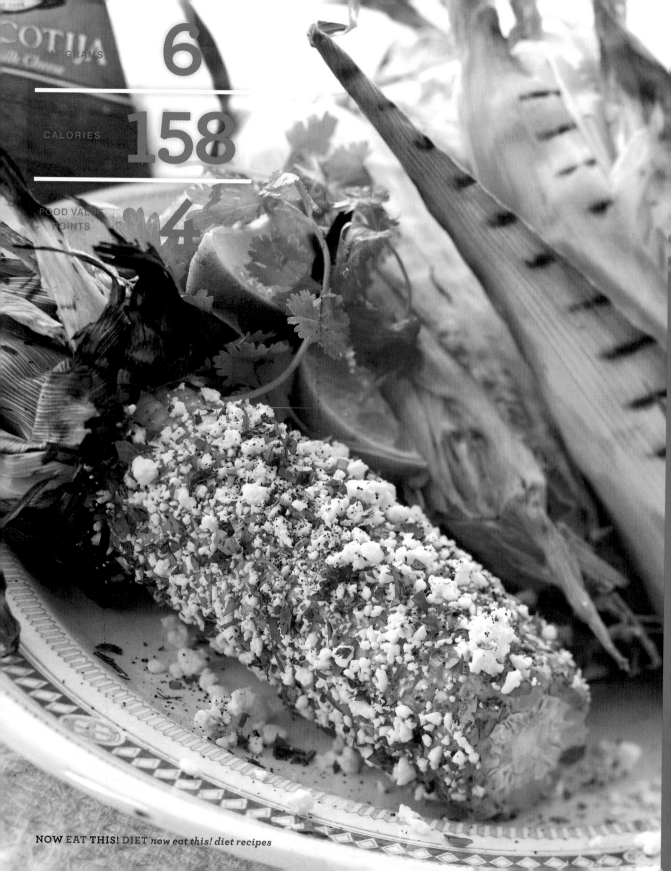

GRAMS **6**

CALORIES **158**

FOOD VALUE POINTS **4**

COTIJA

# Mexican Corn with Chili Mayo

SERVES 4

**FRESH CORN ON THE COB** is so good on its own, you really don't have to do much to it. But if you want to spice up your ears a bit, try my Mexican Corn. It uses cotija cheese, known as the "Parmesan cheese of Mexico." It's a strongly flavored, crumbly cheese that is used like Parmesan in Italian cooking. If you can't find it in your supermarket, try using Parmigiano-Reggiano or feta instead. This recipe makes a delicious addition to quesadillas, tostadas, fajitas, tacos, or burritos. So dig in. Delicious!

## INGREDIENTS

| | |
|---|---|
| 4 | ears corn, in their husks |
| | Butter-flavored cooking spray |
| ¼ | cup fat-free mayonnaise |
| 1 | teaspoon chili powder |
| ½ | cup (about 2 ounces) cotija cheese, grated |
| 2 | tablespoons chopped fresh cilantro |
| 1 | lime, cut into 4 wedges |

PER SERVING
**158** calories **6g** fat ( **3g** sat / **0.8g** mono / **0.6g** poly )
**12mg** cholesterol **367mg** sodium
**23g** carbohydrate **3g** fiber **7g** protein

## METHOD

1 Microwave the corn, two ears at a time, for about 7 minutes on high, turning once. Peel back the husk and test a kernel for tenderness. Microwave again for another minute, if necessary.

2 Heat a grill pan over high heat.

3 Cut an inch off the top of the cobs. Grasp the husk, along with the silk, and peel the husks off the cob like you'd peel the skin off a banana. Continue peeling back the husk around the rest of the cob so that you create a handle with the husk.

4 Spray the corn with cooking spray and place on the hot grill pan. Grill until the kernels begin to develop grill marks, about 2 to 3 minutes. Turn the cobs occasionally.

5 Meanwhile, in a small bowl, mix the mayonnaise and chili powder together. Using a pastry brush, brush the mayonnaise mixture onto each cob. Sprinkle the cheese and cilantro over the cobs.

6 Serve immediately with lime wedges.

**✳ CALORIE SAVER**

Omit the cheese and save **51** calories per serving.

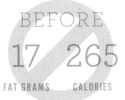

BEFORE
17 265
FAT GRAMS CALORIES

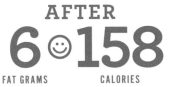

**AFTER**
6 ☺ **158**
FAT GRAMS CALORIES

*savory snacks*

# Curried Chicken Skewers

**THIS RECIPE IS** my version of satay, skewered strips of chicken normally marinated in coconut-milk curry. Mine are marinated in Greek yogurt instead. They come together with almost no effort, are easily customized, and even can be done in batches to allow you to replenish the offering. Chicken skewers beat chicken nuggets any day. ✱TIP: Char them until almost blackened on a very hot grill, don't overcook them, and they will be juicy and moist.

## INGREDIENTS

| | |
|---|---|
| 3 | tablespoons yellow curry paste, such as Karee |
| ½ | cup nonfat Greek yogurt, such as 0% Fage Total |
| | Salt |
| 1 | pound chicken tenders |
| | Nonstick cooking spray |
| | Metal or wooden skewers |
| 2 | limes, cut into quarters |

**PER SERVING**
**159** calories **4g** fat ( **0.7g** sat / **1g** mono / **0.5g** poly )
**73mg** cholesterol **422mg** sodium
**5g** carbohydrate **0.5g** fiber **25g** protein

## METHOD

1 Preheat the oven to 425°F.

2 In a medium bowl, add the curry paste, yogurt, and salt if desired. Stir together until well combined. Add the chicken and toss to coat. Let stand for 30 minutes at room temperature, or refrigerate overnight.

3 Heat a grill pan over high heat. When the pan is hot, remove it from the stove just while you spray it with the nonstick cooking spray. Thread the chicken onto metal or wooden skewers. Place on the grill pan and grill until the meat is slightly charred and cooked through, about 3 minutes each side. Transfer the skewers to a baking sheet and cook for an extra 2 minutes in the oven.

4 Serve with lime wedges.

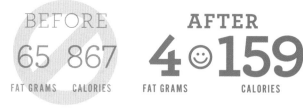

BEFORE
65 867
FAT GRAMS    CALORIES

AFTER
4 ☺ 159
FAT GRAMS    CALORIES

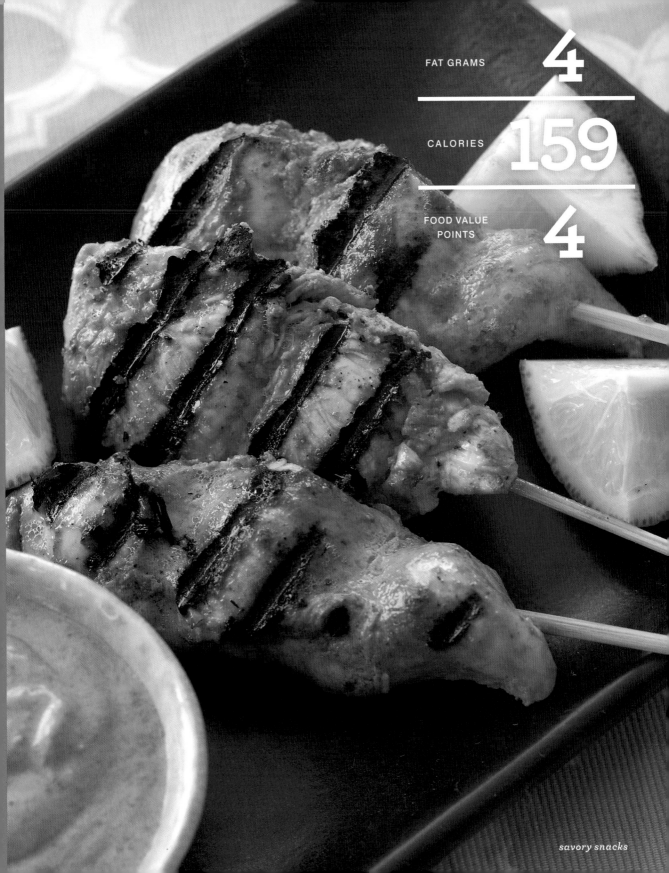

FAT GRAMS **4**

CALORIES **159**

FOOD VALUE POINTS **4**

*savory snacks*

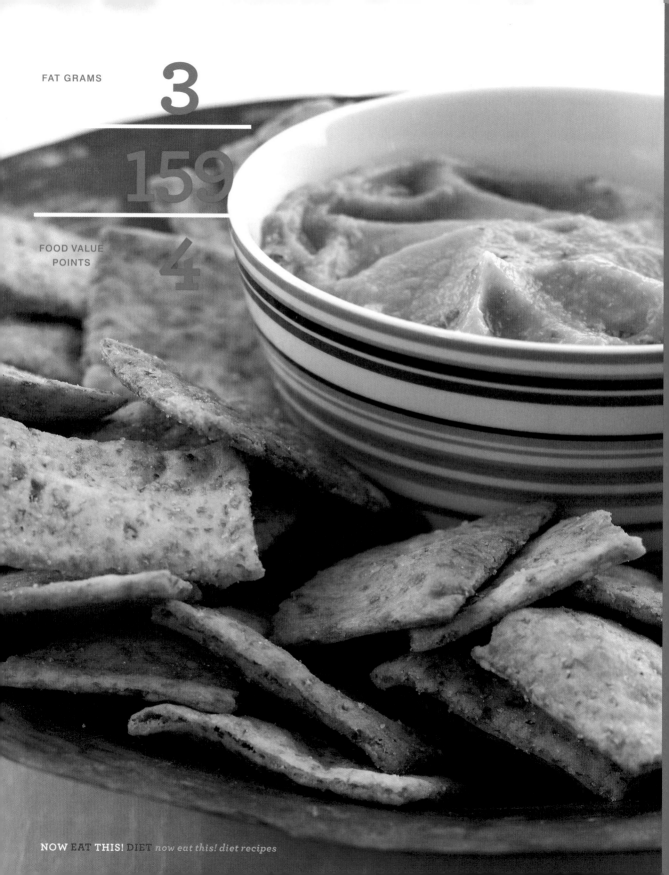

FAT GRAMS

**3**

CALORIES

**159**

FOOD VALUE
POINTS

**4**

# Pita Chips with Charred Eggplant Dip

SERVES 4

**WINGS, NACHOS, AND CHEESE** balls may strike many people as the quintessential snack foods. But what about charred eggplant dip, also known as baba ghanoush? (That's a Middle Eastern eggplant-based spread, not a defensive lineman for the NFL.) It's a superhealthy dip that's gaining in popularity. I make mine without sesame tahini, which packs in 200 calories for 2 tablespoons. Instead, I use white beans to thicken the dip without adding too many fat grams.

## INGREDIENTS

| | |
|---|---|
| 1 | large eggplant |
| ⅓ | cup cannellini beans, drained and rinsed |
| 1 | garlic clove, coarsely chopped |
| 5 | teaspoons lemon juice |
| | Pinch of ground cumin |
| | Salt |
| | Freshly ground black pepper |
| 3 | teaspoons chopped fresh flat-leaf parsley |
| 4 | ounces whole wheat baked pita chips (28 chips; 7 chips per serving), such as 365 Everyday Value |

PER SERVING
**159** calories **3g** fat ( **0g** sat / **0g** mono / **0g** poly )
**0mg** cholesterol **232mg** sodium
**28g** carbohydrate **8g** fiber **6g** protein

## METHOD

1 Place the eggplant on the grate of a gas burner over a high flame. Char the eggplant, turning it every few minutes, until the skin is blackened and the flesh is cooked through; this should take about 12 minutes. (Alternatively, you can char the eggplant on a barbecue grill, on a grill pan, or on a baking sheet under the broiler of a gas or electric oven.) Allow the eggplant to cool slightly, and then cut it in half. Scrape out the flesh, being careful not to incorporate the blackened skin, into the bowl of a food processor.

2 Add the beans, garlic, lemon juice, and cumin to the food processor bowl. Puree until smooth. Season with salt and pepper to taste.

3 Transfer the mixture to a serving bowl. Sprinkle parsley over the mixture and serve with pita chips.

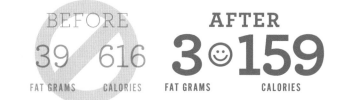

BEFORE
39 616
FAT GRAMS  CALORIES

AFTER
3 ☺ 159
FAT GRAMS  CALORIES

*savory snacks*

# South of the Border Loaded Potato Skins

SERVES 4

**EVER ORDER STUFFED POTATO SKINS** as an appetizer at a dinner-house chain? Estimated damage in a typical 12-ounce (8-skin) serving: some 600 to 1,100 calories and 40 to 80 grams of fat, most of them artery-clogging. But don't panic. There's no reason to stop eating potato skins—as long as they are the ones in my recipe. They're light because of reduced-fat ingredients like cheddar cheese and sour cream.

## INGREDIENTS

| | |
|---|---|
| 2 | medium russet potatoes (about 8 ounces each), scrubbed |
| | Nonstick cooking spray |
| | Salt |
| | Freshly ground black pepper |
| ¾ | cup mild or spicy salsa, such as Pace |
| 1 | cup (about 1 ounce) coarsely crumbled baked corn chips, such as Guiltless Gourmet |
| 1 | cup shredded (about 3½ ounces) 50% reduced-fat cheddar cheese, such as Cabot |
| 1 | tablespoon finely chopped jalapeño pepper (leave the seeds in if you like it hot) |
| ¼ | cup reduced-fat sour cream, such as Breakstone's |
| 2 | tablespoons chopped fresh cilantro |

PER SERVING
**159** calories **8g** fat ( **4g** sat / **0.5g** mono / **1g** poly )
**21mg** cholesterol **622mg** sodium
**15g** carbohydrate **2g** fiber **10g** protein

## METHOD

1 Preheat the oven to 475°F. Line a baking sheet with foil, and set it aside.

2 Prick the surface of the potatoes several times with a fork. Microwave the potatoes on high until they are completely cooked through, about 12 minutes, turning them halfway through. Let the potatoes cool until you can handle them.

3 Cut each potato in half lengthwise. Using a small spoon, scoop out and discard (or reserve for another use) the flesh of the potatoes, leaving a very thin wall of flesh— less than ¼ inch thick—attached to the skin.

4 Put the potato shells on the prepared baking sheet, hollowed side up. Spray them inside and out with cooking spray, and season with salt and pepper to taste. Bake the potato shells until they are golden brown and beginning to crisp, about 10 minutes. If the bottoms of the shells start to brown too much, flip the shells over and continue baking.

5 Spoon 2 tablespoons of salsa into each shell. Scatter the crumbled chips over the salsa. Toss the cheese and jalapeño together in a small bowl and top the chips with the cheese mix. Bake until the cheese is bubbly, about 8 minutes.

6 Serve the potatoes topped with dollops of sour cream and the remaining salsa and a sprinkling of cilantro.

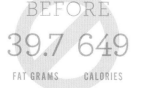

BEFORE
39.7 649
FAT GRAMS    CALORIES

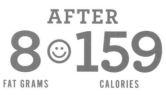

AFTER
8 ☺ 159
FAT GRAMS    CALORIES

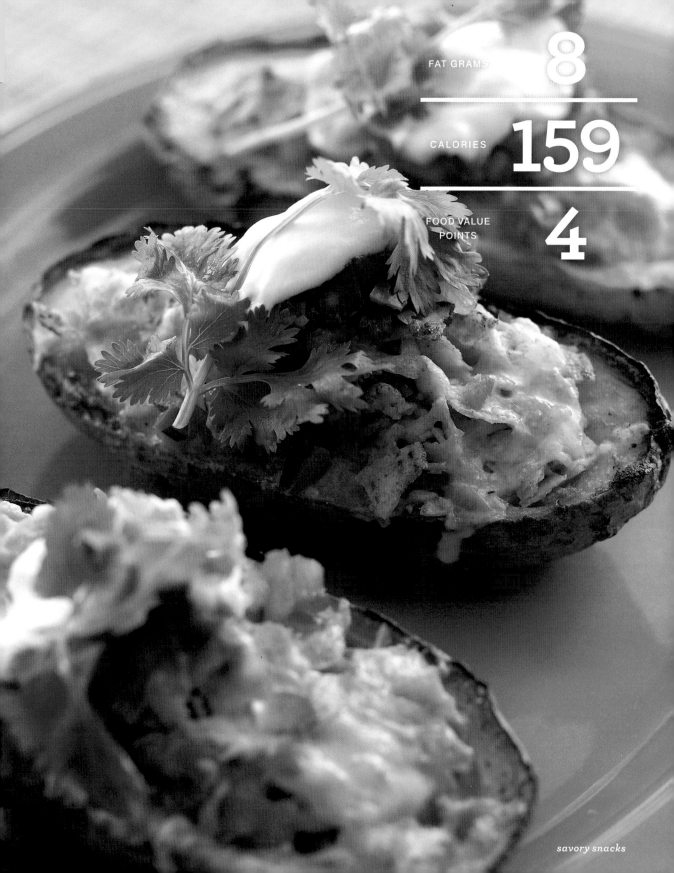

# Tuna Croquettes with Dill Relish

SERVES 4
(3 croquettes per serving)

**I LOVE THESE** simple snacks made with tuna. You just mash up some tuna, mix in onions, relish, fat-free mayo, fresh herbs, and whole wheat panko bread crumbs, and then bake in the oven. Any dried-out leftovers are excellent for table hockey. But don't worry; there won't be any leftovers. **✱ TIP**: If you're worried about consuming tuna because of mercury content, the FDA says it's okay to eat up to 6 ounces of albacore tuna per week. I prefer albacore tuna over chunk light because the texture is not as mushy. But you can use chunk light if you prefer. Always use tuna packed in water, not in oil, so you don't have all the added calories.

## INGREDIENTS

|   | |
|---|---|
|  | Nonstick cooking spray |
| 1 | (12-ounce) can albacore tuna packed in water, drained |
| ¼ | cup chopped yellow onion |
| 1 | tablespoon chopped fresh flat-leaf parsley |
| 1 | tablespoon chopped fresh dill, plus 12 sprigs |
| 1 | teaspoon lemon zest |
| ¼ | cup plus 2 teaspoons no-sugar-added sweet relish, such as Mt. Olive |
| ½ | cup fat-free mayonnaise |
|  | Salt |
|  | Frsshly ground black pepper |
| ½ | cup whole wheat panko bread crumbs, such as Ian's All-Natural |

## METHOD

1 Preheat the oven to 450°F. Spray a 12-cup mini-muffin pan with cooking spray, and set it aside.

2 In a medium bowl, combine the tuna, onion, parsley, dill, lemon zest, ¼ cup relish, and ¼ cup mayonnaise. Season with salt and pepper to taste.

3 Put the panko in a shallow dish. Divide the tuna mixture into 12 equal portions, and roll each portion into a ball. Roll the tuna balls in the panko to coat completely.

4 Place the croquettes into the cups of the prepared muffin pan. Spray the tops of the croquettes with cooking spray. Bake until the breading is golden and the croquettes are hot throughout, about 4 to 5 minutes.

5 While the croquettes are baking, add the remaining relish and mayonnaise to a small bowl. Stir together and set aside.

6 Gently lift the croquettes out of the muffin pan with a fork or a mini offset spatula. Serve immediately with the sauce. Garnish with dill sprigs.

**PER SERVING**
**160**calories **3g**fat ( **0g**sat / **0.8g**mono / **0g**poly )
**41mg**cholesterol **565mg**sodium
**14g**carbohydrate **2g**fiber **22g**protein

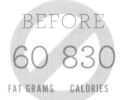

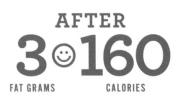

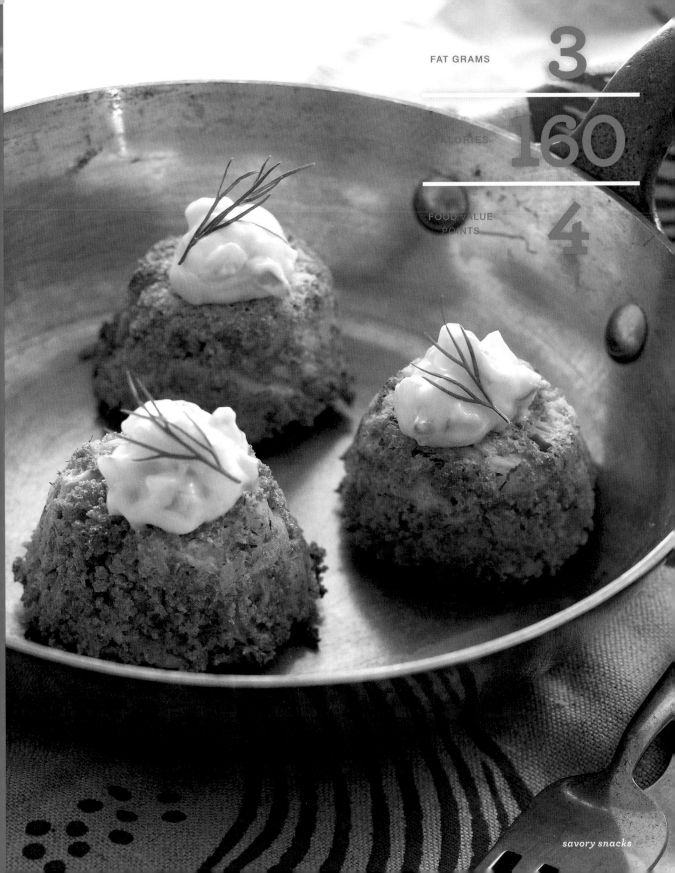

FAT GRAMS **3**

CALORIES **160**

FOOD VALUE POINTS **4**

*savory snacks*

# Crunchy Tomato Bread

**I'M HAPPY TO REPORT THE LATEST,** greatest news: Bread has been vindicated. A bunch of new studies on carbs show that not eating them can make you moody, angry, and hostile. Rejoice! Now we know what millions of Italians have known for years without having to research anything.

On the heels of this news, I give you my Crunchy Tomato Bread. Italians call a toast like this bruschetta (pronounced *broo-SKEH-tah*) from the word *bruscare,* meaning to roast over the coals (except here you use a toaster). This bread is perfect served as a snack or an appetizer. It does wonders to comfort the beast of hunger while you're deciding what's for dinner. I like to use canned plum tomatoes. They have an intense flavor that fresh ones cannot match. Look for them around the pasta sauce section in the supermarket.

## INGREDIENTS

| | |
|---|---|
| 8 | ounces whole wheat baguette |
| 1 | garlic clove |
| 1 | cup canned peeled plum tomatoes, roughly chopped |
| ½ | teaspoon dried oregano |
| | Pinch of red pepper flakes |
| ¼ | cup grated Parmigiano-Reggiano |
| 1 | teaspoon extra-virgin olive oil |
| | Salt |
| | Freshly ground black pepper |

## METHOD

1 Cut the bread in half lengthwise. Place it in the toaster oven and toast.

2 Rub the toasted halves with the clove of garlic. Divide the tomatoes in half, and distribute them over the bread pieces. Sprinkle the oregano, red pepper flakes, and cheese over the bread. Top with a few drops of olive oil, and then season with salt and pepper to taste.

3 Transfer the bread back to the toaster oven and toast until the tomatoes are warmed through and the cheese is melted, about 5 minutes.

4 Slice into 8 separate pieces. Serve immediately.

PER SERVING
**168** calories **3g** fat ( **1g** sat / **1.3g** mono / **0g** poly )
**4mg** cholesterol **394mg** sodium
**28g** carbohydrate **4g** fiber **8g** protein

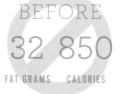

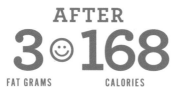

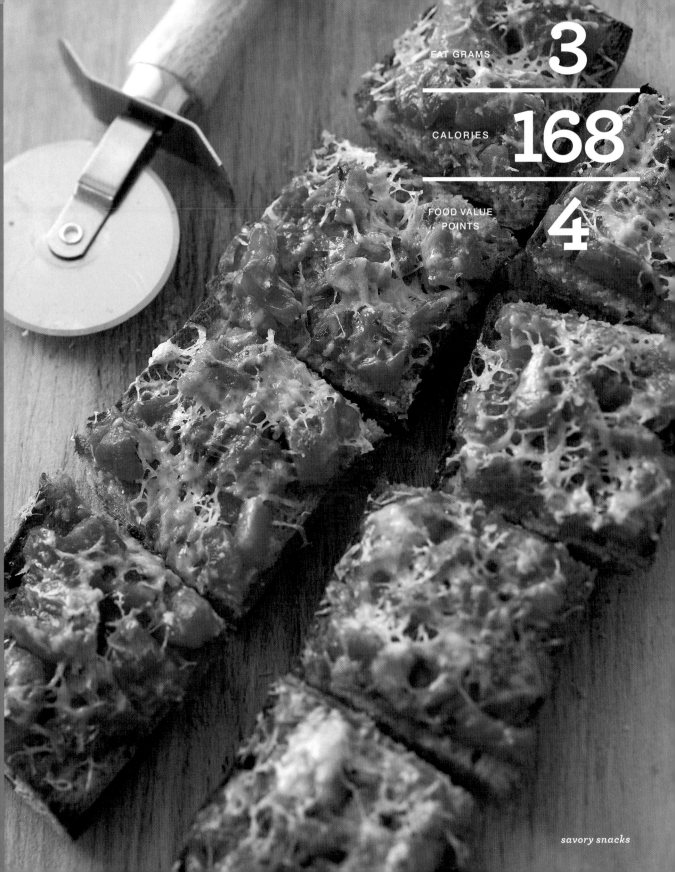

FAT GRAMS **3**

CALORIES **168**

FOOD VALUE POINTS **4**

*savory snacks*

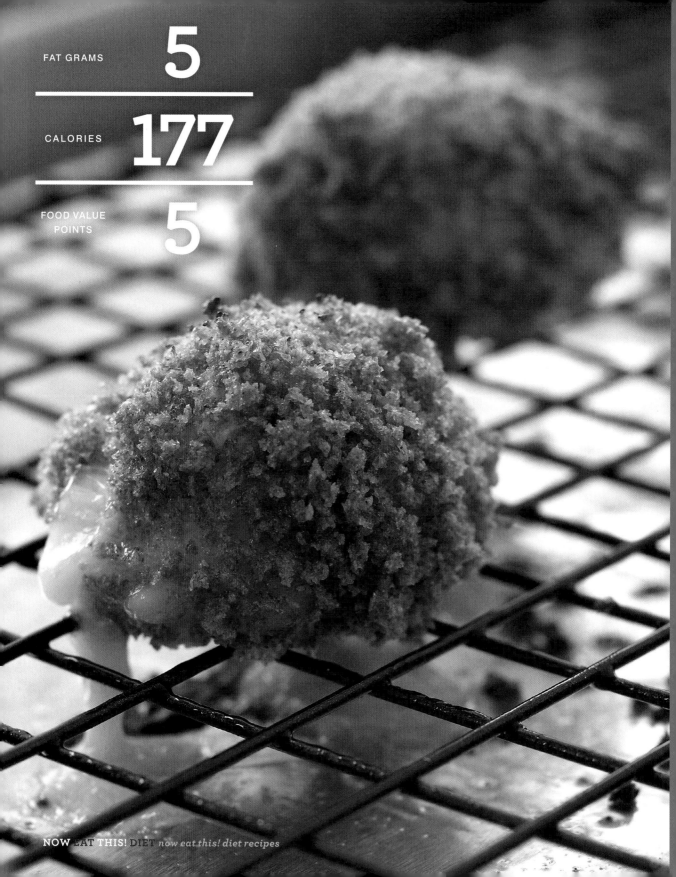

FAT GRAMS **5**

CALORIES **177**

FOOD VALUE
POINTS **5**

# "Fried" Cheese Balls

**YOU THINK I MUST BE KIDDING,** right? The to-die-for stuff you wash down with a few beers at a sports bar? Isn't this the kind of snack that can induce an angioplasty? No, no, and no. These things don't even go near a deep fat fryer. They're "oven fried," and hardly a drop of oil is used.

## INGREDIENTS

| | |
|---|---|
| 1 | cup frozen chopped onions and peppers, defrosted |
| 4 | ounces (about 1 cup) shredded 50% cheddar cheese, such as Cabot |
| 1 | teaspoon cornstarch |
| | Salt |
| | Freshly ground black pepper |
| ½ | cup whole wheat flour |
| 1½ | cups whole wheat panko bread crumbs, such as Ian's All-Natural |
| 2 | large egg whites |
| | Nonstick cooking spray |
| ½ | cup unsweetened applesauce |
| 1 | teaspoon chopped pickled jalapeños |
| 1 | teaspoon Dijon mustard |

PER SERVING
**177** calories **5g** fat ( **3g** sat / **0g** mono / **0g** poly )
**15mg** cholesterol **247mg** sodium
**23g** carbohydrate **3g** fiber **13g** protein

## METHOD

1  In a medium bowl, mix the pepper and onion mixture with the cheese and cornstarch. Season with salt and pepper to taste. Form the mixture into 8 balls, squeezing out any excess liquid. (The balls will seem loose.) Transfer the balls to a plate and freeze for at least 15 minutes.

2  Preheat the oven to 450°F. Place a wire rack on a foil-lined baking sheet, and set it aside.

3  Put the flour in a shallow dish. Put the panko in another shallow dish. In a medium bowl, whip the egg whites with a whisk until they are extremely foamy but not quite holding peaks.

4  Working in batches, dredge the cheese balls in the flour, shaking off any excess. Add the cheese balls to the egg whites and toss to coat them completely. Add the cheese balls, a few pieces at a time, to the bowl of panko and coat completely.

5  Spread the balls on the wire rack. Spray them lightly with cooking spray. Bake the cheese balls until the breading is golden and crispy, about 5 to 7 minutes.

6  Meanwhile, combine the applesauce, jalapeños, and mustard in a small bowl. Season with salt and pepper to taste.

7  Serve the cheese balls immediately with the sauce.

**✶ CALORIE SAVER**
Omit the sauce and save **14** calories per serving.

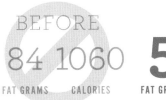

BEFORE
84 1060
FAT GRAMS    CALORIES

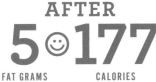

**AFTER**
5 ☺ **177**
FAT GRAMS    CALORIES

# Mama's Mini Meatball Bites

**THIS DISH IS A SNACK-SIZE** version of my mother's signature dish, fondly known as Mama's Meatballs. While you won't find them atop a mound of begging-to-be-swirled spaghetti, you'll still be wowed by their full-on flavor. In fact, they might even inspire you to stick to all your New Year's resolutions. I lowered the fat in this dish by using ground turkey. Make sure you buy "ground turkey breast," which contains the white meat and no skin. Regular "ground turkey" is made from dark and white meats and some skin.

## INGREDIENTS

Nonstick cooking spray

1 small eggplant

2 tablespoons low-fat, low-sodium chicken broth

¼ small yellow onion

1 garlic clove

1 large egg white

12 ounces lean ground turkey breast

¼ cup chopped fresh flat-leaf parsley

6 tablespoons grated Parmigiano-Reggiano cheese

Salt

Freshly ground black pepper

¾ cup low-fat marinara sauce

### PER SERVING
**177** calories **5g** fat ( **1.7g** sat / **1g** mono / **0.7g** poly )
**41mg** cholesterol **379mg** sodium
**8.5g** carbohydrate **1.6g** fiber **26g** protein

## METHOD

1 Preheat the oven to 450°F. Spray a 12-cup mini-muffin pan with cooking spray, and set it aside.

2 Place the eggplant on the grate of a gas burner over a high flame. Char the eggplant, turning it every few minutes, until the skin is blackened and the flesh is cooked through; this should take about 12 minutes. (Alternatively, you can char the eggplant on a barbecue grill, on a grill pan, or on a baking sheet under the broiler of a gas or electric oven.) Allow the eggplant to cool slightly, and then cut it in half. Scrape out the flesh, being careful not to incorporate the blackened skin. Measure out ¼ cup of the flesh; reserve the remaining eggplant for another use.

3 In a blender, combine the cooked eggplant, chicken broth, onion, garlic, and egg white. Puree until the mixture is smooth. In a large bowl, combine the pureed mixture with the ground turkey, parsley, and 2 tablespoons of the cheese. Season lightly with salt and pepper. Set aside.

4 Spoon about half of the marinara sauce into the cups of the prepared muffin pan; then drop rounded tablespoons (about 2 ounces each) of the meat mixture into the cups. Top the meat with the remaining marinara sauce. (The cups will look overfilled, but the meat will shrink when cooked through.) Bake until the meatballs are done, about 15 to 20 minutes.

5 Sprinkle the remaining cheese on top, and serve.

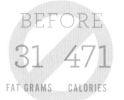

BEFORE
31 471
FAT GRAMS CALORIES

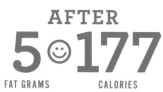

AFTER
5 ☺ 177
FAT GRAMS CALORIES

* CALORIE SAVER
Omit the Parm cheese and save **32** calories per serving.

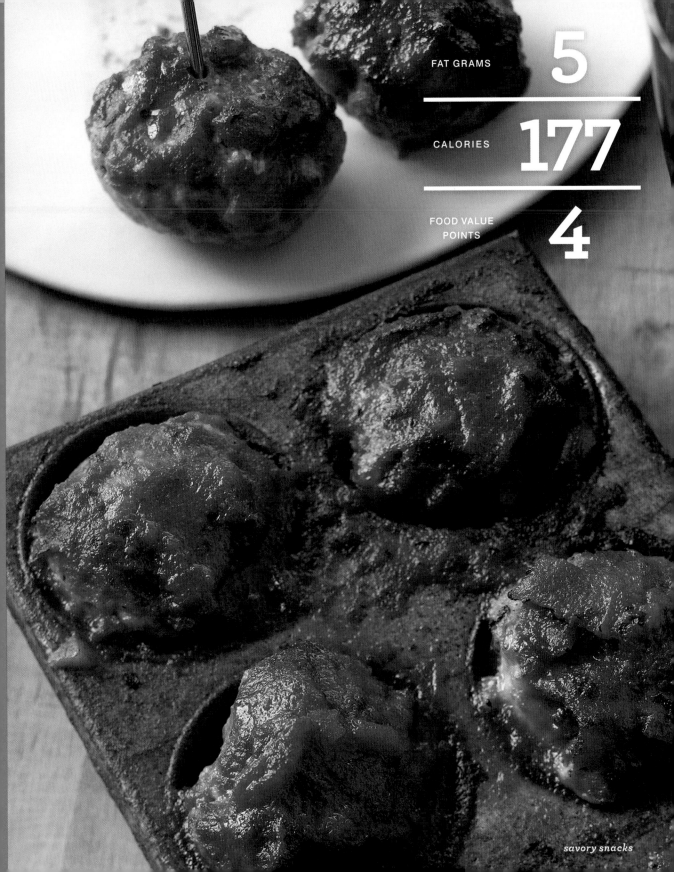

FAT GRAMS **5**

CALORIES **177**

FOOD VALUE POINTS **4**

*savory snacks*

# Eggplant and Roasted Red Pepper Torta

SERVES 4

**IF I COULD HAVE** only one Mexican food for the rest of my life, it would be a torta.

A torta is a Mexican-style sandwich that is normally in a sandwich roll. Mine is an open-faced variation using low-carb tortillas. These tortillas are so versatile. A lot of carb-busters recommend replacing sliced bread with tortillas for sandwiches. Don't skip the lemon juice in this snack! It makes the dish brighter and fresher. And for the vegetarians in the room, this dish is completely meat-free.

## INGREDIENTS

   Nonstick cooking spray
½  medium eggplant
   Salt
   Freshly ground black pepper
2  (9-inch) low-carb tortillas, such as La Tortilla Factory
5  ounces (1¼ cups) shredded part-skim mozzarella cheese
½  cup jarred roasted red peppers, such as Cento Roasted Peppers
2  tablespoons chopped fresh flat-leaf parsley
1  tablespoon chopped fresh mint
   Juice of ½ lemon

PER SERVING
**183**calories **9g**fat ( **4g**sat / **2.7g**mono / **0.8g**poly )
**19mg**cholesterol **447mg**sodium
**17g**carbohydrate **9g**fiber **14g**protein

## METHOD

1 Preheat the oven to 425°F. Heat a grill pan over high heat. Line a baking sheet with foil.

2 Slice the eggplant crosswise into ½-inch slices. When the pan is hot, remove it from the stove and coat it with cooking spray. In batches, lay the eggplant slices on the pan and season with salt and pepper to taste. Grill until the eggplant slices are soft and pliable, about 5 to 6 minutes each side. Remove from heat and set aside. Repeat with remaining eggplant until finished.

3 Place the tortillas on the baking sheet and spray them on both sides with cooking spray. Toast the tortillas in the oven until they are brown and crispy, about 3 minutes each side.

4 Scatter half of the cheese on both tortillas. Divide the eggplant and red peppers over the tortillas and then scatter the chopped parsley and mint over the vegetables. Divide the remaining mozzarella cheese and scatter over the vegetables. Sprinkle the lemon juice over the vegetables and cheese. Season with salt and pepper to taste. Transfer the baking sheet to the oven and bake till the cheese is melted and the vegetables are hot throughout, about 8 minutes.

5 Using a spatula, carefully lift one of the tortillas and place it on top of the other tortilla. Transfer the torta to a cutting board and cut into wedges. Serve immediately.

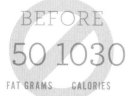

BEFORE
50 1030
FAT GRAMS    CALORIES

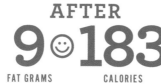

AFTER
9 ☺ 183
FAT GRAMS    CALORIES

**✳ CALORIE SAVER**

Cut the cheese in half and save **54** calories per serving.

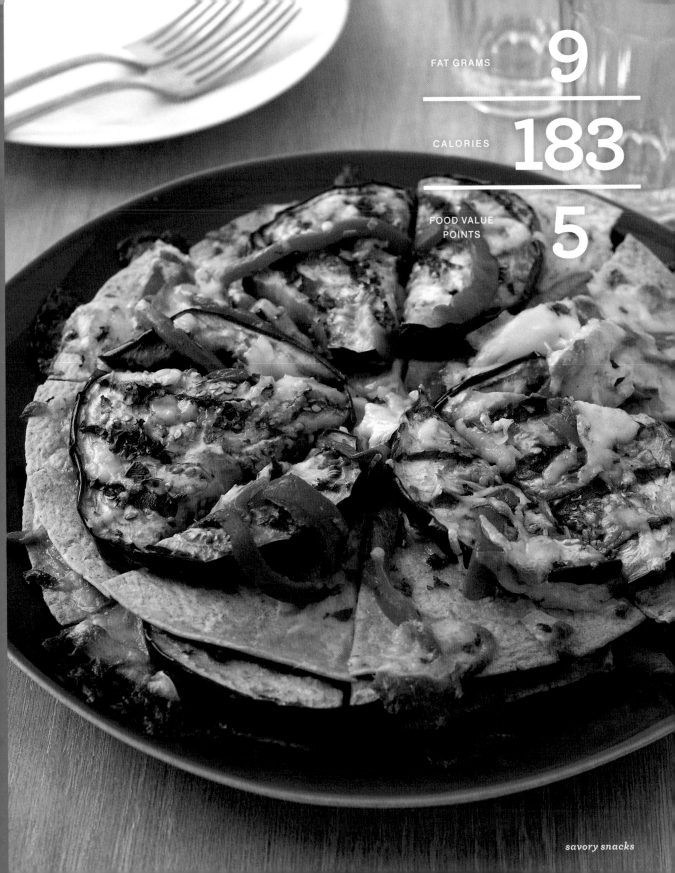

FAT GRAMS **9**

CALORIES **183**

FOOD VALUE POINTS **5**

*savory snacks*

# Hogs Undercover

SERVES 4

**EVEN THE NAME** of this holiday entertaining favorite sounds unhealthy: Hogs Undercover, also known as "pigs in a blanket." As tasty as they are, the traditional version of this popular appetizer takes the already-suspect hot dog and sends it over a nutritional cliff by wrapping it in fatty puff pastry. Mindlessly scarf down just three or four of these at a party, and you could swallow 500 calories or more. But with the right ingredients, namely, whole wheat pizza dough and Italian chicken-turkey sausage, it's possible to make a healthier version. You can find whole wheat pizza dough in the freezer or refrigerated section of the supermarket, or you can use the recipe for my whole wheat pizza dough (page 166). So no matter what you call them . . . call me when they're done.

## INGREDIENTS

Nonstick cooking spray

6   ounces whole wheat pizza dough, from page 166 or such as Papa Sal's

2   sweet Italian chicken and turkey sausages, such as Applegate Farms

1   teaspoon grated Parmigiano-Reggiano

1   teaspoon grated Romano cheese

1   cup low-fat marinara sauce, such as Victoria or Trader Joe's

### PER SERVING

**189** calories **5g** fat ( **1g** sat / **0g** mono / **0g** poly )
**36mg** cholesterol **716mg** sodium
**26g** carbohydrate **2g** fiber **11g** protein

## METHOD

1  Preheat the oven to 400°F. Line a baking sheet with foil. Coat lightly with nonstick cooking spray and set aside.

2  Divide the pizza dough into four equal pieces. Using a rolling pin, roll the dough into 2 x 4-inch rectangles.

3  Cut the sausages in half crosswise, and then wrap the dough securely around them.

4  Place the rolled sausages, seam side down, on the prepared baking sheet and sprinkle the cheeses on top. Spray them lightly with cooking spray, and bake until they are golden brown, about 15 minutes.

5  Meanwhile, heat the marinara sauce in a small microwave-safe bowl in the microwave.

6  Serve the sausages with the sauce for dipping.

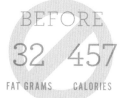

BEFORE
32 457
FAT GRAMS   CALORIES

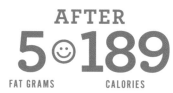

AFTER
5 ☺ 189
FAT GRAMS   CALORIES

**\* CALORIE SAVER**

Omit the marinara sauce and save **30** calories per serving.

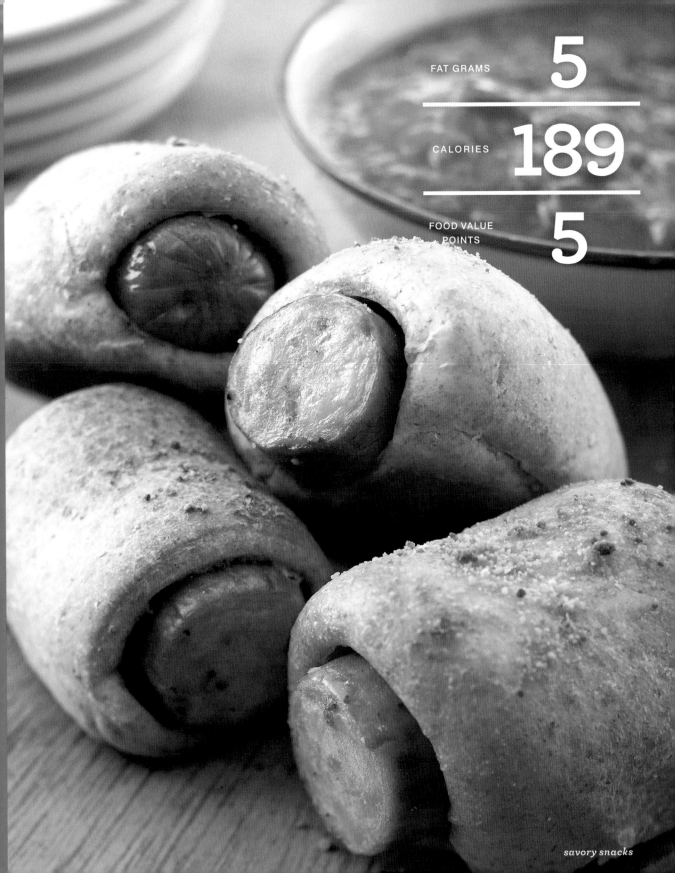

FAT GRAMS
**5**

CALORIES
**189**

FOOD VALUE
POINTS
**5**

*savory snacks*

# Chicken Tenders with Ranch Dressing

**MY RECIPE FOR** chicken tenders is a far cry from the fast-food mainstay. I'm talking legitimate chicken here: meaty tenders lightly breaded with whole wheat panko bread crumbs and *not* bone, skin, beak, and fat ground together in a giant blender until who knows what you're eating. They're plump, delicious, hot, and so succulent that adults gobble them up as fast as kids do.

## INGREDIENTS

| | |
|---|---|
| 1 | cup whole wheat flour |
| 2½ | cups whole wheat panko bread crumbs, such as Ian's All-Natural |
| ½ | teaspoon poultry seasoning, such as Spice Hunter |
| 4 | large egg whites |
| 8 | ounces (about 8) chicken tenders |
| | Salt |
| | Freshly ground black pepper |
| | Nonstick cooking spray |
| 3 | teaspoons ranch salad dressing and seasoning mix, such as Hidden Valley |
| 6 | tablespoons (about 3 ounces) reduced-fat sour cream, such as Breakstone's |
| 6 | tablespoons (about 3 ounces) low-fat buttermilk |

PER SERVING

**198** calories **5g** fat ( **2g** sat / **1.4g** mono / **0g** poly )
**46mg** cholesterol **352mg** sodium
**19g** carbohydrate **2g** fiber **19g** protein

## METHOD

1 Preheat the oven to 450°F. Place a wire rack on a foil-lined baking sheet, and set it aside.

2 Put the flour in a shallow dish. Mix the panko and poultry seasoning together in another shallow dish. In a medium bowl, whip the egg whites with a whisk until they are extremely foamy, but not quite holding peaks.

3 Season the chicken with salt and pepper to taste. Working in batches, dredge the chicken tenders in the flour, shaking off any excess. Add the chicken to the egg whites and toss to coat them completely. Add the chicken, a few pieces at a time, to the bowl of panko and coat completely.

4 Spread the chicken out on the wire rack. Season the chicken well with salt and pepper, and spray lightly with cooking spray. Bake the tenders until the breading is golden and crispy and the chicken is cooked through, about 10 minutes.

5 Meanwhile, in a small bowl, mix the salad dressing mix with the sour cream and buttermilk.

6 Serve the chicken tenders with the ranch dressing.

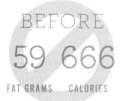

BEFORE
59 666
FAT GRAMS    CALORIES

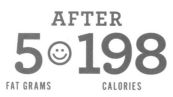

AFTER
5 ☺ 198
FAT GRAMS    CALORIES

**✳ CALORIE SAVER**
Omit the salad dressing, sour cream, and buttermilk and save **45** calories per serving.

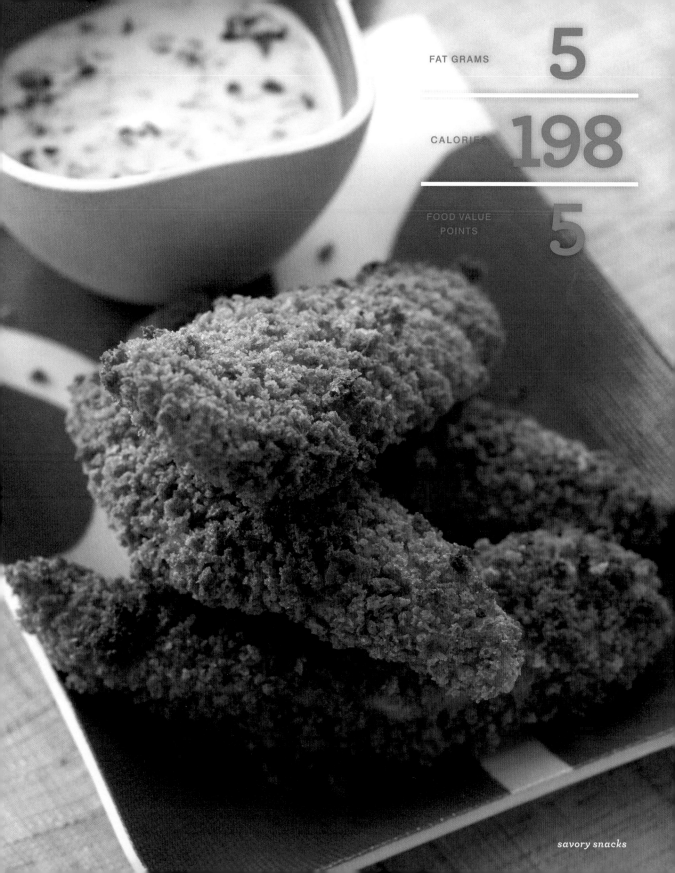

FAT GRAMS 5

CALORIES 198

FOOD VALUE POINTS 5

*savory snacks*

# Shrimp and Cheddar Tostada with Salsa Verde

SERVES 4

**A TOSTADA IS BASICALLY A** flat tortilla with various fillings piled on it—in this case, we're piling on shrimp and cheese. To save time, look for already-prepared shrimp or shrimp cocktail in the seafood department. Alternatively, you can use precooked frozen shrimp. To pull the shrimp tails off, grasp the body of the shrimp with one hand and with the thumb and index finger of your other hand squeeze and twist the tail off. Tostadas usually require the tortillas to be fried, but this one is baked till brown and crispy, saving you fat and calories.

## INGREDIENTS

Nonstick cooking spray

2   (9-inch) low-carb tortillas, such as La Tortilla Factory

¾   pound precooked large shrimp, peeled and deveined, tails removed

½   teaspoon garlic powder

½   cup jarred tomatillo salsa

Pinch of red hot pepper flakes

¼   cup chopped fresh cilantro

Salt

Freshly ground black pepper

3   ounces (about ¾ cup) shredded 75% reduced-fat cheddar, such as Cabot

## METHOD

1   Preheat the oven to 425°F. Line a baking sheet with aluminum foil and coat with cooking spray.

2   Place the tortillas on the baking sheet, and spray them on both sides with cooking spray. Toast the tortillas in the oven until they are brown and crispy, about 3 minutes each side.

3   Meanwhile, in a medium bowl, toss the shrimp with garlic powder, salsa, red pepper flakes, and 2 tablespoons cilantro. Season with salt and pepper to taste.

4   Scatter half the cheese on the tortillas and then equally divide the shrimp onto the tortillas. Top with the remaining cheese, and then bake in the oven till the cheese is melted and the shrimp is warmed through, about 8 minutes. (Watch carefully to make sure the tortillas do not burn.)

5   Sprinkle the remaining cilantro over the tostadas and transfer them to a cutting board. Cut into wedges and serve immediately.

PER SERVING
**200** calories **5g** fat ( **1g** sat / **1.3g** mono / **0.5g** poly )
**180mg** cholesterol **723mg** sodium
**12g** carbohydrate **6g** fiber **32g** protein

BEFORE
70 1089
FAT GRAMS    CALORIES

AFTER
5 ☺ 200
FAT GRAMS    CALORIES

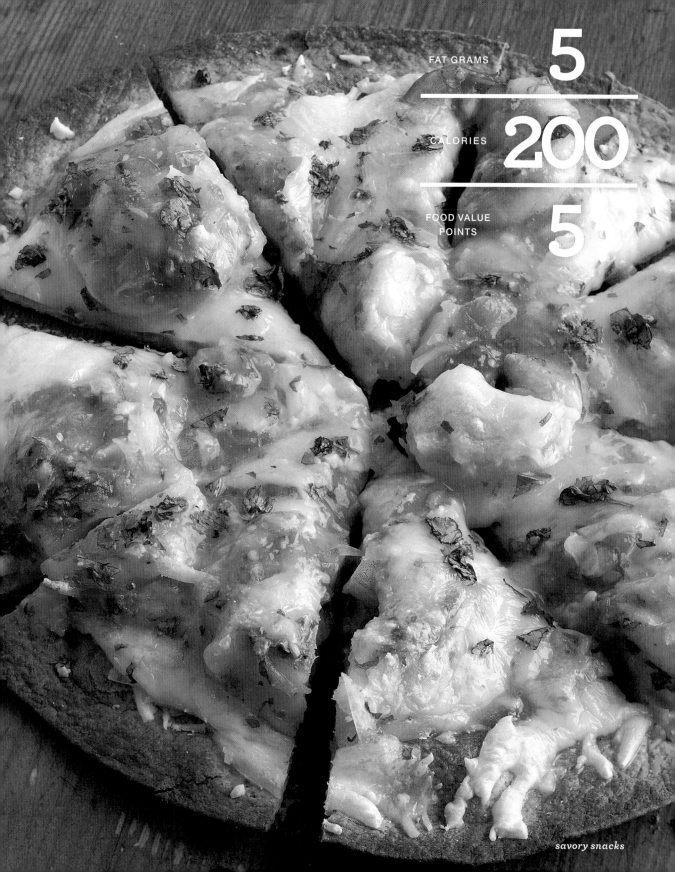

FAT GRAMS

5

CALORIES

200

FOOD VALUE
POINTS

5

*savory snacks*

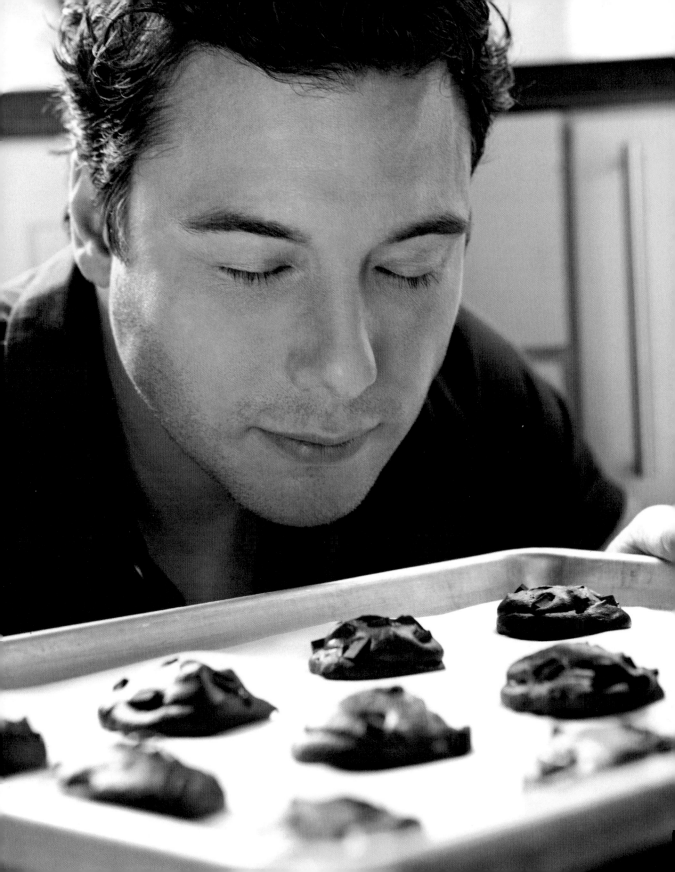

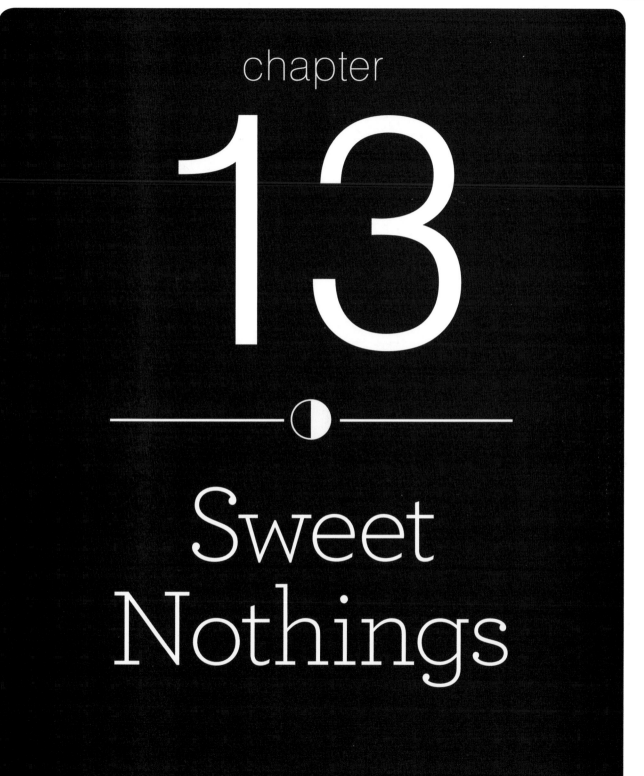

chapter

# 13

## Sweet Nothings

# PBJ Cookies

MAKES 20 COOKIES
(55 calories each)

**WHEN I THINK OF GREAT DUOS,** several pop into mind: Batman and Robin, Dean Martin and Jerry Lewis, Brooks and Dunn, and the best of all, peanut butter and chocolate. If you love peanut butter and chocolate, now you can get your fix but without the calories. (I didn't take out all the calories; I left in 55.) Everyone knows that these are two tastes that go great together, but this confection takes the combo to a whole new level of healthy decadence. While there isn't any jelly in the cookie, I got my fruity sweetness from dried cranberries. Feel free to use mini peanut butter chips in these cookies if you can find them.

## INGREDIENTS

Nonstick cooking spray

¼ cup dried cranberries

½ teaspoon vanilla extract

⅓ cup unsweetened cocoa powder, sifted

1 cup canned white cannellini beans, rinsed and drained

¼ cup reduced-fat peanut butter, such as Better'n Peanut Butter

2 tablespoons agave nectar

3 large egg whites

4 packets (about 4 grams) powdered stevia, such as SweetLeaf

¼ cup puffed millet cereal, such as Arrowhead Mills

¼ cup peanut butter chips

PER SERVING

**55**calories **1g**fat ( **1g**sat / **0g**mono / **0g**poly )
**0mg**cholesterol **69mg**sodium
**9g**carbohydrate **1g**fiber **3g**protein

## METHOD

1 Preheat the oven to 375°F. Line 2 baking sheets with parchment paper and spray lightly with cooking spray. Set aside.

2 In a small bowl, add the cranberries. Pour in hot water to cover and allow to soak.

3 Meanwhile, in the bowl of a food processor, combine the vanilla, cocoa, cannellini beans, peanut butter, and agave. Blend until the mixture is smooth, about 3 minutes, scraping down the side of the bowl halfway through blending.

4 In the bowl of a mixer fitted with a whip attachment, beat the egg whites until they form soft peaks. Gradually beat in the stevia. Continue to beat the whites until they are creamy and nearly stiff. Add one-third of the egg-white mixture to the cocoa-bean mixture in the food processor. Blend to combine, about 30 seconds. In 2 batches, fold the lightened cocoa mixture into the egg whites until they are almost fully combined.

5 Drain the liquid from the cranberries and then add the cranberries to the batter. Add the millet. Fold the batter until the cranberries and millet are evenly dispersed and the cocoa mixture is completely incorporated.

6 Drop mounded spoonfuls of the batter onto the prepared sheets. Spread the batter out to form cookies about 2 inches in diameter. Sprinkle the peanut butter chips on top of the cookies.

7 Bake for 12 to 14 minutes, rotating the pans one turn halfway through baking. Using a metal spatula, transfer the cookies to wire racks to cool.

BEFORE
**15** **397**
FAT GRAMS CALORIES

AFTER
**1** ☺ **55**
FAT GRAMS CALORIES

**✱ CALORIE SAVER**

Omit the cranberries and peanut butter chips and save **21** calories per serving.

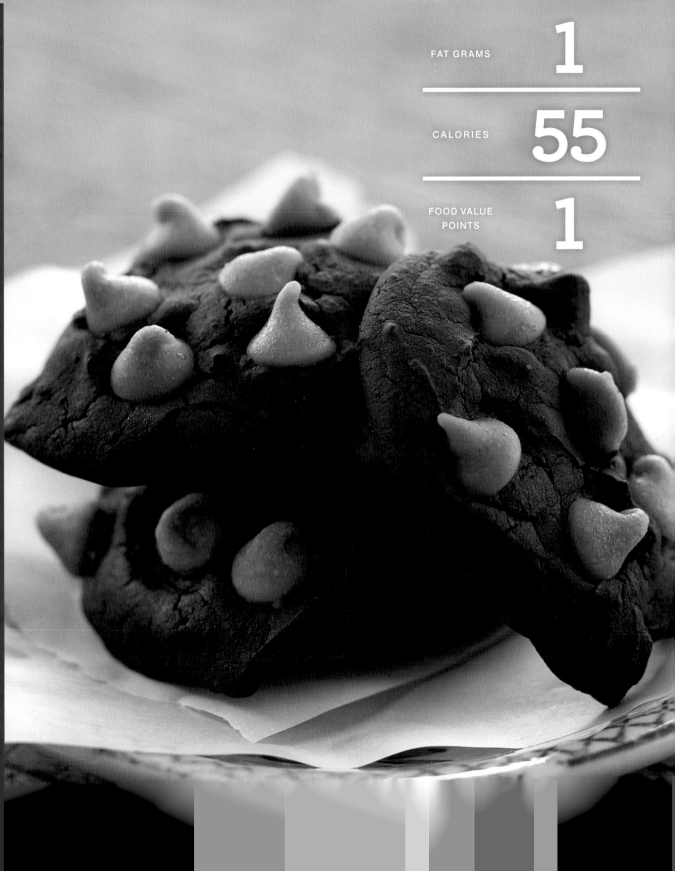

# Double Chocolate Chip Cookies

MAKES 12 LARGE COOKIES
(74 calories each)

**DID YOU EVER WISH** that chocolate chip cookies loved you as much as you love them? Well, here's a cookie that will. The puffed millet adds crunch and volume to the cookies without adding many calories. There's not a bit of flour in these cookies; I used white cannellini beans as a replacement. Everyone in your family will love these cookies, too, dieters or not. Expect them to not-so-mysteriously disappear from your house at an alarming rate … along with your weight.

## INGREDIENTS

|  | |
|---|---|
|  | Nonstick cooking spray |
| ½ | teaspoon vanilla extract |
| ⅓ | cup unsweetened cocoa powder, sifted |
| 1 | cup canned white cannellini beans, rinsed and drained |
| 2 | tablespoons agave nectar |
| 3 | large egg whites |
| 4 | packets (about 4 grams) powdered stevia, such as SweetLeaf |
| ¼ | cup puffed millet cereal, such as Arrowhead Mills |
| ¼ | cup mini chocolate chunks |
| 2 | tablespoons turbinado sugar, such as Sugar in the Raw |

### PER SERVING

**74** calories **2g** fat ( **1g** sat / **0g** mono / **0g** poly )
**0mg** cholesterol **71mg** sodium
**13g** carbohydrate **2g** fiber **3g** protein

## METHOD

1 Preheat the oven to 375°F. Line 2 baking sheets with parchment paper and spray lightly with cooking spray. Set aside.

2 In the bowl of a food processor, combine the vanilla, cocoa, cannellini beans, and agave, and blend the mixture until smooth, about 3 minutes, scraping down the sides of the bowl halfway through blending.

3 In the bowl of a mixer fitted with a whip attachment, beat the egg whites until they form soft peaks. Gradually beat in the stevia. Continue to beat the whites until they are creamy and nearly stiff. Add one-third of the egg-white mixture to the cocoa-bean mixture in the food processor. Blend to combine, about 30 seconds. In 2 batches, fold the lightened cocoa mixture into the egg whites until they are almost fully combined. Add the millet to the batter. Fold the batter until the millet is evenly dispersed and the cocoa mixture is completely incorporated.

4 Drop mounded spoonfuls of batter onto the prepared sheets. Spread the batter out to form cookies about 2½ inches in diameter. Sprinkle the chocolate chips and turbinado sugar on top of the cookies.

5 Bake for 12 to 14 minutes, rotating the pans one turn halfway through baking. Using a metal spatula, transfer the cookies to wire racks to cool.

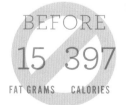

BEFORE
**15** FAT GRAMS **397** CALORIES

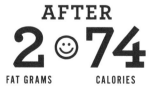

**AFTER**
**2** FAT GRAMS ☺ **74** CALORIES

**\* CALORIE SAVER**
Omit the turbinado sugar and save **8** calories per cookie.

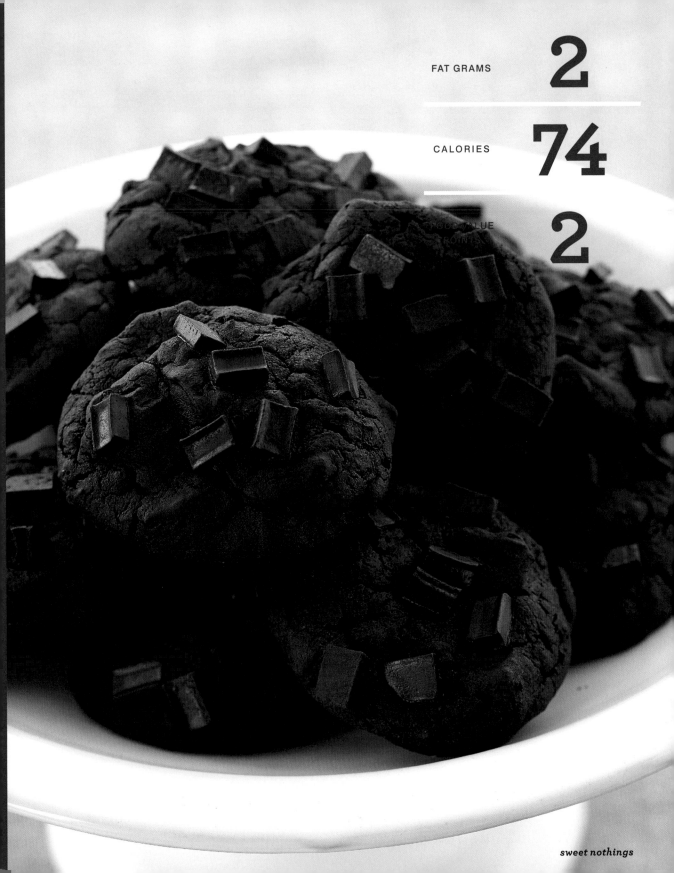

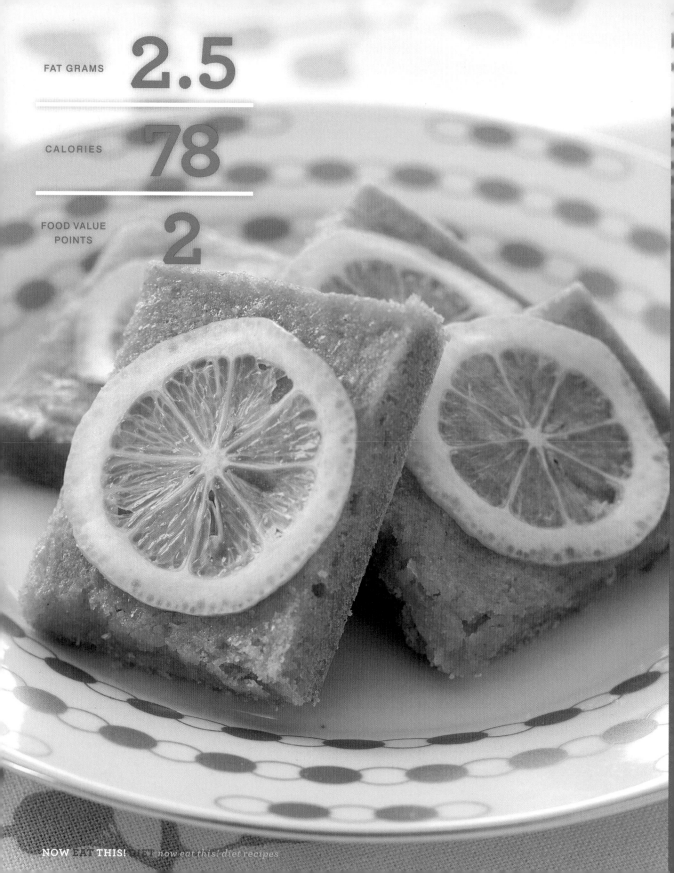

FAT GRAMS **2.5**

CALORIES **78**

FOOD VALUE POINTS **2**

# Decadent Lemon Bars

**THE BETTY CROCKER COOKBOOK** popularized lemon bars in the early sixties. Afterward, recipes popped up everywhere. An adaptation of these always popular bars, mine pairs lemon zest and lemon juice with natural sweeteners to form an elegant, tangy treat.

## INGREDIENTS

| | |
|---|---|
| | Nonstick cooking spray |
| 1 | cup whole wheat pastry flour |
| 7 | packets (7 grams) powdered stevia, such as SweetLeaf |
| 2 | tablespoons canola oil |
| 3 | large egg whites |
| ¼ | cup agave nectar |
| 1½ | tablespoons grated lemon zest |
| 1 | teaspoon baking powder |
| ½ | teaspoon salt |
| ⅔ | cup lemon juice, fresh squeezed |
| 1 | small lemon |

PER SERVING
**78** calories **2.5g** fat ( **0g** sat / **1.5g** mono / **0.7g** poly )
**0mg** cholesterol **135mg** sodium
**13g** carbohydrate **1g** fiber **2g** protein

## METHOD

1 Preheat the oven to 350°F. Spray an 8 x 8 x 2-inch baking dish with cooking spray.

2 In a large bowl, add ¾ cup of the pastry flour and 2 packets of the stevia. Stir to combine. Add the oil and continue to mix until well combined. The mixture should be rather crumbly and dry. Transfer the mixture to the baking dish and press into the bottom of the pan. Bake in the oven until golden brown, about 8 to 9 minutes.

3 In a large mixing bowl, add the egg whites, agave, and lemon zest. Mix together with a whisk until all of the ingredients are incorporated.

4 In a small bowl, add the remaining flour, baking powder, remaining stevia, and salt. Stir together, and then add to the egg white mixture. Mix well, and then beat in the lemon juice.

5 Pour the mixture into the crust and bake until the top layer is firm, about 10 minutes.

6 Meanwhile, slice the lemon on a mandoline into paper-thin circles.

7 Cool the bars, then cut into 12 even squares and place one lemon slice on top of each.

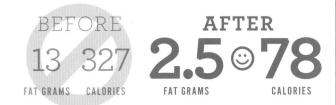

BEFORE
13 327
FAT GRAMS CALORIES

AFTER
2.5 ☺ 78
FAT GRAMS CALORIES

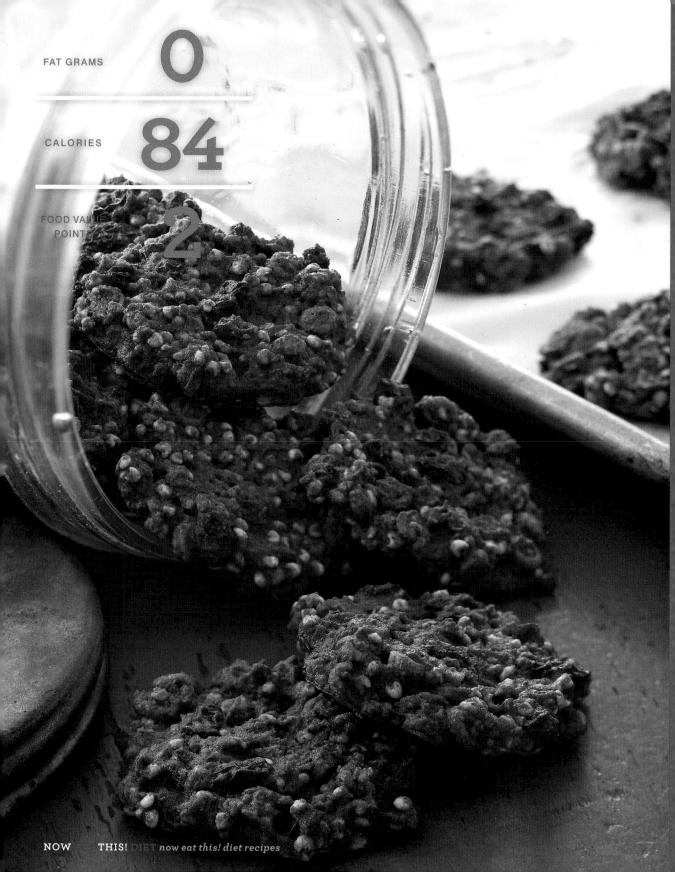

# Oatmeal Raisin Cookies

MAKES 12 COOKIES
(84 calories each)

**IF YOU ADORE** oatmeal raisin cookies, crave them like mad, you no longer have to fight the urge. You can heed the call by whipping up a batch of these. It took about a week of experimenting with many different ingredients to get this super low-in-fat, low-calorie result. You're still getting the heart benefits of oats in this cookie, but in the form of cereal. It also adds good crunch and texture to the cookies. *TIP: Use apple butter to cut the fat in baked goods. As a rule of thumb, as much as half the fat, be it butter, oil, or shortening, can be cut in some recipes by substituting apple butter. You can cut the sugar as well, because apple butter is naturally sweet. The cookies will seem loose when you spoon them onto the baking sheet, but they will firm up after baking and cooling.

## INGREDIENTS

Nonstick cooking spray

¼ cup agave nectar

1 teaspoon vanilla extract

½ cup no-sugar-added apple butter

½ cup liquid egg substitute

1 teaspoon ground cinnamon

2 cups toasted whole-grain oat cereal, such as Cheerios

1 cup puffed millet cereal, such as Arrowhead Mills

½ cup raisins

PER SERVING
**84**calories **0g**fat ( **0g**sat / **0g**mono / **0g**poly )
**0mg**cholesterol **52mg**sodium
**20g**carbohydrate **1g**fiber **2g**protein

## METHOD

1 Preheat the oven to 350°F. Line a baking sheet with parchment paper and spray lightly with cooking spray.

2 In a large bowl, add the agave, vanilla, apple butter, egg substitute, and cinnamon. Stir together until well blended.

3 Place half of the oat cereal in a reusable plastic bag, and crush with a rolling pin. Add the crushed cereal, remaining cereal, millet, and raisins to the apple-butter mixture. Stir together.

4 Spoon the cookie mixture onto the prepared baking sheets, and bake until they are lightly browned, about 15 minutes. Let cool for 5 minutes before transferring to a wire rack.

**✳ CALORIE SAVER**
Omit the raisins and save **21** calories per serving.

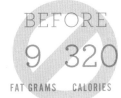

BEFORE
9 320
FAT GRAMS CALORIES

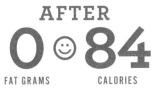

AFTER
0 ☺ 84
FAT GRAMS CALORIES

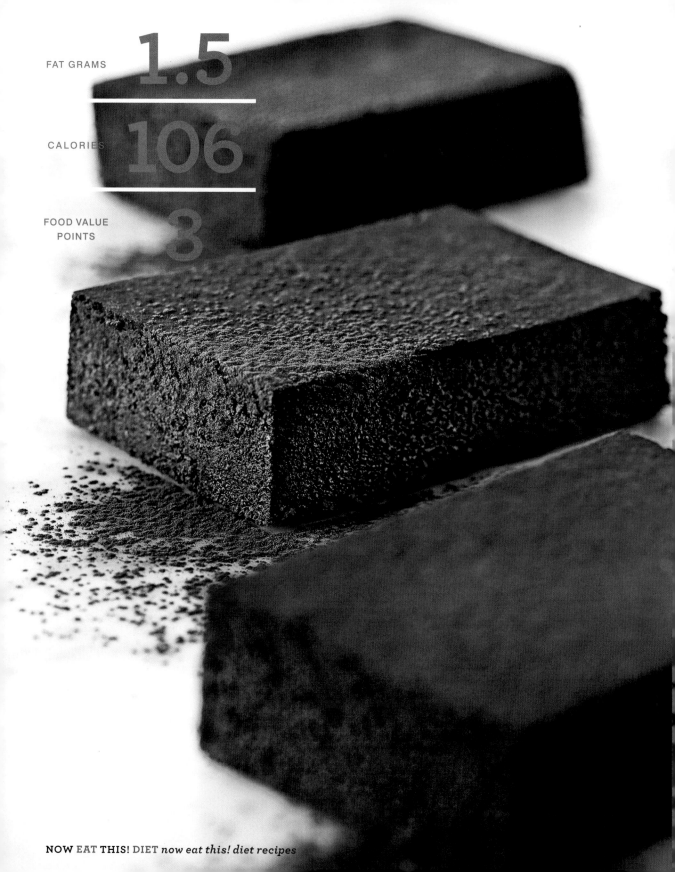

FAT GRAMS 1.5

CALORIES 106

FOOD VALUE POINTS 3

NOW EAT THIS! DIET *now eat this! diet recipes*

# Red Velvet Chocolate Squares

MAKES 12 BARS
(106 calories each)

**THE RECIPE FOR** red velvet cake has been around since the 1920s, when the cake was the signature dessert at the Waldorf-Astoria Hotel in New York City. The cake captured my heart—and it plays hard to get. It took me forever to come up with a magical adaptation that would capture the richness of its namesake. These bars get their health benefits, velvety texture, and deep red color from a paste made of beets, red beans, cocoa powder, and red food coloring. I took a slight departure from the traditional red velvet cake flavor by adding a touch of almond extract, and that, my friends, is where the magic happened.

Cold Is Best I've experimented with these squares many times in my kitchen. What I discovered is that, unlike most baked items, these squares and the Fudgy Fruit and Nut Bars (page 265) taste best after being refrigerated for at least three hours. Chilling the bars coalesces the flavor and stabilizes the texture. So please: Enjoy them cold, and you'll enjoy them more.

## INGREDIENTS

Butter-flavored nonstick cooking spray

½ cup chopped canned beets, drained

7 ounces (about 1 cup) canned red beans, drained and rinsed

½ cup unsweetened cocoa powder

¾ cup liquid egg substitute

3 tablespoons whole wheat pastry flour

¾ cup agave nectar

1 tablespoon unsalted butter, melted

1 teaspoon vanilla extract

½ teaspoon almond extract

2 teaspoons natural red food coloring

PER SERVING
**106** calories **1.5g** fat ( **1g** sat / **0g** mono / **0g** poly )
**2.5mg** cholesterol **62mg** sodium
**22g** carbohydrate **2g** fiber **3g** protein

## METHOD

1 Preheat the oven to 350°F. Spray an 8 x 8 x 2-inch baking dish with cooking spray.

2 Combine the beets, beans, cocoa powder, egg substitute, and flour in the bowl of a food processor. Process until the mixture is smooth, about 2 minutes, scraping down the bowl halfway through.

3 Add the agave, butter, vanilla, almond extract, and food coloring. Process until all of the ingredients are combined, about 1 minute.

4 Pour the batter into the prepared baking dish, and smooth the top with a spatula. Bake for 20 minutes, turning the dish halfway through the baking time. Turn down the temperature of the oven to 300°F and bake for another 5 to 8 minutes, until a toothpick inserted in the center comes out with a little bit of soft batter clinging to it. It should not come out clean, if it does it's overcooked.

5 Let the brownies cool completely in the baking dish on a wire rack. Then put them in the fridge for at least 3 hours. When they're cold, cut them into 12 squares and serve. Refrigerate any leftovers.

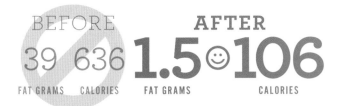

BEFORE
39 636
FAT GRAMS  CALORIES

AFTER
1.5 ☺ 106
FAT GRAMS  CALORIES

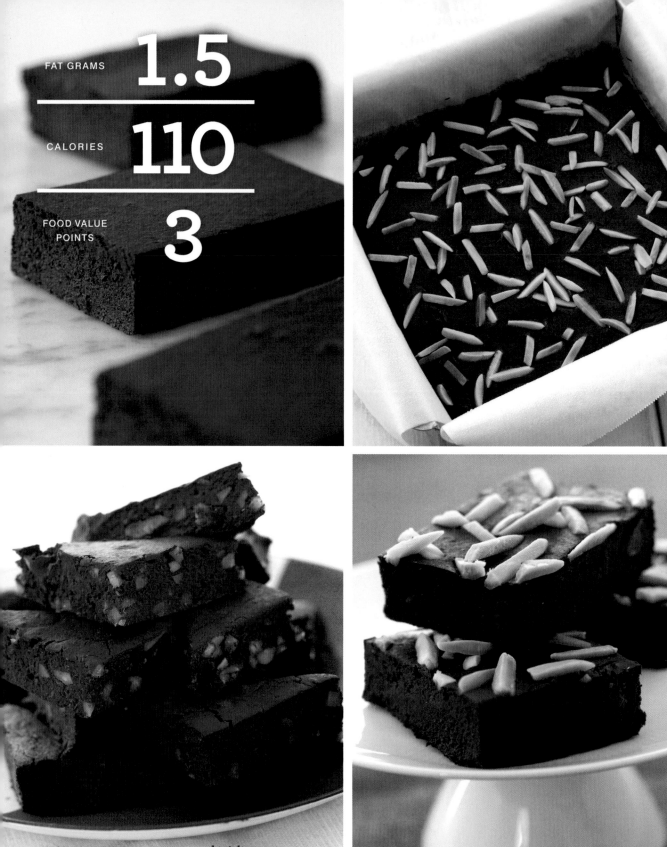

FAT GRAMS **1.5**

CALORIES **110**

FOOD VALUE POINTS **3**

NOW EAT THIS! DIET *now eat this! diet recipes*

# Fudgy Fruit and Nut Bars

MAKES 12 BARS
(110 calories each)

**CALLING ALL CHOCOHOLICS:** This richly flavored treat is a cross between a brownie and fudge. What could be better? And by the way, you read the recipe correctly. I use black beans in this recipe. Does that conjure up memories of last night's burrito? Don't worry. The beans add texture and moisture. And unlike a burrito, they're even better the next day. ✳TIP: **The brownies will seem underdone when you take them out of the oven, but they will firm up once they cool.** The result is a very moist and fudgelike brownie. For added texture, top the brownies with ½ cup of chopped walnuts or slivered almonds before putting them in the oven. Alternatively, you can stir ¼ cup nuts and ¼ cup raisins into the batter before baking. If you have kitchen scales, weigh the beans instead of using the weight on the can, which is not always accurate.

## INGREDIENTS

Butter-flavored nonstick cooking spray

15 ounces canned black beans, rinsed and drained

½ cup unsweetened cocoa powder

1 teaspoon espresso powder

¾ cup liquid egg substitute

3 tablespoons whole wheat pastry flour

¾ cup agave nectar

1 tablespoon unsalted butter, melted

1 teaspoon vanilla extract

PER SERVING
110 calories 1.5g fat ( 1g sat / 0.5g mono / 0g poly )
2.5mg cholesterol 103mg sodium 24g carbohydrate 3g fiber 4g protein

PER SERVING (with ½ cup walnuts)
142 calories 5g fat ( 1.2g sat / 0.9g mono / 2.4g poly )
2.5mg cholesterol 103mg sodium 26g carbohydrate 3g fiber 4.5g protein

PER SERVING (with ¼ cup raisins and ¼ cup walnuts)
136 calories 3g fat ( 1g sat / 0.7g mono / 1.2g poly )
2.5mg cholesterol 104mg sodium 27g carbohydrate 3g fiber 4g protein

PER SERVING (with almonds)
136 calories 4g fat ( 1g sat / 1.8g mono / 0.6g poly )
2.5mg cholesterol 103mg sodium 25g carbohydrate 4g fiber 5g protein

PER SERVING (with raisins and almonds)
133 calories 3g fat ( 1g sat / 1g mono / 0g poly )
2.5mg cholesterol 104mg sodium 27g carbohydrate 3g fiber 4g protein

PER SERVING (with raisins)
131 calories 1.5g fat ( 1g sat / 0.5g mono / 0g poly )
2.5mg cholesterol 104mg sodium 30g carbohydrate 3g fiber 4g protein

## METHOD

1 Preheat the oven to 350°F. Spray an 8 x 8 x 2-inch baking dish with cooking spray.

2 Combine the beans, cocoa powder, espresso powder, egg substitute, and flour in the bowl of a food processor. Process until the mixture is smooth, about 2 minutes, scraping down the bowl halfway through.

3 Add the agave, butter, and vanilla. Process until all of the ingredients are combined, about 1 minute.

4 Pour the batter into the prepared baking dish, and smooth the top with a spatula. Bake for 20 minutes, turning the dish halfway through the baking time. Turn down the temperature of the oven to 300°F and bake for another 5 to 8 minutes, until a toothpick inserted in the center comes out with a little bit of soft batter clinging to it. It should not come out clean, if it does it's overcooked.

5 Let the bars cool completely at room temperature in the baking dish on a wire rack. Then put them in the fridge for at least 3 hours. When they're cold, cut them into 12 squares and serve. Refrigerate any leftovers.

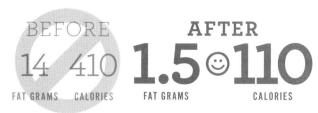

BEFORE
14  410
FAT GRAMS  CALORIES

AFTER
1.5 ☺ 110
FAT GRAMS  CALORIES

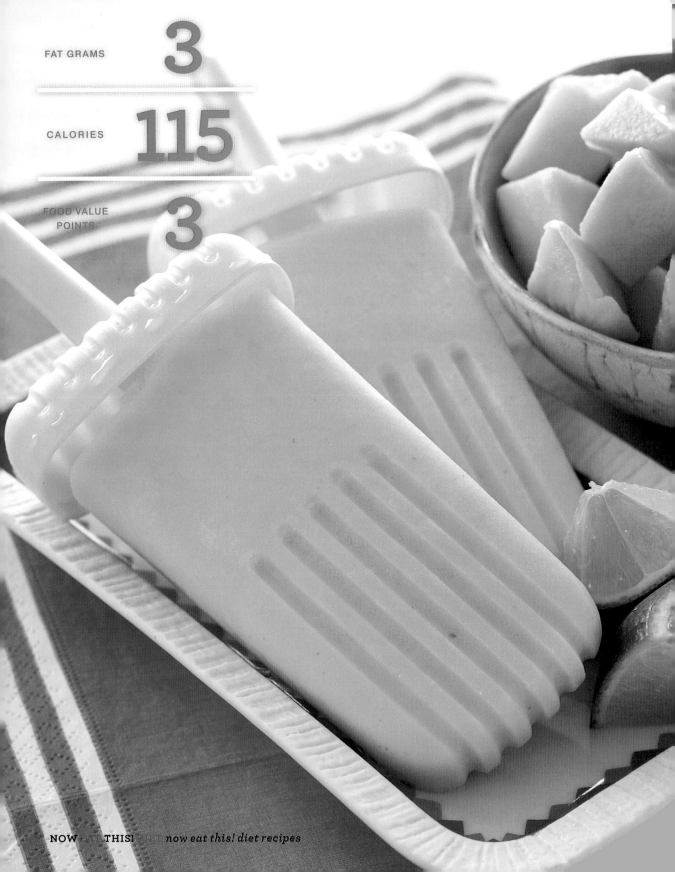

# Coconut Cream Mango Pops

MAKES 6 POPS
(115 calories each)

**LOOKING FOR EXCUSES** to take things out of the freezer and put them back in so you can stand in front of the open door to cool down on a hot summer day? There's a better way to put your freezer to work for you in hot weather. Use it to make these Coconut Cream Mango Pops. They taste like a piña colada on a stick. Plus, they're better for you than most of the treats in the grocery case (less expensive, too). And you can put them together in minutes, then keep a supply in the freezer for snacks and desserts. Now, shut the door! You're wasting energy! ✷ TIP: Don't skimp on the lime zest. Not only does it make the pop look nice, but it has a very intense flavor. When mangoes are out of season, frozen ones are your next best choice.

## INGREDIENTS

| | |
|---|---|
| 1 | cup fresh or frozen mango chunks |
| 8 | ounces light or reduced-fat coconut milk |
| 6 | ounces 2% Greek yogurt, such as Fage Total |
| ½ | teaspoon vanilla extract |
| ½ | teaspoon coconut extract |
| 5 | tablespoons agave nectar |
| 1 | teaspoon lime zest |

## METHOD

1 Combine all the ingredients in a blender, and puree until the mixture is smooth.

2 Pour the mixture into 6 freezer-pop molds. Freeze for at least 4 hours.

3 Dip the freezer pop molds in warm water for 3 seconds to unmold them.

PER SERVING
**115**calories **3g**fat ( **2g**sat / **0g**mono / **0g**poly )
**2mg**cholesterol **17mg**sodium
**21g**carbohydrate **1g**fiber **3g**protein

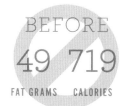

BEFORE
49 719
FAT GRAMS    CALORIES

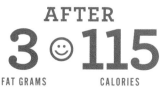

AFTER
3 ☺ 115
FAT GRAMS    CALORIES

*sweet nothings*

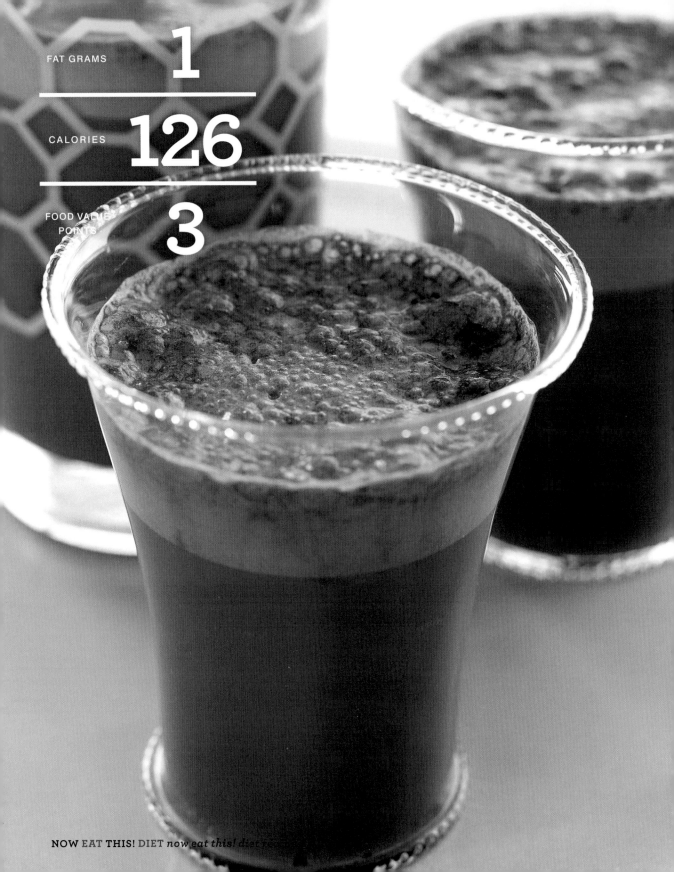

FAT GRAMS **1**

CALORIES **126**

FOOD VALUE POINTS **3**

# Chocolate Malted Milk Shake

SERVES 1

**NOTHING CONJURES** the small-town America of Norman Rockwell like a malted milk shake served in an old-fashioned soda glass and slurped through a straw. In 1922 a Walgreen's soda jerk in Chicago invented the malted milk shake by adding ice cream to an already-popular malted milk and chocolate syrup drink. My version is a chocoholic's paradise in a glass—but without the sugar. The secret ingredient here is malt powder, which makes an earthy, nutty contribution to the shake. Please note how many calories I've eradicated with this concoction, so drink up! *TIP: Instead of making this drink in a blender, I decided to shake it up and make it in a cocktail shaker. If you use a blender, don't blend it with ice. Instead, pour the mixture over ice. Look for malted milk powder that does not have sugar listed as the first ingredient.

## INGREDIENTS

½   cup ice cubes

10   ounces skim milk

1   tablespoon malted milk powder, such as Carnation

¼   cup sugar-free chocolate syrup, such as Fox's U-bet

## METHOD

1 In a large cocktail shaker, add the ice, milk, malt powder, and chocolate syrup. Shake until foamy. Strain into a tall glass. Serve immediately.

PER SERVING
**126**calories **1g**fat ( **0.5g**sat / **0g**mono / **0g**poly )
**7mg**cholesterol **222mg**sodium
**19g**carbohydrate **0g**fiber **10g**protein

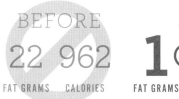

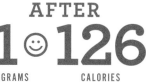

*sweet nothings*

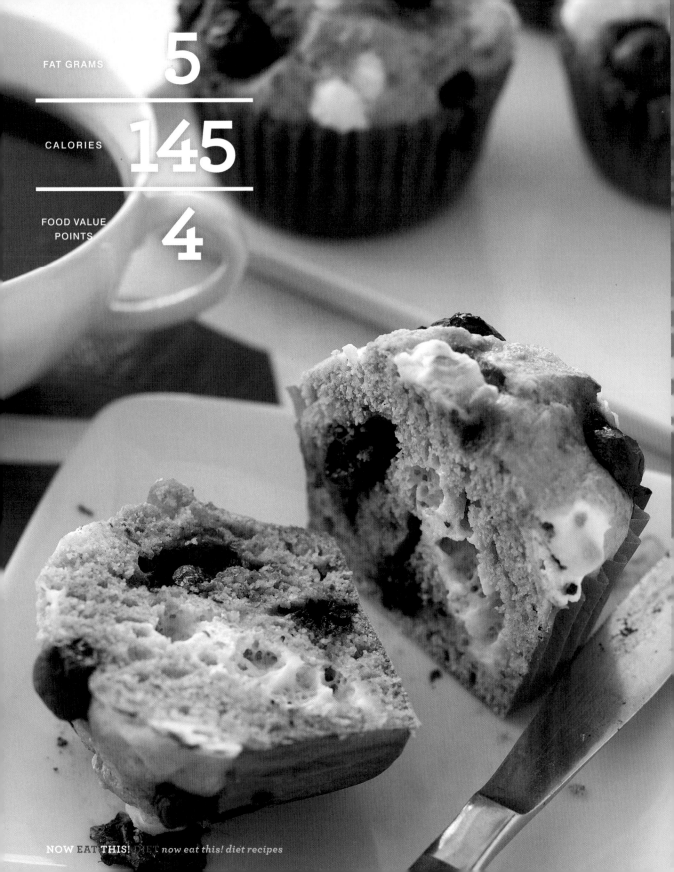

FAT GRAMS **5**

CALORIES **145**

FOOD VALUE POINTS **4**

# Blueberry Cream Muffins

MAKES 12 MUFFINS
(145 calories each)

**EAT THESE MUFFINS** and you won't develop a "muffin top." I'm referring to the flab that gets squeezed out of your waistband when you wear low-cut jeans and quite often has you unbuttoning your pants at restaurants. ✱TIP: If you freeze the cream cheese for 10 minutes, it'll be easier to cut into small pieces.

## INGREDIENTS

Butter-flavored nonstick cooking spray

2 cups plus 2 tablespoons whole wheat pastry flour

1 teaspoon baking powder

½ teaspoon baking soda

4 packets (about 4 grams) powdered stevia, such as SweetLeaf

½ teaspoon salt

½ cup skim milk

½ cup unsweetened applesauce

¼ cup agave nectar

2 tablespoons canola oil

2 teaspoons vanilla extract

½ cup liquid egg substitute

4 ounces reduced-fat cream cheese, cut into small chunks

1 cup frozen blueberries

## METHOD

1 Preheat the oven to 350°F. Line a 12-cup muffin tin with paper baking cups, and lightly coat the cups with cooking spray.

2 In a large mixing bowl, add the flour, baking powder, baking soda, stevia, and salt. Whisk together.

3 In a medium bowl, add the milk, applesauce, agave, oil, vanilla, and egg substitute. Stir together until well incorporated. Add the liquids to the dry ingredients and stir till well combined. Fold in the cream cheese and blueberries.

4 Spoon the mixture into the prepared muffin tin. Bake until a toothpick inserted into the center of the muffins comes out clean, about 18 to 20 minutes.

PER SERVING
**145**calories **5g**fat ( **1g**sat / **1.5g**mono / **0.7g**poly )
**7mg**cholesterol **244mg**sodium
**22g**carbohydrate **2g**fiber **4g**protein

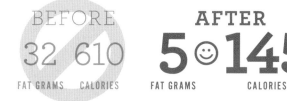

BEFORE
32 610
FAT GRAMS   CALORIES

AFTER
5 ☺ 145
FAT GRAMS   CALORIES

*sweet nothings*

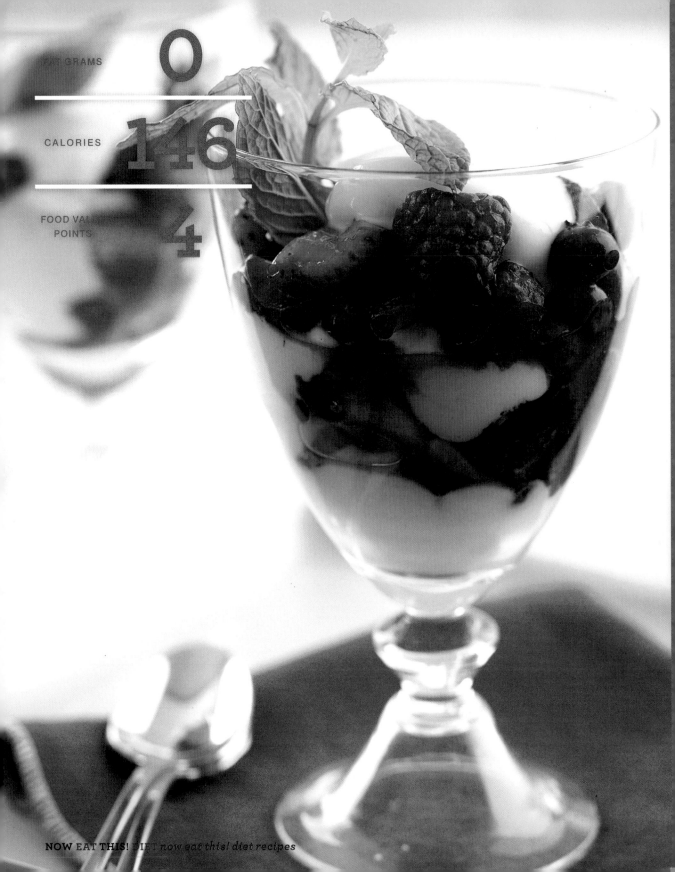

FAT GRAMS

0

CALORIES

146

FOOD VALUE POINTS

4

# Any Berry Parfait

**THIS RECIPE IS KID-FRIENDLY,** diet-friendly, waistline-friendly, convenience-friendly, budget-friendly . . . so friendly that you won't need Facebook anymore. You can use any kind of cut-up fruit to make this parfait. Just make sure it's fresh. **✱ TIP:** To *macerate* means to soak the food in a liquid for a period of time so that the two elements flavor each other. In *marination,* only the marinade flavors the food.

## INGREDIENTS

⅔   cup fresh blueberries

1⅓   cups fresh strawberries, hulled and cut into quarters

4   ounces fresh raspberries

3   packets (3 grams) powdered stevia, such as SweetLeaf

2   tablespoons chopped fresh mint

½   cup pomegranate juice

2   cups nonfat Greek yogurt, such as 0% Fage Total

1   teaspoon vanilla extract

2   tablespoons agave nectar

## METHOD

1 In a medium bowl, toss the fruit with the stevia, mint, and pomegranate juice. Stir till combined. Set aside and allow to macerate for 30 minutes.

2 In a medium bowl, add the yogurt, vanilla, and agave nectar. Stir until thoroughly combined.

3 Spoon ¼ cup of the yogurt mixture into each of 4 parfait glasses. Add a layer of the fruit and another ¼ cup of the yogurt. Top with the remaining fruit and serve.

PER SERVING
**146**calories **0g**fat ( **0g**sat / **0g**mono / **0g**poly )
**0mg**cholesterol **46mg**sodium
**26g**carbohydrate **3g**fiber **11g**protein

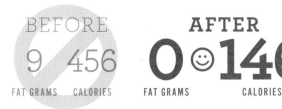

BEFORE
9   456
FAT GRAMS   CALORIES

AFTER
0 ☺ 146
FAT GRAMS   CALORIES

# Chocolate Crème Brûlée

**THIS RECIPE** is not a diet-buster. I know you're thinking that crème brûlée is the biggest no-no in the dessert universe, and normally you'd be correct. But since I replaced the cream with low-fat milk and Greek yogurt, you're in luck. Both create the particularly velvety custard that is so characteristic of crème brûlée. Vanilla beans are relatively hard to find, but the results are well worth the effort. If you can't find them, just use vanilla extract. Be careful to watch the mixture while it's on the stovetop to prevent it from burning.

So enjoy—and pass some more crème brûlée.

## INGREDIENTS

1¼    teaspoons unflavored powdered gelatin

1⅔    cups 2% milk

2    tablespoons plus 1 teaspoon cornstarch

2    tablespoons unsweetened cocoa powder

¼    cup agave nectar

¼    vanilla bean, seeds scraped out and reserved or ½ teaspoon vanilla extract

  Large pinch of salt

2    tablespoons nonfat Greek yogurt, such as 0% Fage Total

2    tablespoons turbinado sugar, such as Sugar in the Raw

### PER SERVING
**158** calories **2g** fat ( **1g** sat / **1g** mono / **0g** poly )
**8mg** cholesterol **174mg** sodium
**30g** carbohydrate **1g** fiber **6g** protein

## METHOD

1  Place the gelatin into a medium bowl. Pour 2 tablespoons of the milk over the gelatin, and set it aside to soften for at least 3 minutes.

2  In a small saucepan, whisk the remaining milk into the cornstarch. Whisk in the cocoa powder, agave, vanilla bean and seeds, and salt. Bring the mixture to a boil over high heat, whisking constantly. When it boils, reduce the heat to low and continue to cook until it has thickened, about 30 seconds. Remove and discard the vanilla bean. Whisk about ⅓ cup of the thickened milk mixture into the softened gelatin to melt it. Then whisk in the remaining milk mixture. Whisk the yogurt into the gelatin-milk mixture.

3  Divide the mixture among 4 (4-ounce) ramekins. Chill, covered, in the refrigerator until completely set and cold, about 2 hours.

4  Pour the sugar into one of the ramekins. Roll it around so that the top is covered with sugar; then pour the leftover sugar into another ramekin. Continue the procedure for all of the ramekins. Discard the remaining sugar. Using a kitchen blowtorch, burn the sugar until it is a deeply caramelized golden brown. Serve immediately.

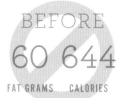

BEFORE
**60** FAT GRAMS **644** CALORIES

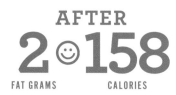

**AFTER**
**2** FAT GRAMS ☺ **158** CALORIES

**✱ CALORIE SAVER**
Omit the the turbinado sugar and save **12** calories per serving.

FAT GRAMS

**2**

CALORIES

**158**

FOOD VALUE
POINTS

**4**

*sweet nothings*

# Silken Chocolate Mousse

**I LIKE COOKING WITH TOFU.** I had no idea. I mean, I've always supported the concept of tofu—healthy, natural, vegetarian—but had never actually worked with the stuff. I didn't eat much of it either. At restaurants, I'd usually say, "Wow, the tofu dish sounds wonderful!" And then order the steak. Just like I'd always heard, tofu doesn't have much of a taste on its own. It basically takes on the flavors of whatever it's combined with. So I got to thinking: Why not pair it with chocolate? In this case, the results were great. The silken tofu here creates a creamy mouthful that will make you forget about the egg yolks and cream in standard mousse recipes. *TIP: Espresso powder brings out the chocolate flavor. Look for it in the coffee section at your supermarket.

## INGREDIENTS

12    ounces silken tofu, such as Nasoya

2     ounces bittersweet (60%) chocolate plus additional for garnish

2     tablespoons unsweetened cocoa powder

2     tablespoons agave nectar

½     teaspoon instant espresso powder

1     teaspoon vanilla extract

1     tablespoon sugar-free chocolate syrup, such as Fox's U-bet

PER SERVING
**161** calories **7g** fat ( **4g** sat / **1g** mono / **0.5g** poly )
**0mg** cholesterol **22mg** sodium
**21g** carbohydrate **1g** fiber **4g** protein

## METHOD

1  Cut the tofu into 1-inch pieces and place in a strainer so that the liquid drains out. Let sit for 10 minutes.

2  With a serrated knife, chop 2 ounces of the chocolate into small chunks. Place the chocolate in a microwave-safe bowl, and microwave on high for 30 seconds. Stir the chocolate. If necessary, continue microwaving in 15-second increments until the chocolate has melted and is smooth.

3  In the bowl of a food processor, add the melted chocolate, tofu, cocoa powder, agave, espresso powder, vanilla, and chocolate syrup. Blend until smooth, stopping once to scrape down the sides.

4  Transfer the mixture into 4 individual cups, and refrigerate. To serve, shave a small amount of chocolate on top of the cups with a vegetable peeler.

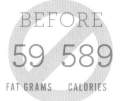

BEFORE
59      589
FAT GRAMS    CALORIES

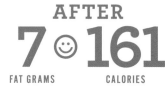

AFTER
7 ☺ 161
FAT GRAMS    CALORIES

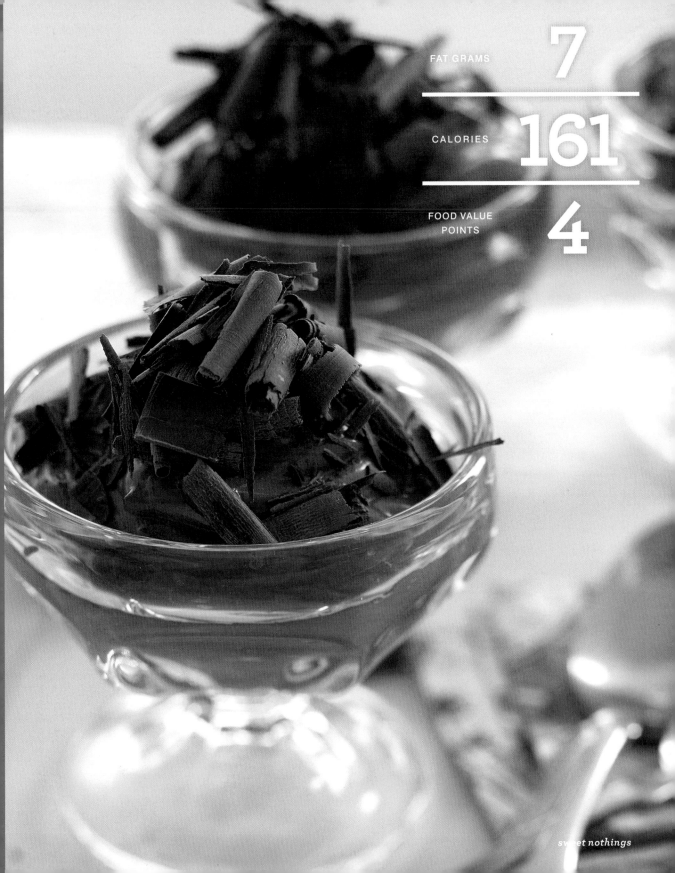

FAT GRAMS
**7**

CALORIES
**161**

FOOD VALUE
POINTS
**4**

*sweet nothings*

# Banana Walnut Muffins

**I REALLY,** really wanted muffins to be an option for you in this diet, but they almost beat me. The algorithm for sweet, moist, flavorful muffins usually means high calories and high fat. This same muffin in a doughnut shop will run you more than 600 belly-fattening calories. I worked on these tirelessly, and I think my revised lower-calorie, lower-fat, and lower-cholesterol recipe is just as tasty and moist as its commercial counterpart. Save leftover bananas to make this treat. Just freeze the bananas and thaw them out when you need them.

## INGREDIENTS

Nonstick cooking spray

2 cups plus 2 tablespoons whole wheat pastry flour

1 teaspoon baking powder

½ teaspoon baking soda

½ teaspoon ground cinnamon

4 packets (4 grams) powdered stevia, such as SweetLeaf

½ teaspoon salt

¾ cup skim milk

¼ cup agave nectar

2 medium ripe bananas, mashed

¼ cup canola oil

1 teaspoon vanilla extract

1 teaspoon banana extract

½ cup liquid egg substitute

12 walnut halves

## METHOD

1 Preheat the oven to 350°F. Line a 12-cup muffin tin with paper baking cups. Lightly spray the cups with cooking spray.

2 In a large mixing bowl, add the flour, baking powder, baking soda, cinnamon, stevia, and salt. Whisk together until well combined. Set aside.

3 In a medium bowl, add the milk, agave, banana, oil, vanilla, banana extract, and egg substitute. Stir together until well incorporated. Fold the wet ingredients into the dry ingredients and stir till well combined.

4 Spoon the mixture into the prepared muffin tin. Top each muffin with a walnut half. Bake until a toothpick inserted into the center of the muffins comes out clean, about 15 to 18 minutes.

PER SERVING
**163** calories **6g** fat ( **0.5g** sat / **3g** mono / **2.3g** poly )
**0mg** cholesterol **217mg** sodium
**24g** carbohydrate **2g** fiber **4g** protein

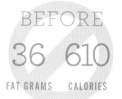

BEFORE
36 610
FAT GRAMS    CALORIES

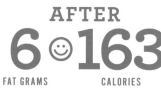

AFTER
6 ☺ 163
FAT GRAMS    CALORIES

**＊ CALORIE SAVER**
Omit the walnuts and save **13** calories per serving.

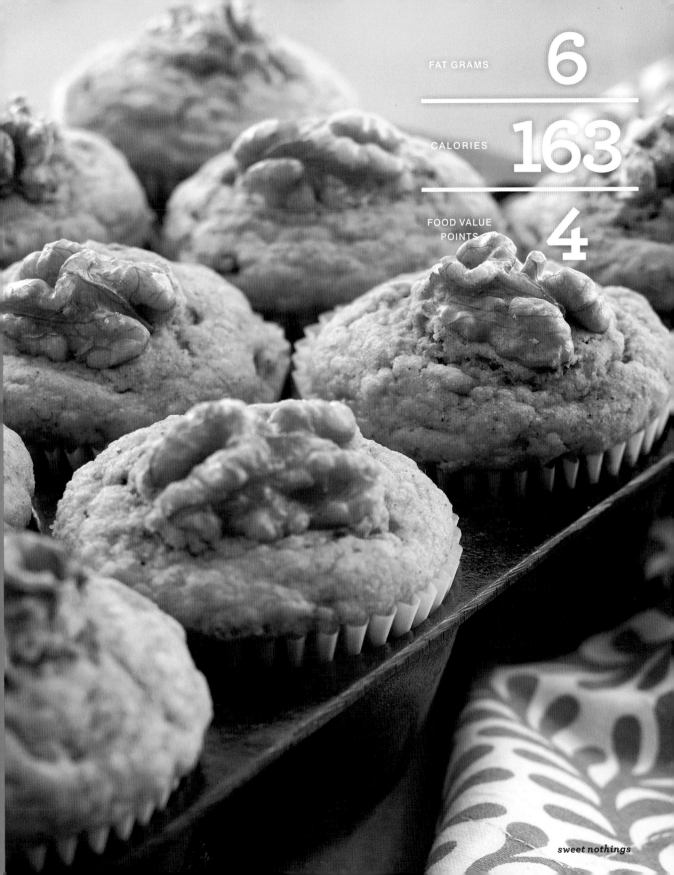

FAT GRAMS 6

CALORIES 163

FOOD VALUE POINTS 4

*sweet nothings*

# Apple Cinnamon Cranberry Cobbler

SERVES 8

**THE COBBLER** probably originated with the early settlers of America, who were very good at improvising. They took seasonal fruits and berries, whatever fresh ingredients were readily at hand, and mixed them up with flour and sugar. With this recipe, I've improvised, too—by cutting the sugar and bad carbs considerably. So be a cobbler gobbler and jump mouthfirst into this piping-hot bowl of cobbler. ✳TIP: Feel free to experiment with other apples, such as Granny Smith, Rome Beauty, Cortland, Pippin, and Winesap.

## INGREDIENTS

|   | |
|---|---|
| | Nonstick cooking spray |
| 5 | Golden Delicious apples, peeled, cored, and cut into large slices |
| 1 | tablespoon lemon juice |
| 1 | tablespoon cornstarch |
| ½ | teaspoon ground ginger |
| ½ | teaspoon cinnamon |
| ¼ | cup dried cranberries |
| ¼ | cup plus 2 tablespoons agave nectar |
| ¾ | cup Bisquick Heart Smart baking mix |
| ¼ | cup skim milk |
| 2 | tablespoons turbinado sugar, such as Sugar in the Raw |

## METHOD

1 Preheat the oven to 425°F. Spray 8 (3½ x 2-inch, four-ounce) ramekins with cooking spray, and set aside.

2 In a medium bowl mix together the apples, lemon juice, cornstarch, ¼ teaspoon ginger, ¼ teaspoon cinnamon, cranberries, and ¼ cup agave. Pour the fruit into the prepared ramekins.

3 In a medium bowl, combine the remaining 2 tablespoons agave nectar, baking mix, remaining ginger and cinnamon, and milk. Stir until the mixture is well mixed and has the consistency of biscuit dough, adding more milk if necessary. Drop spoonfuls of the dough evenly over the fruit. Sprinkle sugar over the dough.

4 Bake the individual cobblers until the fruit is tender and the biscuit topping is golden brown, about 20 minutes. Let them rest for 5 minutes before serving.

PER SERVING
**165**calories **1g**fat ( **0g**sat / **0.5g**mono / **0g**poly )
**0mg**cholesterol **126mg**sodium
**40g**carbohydrate **2g**fiber **1g**protein

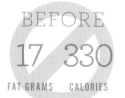

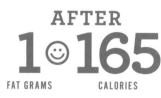

**✳ CALORIE SAVER**

Omit the cranberries and turbinado sugar and save **23**calories per serving.

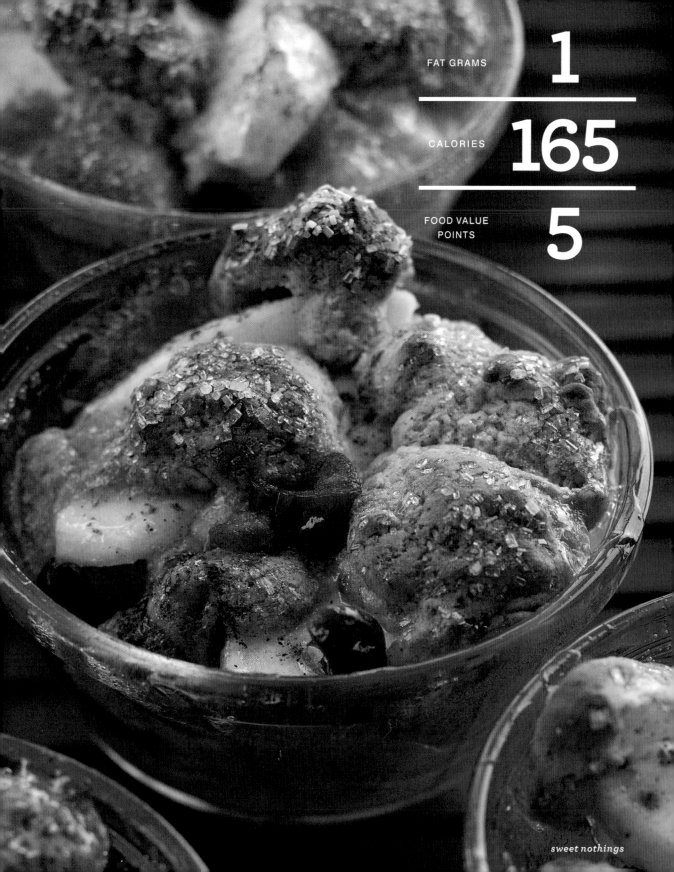

FAT GRAMS

1

CALORIES

165

FOOD VALUE
POINTS

5

*sweet nothings*

# Dark Chocolate–Dipped Figs

SERVES 4
(3 figs per serving)

**I DON'T WANT TO** ruin anyone's Valentine's Day, but honestly, what is it about? Sugar and spice and chocolate hearts, of course. Then comes Easter—is anyone thinking chocolate bunnies here? And what would Mother's Day be without a big box of chocolates? But sometimes the last thing a dieter wants on these holidays is fattening chocolate, so I have a suggestion: Make my chocolate-dipped figs for your loved one. There is just something special about chocolate that induces a feeling of pleasure for a lot of people. And figs are an added treat. Fresh figs are available during late summer and early fall. You can easily substitute dried figs for fresh ones in this recipe. Figs are high in fiber, which is important for digestive health, and also contain other important nutrients such calcium, potassium, and iron. Another big plus is that they contain disease-fighting antioxidants.

## INGREDIENTS

2   ounces high-quality bittersweet 60%–70% chocolate, chopped in small pieces

12   medium fresh figs

PER SERVING
**182**calories **4.5g**fat ( **3.6g**sat / **0g**mono / **0g**poly )
**0mg**cholesterol **17mg**sodium
**38g**carbohydrate **4g**fiber **1g**protein

## METHOD

1   Place the chocolate in a microwave-safe bowl, and microwave on high for 15 seconds. If the chocolate is not melted, stir and microwave again for 10 seconds, watching closely so it does not burn. Stir until chocolate is smooth and melted.

2   Holding the stem of the figs, dip the figs into the chocolate so that the bottom third of the figs is covered in chocolate. (You may have to tilt the bowl.)

3   Place the figs on waxed paper until the chocolate sets.

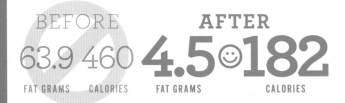

BEFORE
63.9 460
FAT GRAMS   CALORIES

AFTER
4.5 ☺ 182
FAT GRAMS   CALORIES

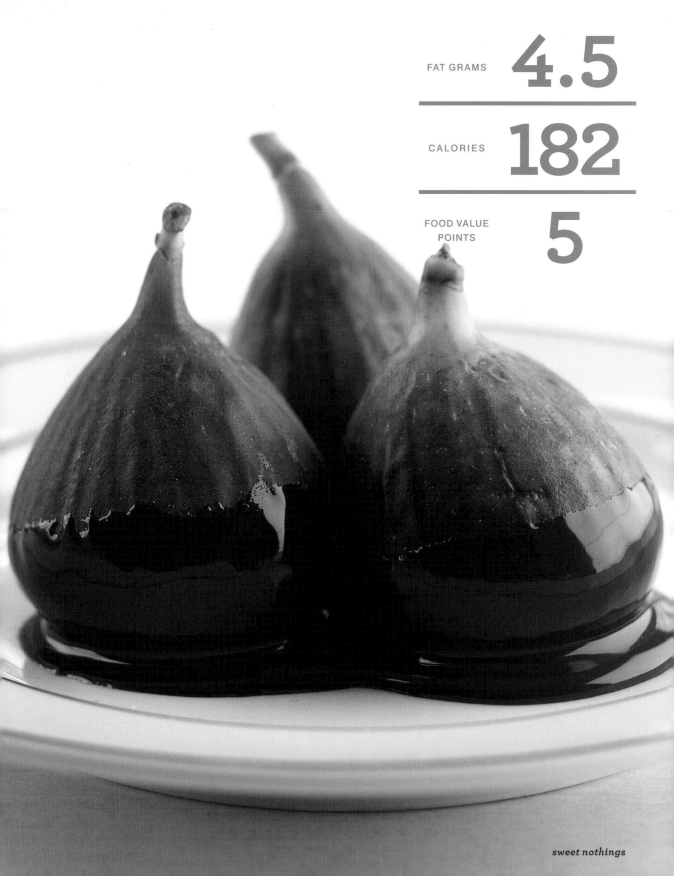

FAT GRAMS **4.5**

CALORIES **182**

FOOD VALUE
POINTS **5**

*sweet nothings*

# Chocolate Fondue

**YES, I'M A 'DUER.** Especially when it comes to chocolate fondue. What could be more romantic than taking turns dipping fresh strawberries and pieces of bananas into a creamy pool of dark chocolate? The Swiss even make a game of it by saying that anyone who drops their morsel of food into the pot has to kiss someone at the table. How fun is that?

## INGREDIENTS

| | |
|---|---|
| 2 | tablespoons unsweetened cocoa powder |
| 1 | cup skim milk |
| 2 | tablespoons agave nectar |
| ½ | teaspoon vanilla extract |
| 2 | teaspoons cornstarch |
| 1½ | ounces bittersweet (60%) chocolate |
| 1 | pint fresh strawberries, hulled and halved |
| 2 | medium bananas, sliced into bite-size pieces |

## METHOD

1 In a small saucepan over medium heat, combine the cocoa powder, ½ cup milk, agave, and vanilla. Continually whisk the mixture until the cocoa powder is dissolved. In a small bowl, add the cornstarch and the remaining milk. Stir together until the cornstarch is dissolved, and then add to the saucepan. Bring the mixture to a boil, continually whisking. Turn down the heat, and then add the chocolate. Whisk until combined. Turn off the heat.

2 Transfer the chocolate mixture to a fondue pot, and serve with strawberries and bananas.

PER SERVING
**192**calories **4g**fat ( **3g**sat / **0g**mono / **0g**poly )
**1mg**cholesterol **39mg**sodium
**39g**carbohydrate **3g**fiber **4g**protein

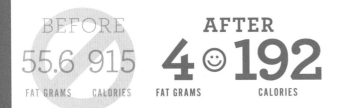

BEFORE
55.6 915
FAT GRAMS    CALORIES

AFTER
4 ☺ 192
FAT GRAMS    CALORIES

FAT GRAMS

4

CALORIES

192

FOOD VALUE
POINTS

5

*sweet nothings*

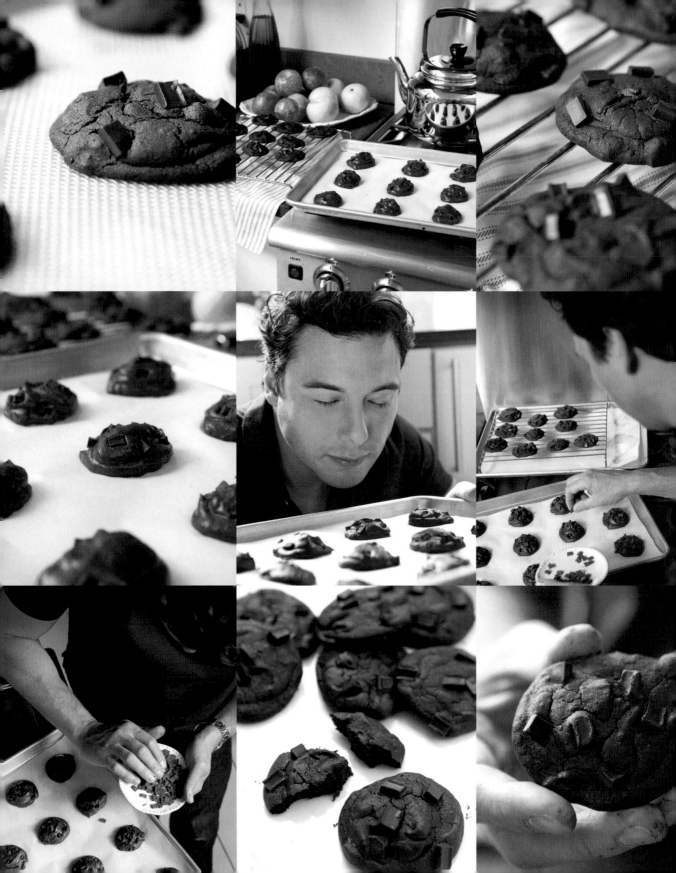

# ONLINE SOURCES FOR SELECT INGREDIENTS

**AGAVE NECTAR**
www.amazon.com (search for agave nectar)

**APPLEGATE FARMS SWEET ITALIAN CHICKEN AND TURKEY SAUSAGE (LINKS)**
store.applegatefarms.com
Netgrocer.com

**BETTER'N PEANUT BUTTER REDUCED-FAT PEANUT BUTTER**
www.amazon.com
(search for Better'n Peanut Butter)
mybrands.com (search for Better'n Peanut Butter)

**BIONATURAE ORGANIC WHOLE WHEAT RIGATONI PASTA**
Netgrocer.com
www.amazon.com (search for Bionaturae Organic Whole Wheat Rigatoni Pasta)

**BISQUICK HEART SMART BAKING MIX**
Netgrocer.com

**BORDEN'S 2% MILK REDUCED-FAT SHARP SINGLES**
Netgrocer.com

**BREAKSTONE'S REDUCED-FAT SOUR CREAM**
Netgrocer.com

**CABOT REDUCED-FAT CHEDDAR CHEESE (50% AND 75%)**
www.shopcabot.com
Netgrocer.com

**CENTO SAUTÉED SWEET PEPPERS WITH ONIONS**
www.fineproductsinternational.com

**COTIJA CHEESE**
Netgrocer.com (Queso Del Valle brand)
www.amazon.com (search for cotija cheese)

**DELALLO WHOLE WHEAT NO-BAKE LASAGNA NOODLES**
www.amazon.com
(search for DeLallo Organic Whole Wheat Lasagna)

**DESIGNER WHEY FRENCH VANILLA WHEY PROTEIN POWDER**
www.theconsumerlink.com
(search for Designer Whey)

**FAGE TOTAL YOGURT**
www.amazon.com (search for Fage Total)

**FOX'S U-BET SUGAR-FREE CHOCOLATE SYRUP**
www.webstaurantstore.com (search for Fox's U-bet Sugar-Free Chocolate Syrup)

**GUILTLESS GOURMET BAKED BLUE CORN CHIPS**
guiltlessgourmet.elsstore.com
Netgrocer.com
www.amazon.com (search for Guiltless Gourmet Baked Blue Corn Chips)

**HEINZ REDUCED-SUGAR KETCHUP**
www.amazon.com
(search for Heinz Reduced-Sugar Ketchup)

**HOUSE FOODS TOFU SHIRATAKI NOODLES**
www.amazon.com
(search for House Foods Tofu Shirataki Noodles)
www.asianfoodgrocer.com

**HUY FONG GARLIC-CHILI SAUCE**
www.amazon.com
(search for Huy Fong Garlic-Chili Sauce)

**IAN'S ALL-NATURAL WHOLE WHEAT PANKO**
www.vitacost.com (search for Ians Natural Foods Panko Breadcrumbs Whole Wheat Style)

**KAREE CURRY PASTE (YELLOW)**
www.amazon.com
(search for Karee Curry Paste – yellow)

**MATCHA GREEN TEA POWDER**
www.amazon.com
(search for matcha green tea powder)
www.teavana.com

**MT. OLIVE NO-SUGAR-ADDED SWEET RELISH**
Netgrocer.com

**NATURAL RED FOOD COLORING**
www.amazon.com (search for Natural Food Colorings, India Tree Natural Decorating Colors)

**NO-SUGAR-ADDED APPLE BUTTER**
Netgrocer.com (Manischewitz brand)
www.amazon.com (Search for Walden Farms, Jake and Amos, or Amish Made.)

**PAPA SAL'S WHOLE WHEAT PIZZA DOUGH**
Netgrocer.com
shop.mywebgrocer.com

**PUFFED KAMUT (ARROWHEAD MILLS)**
arrowheadmills.elsstore.com
www.amazon.com
(search for Arrowhead Mills Puffed Kamut)

**PUFFED MILLET (ARROWHEAD MILLS)**
arrowheadmills.elsstore.com
www.amazon.com
(search for Arrowhead Mills Puffed Millet)
Netgrocer.com

**RUBSCHLAGER EUROPEAN WHOLE-GRAIN BREAD**
www.amazon.com (search for Rubschlager EuropeanWhole-Grain Bread)

**STEEL'S GOURMET AGAVE NO-SUGAR-ADDED CRANBERRY SAUCE**
www.steelsgourmet.com

**SUGAR IN THE RAW**
www.sugarintheraw.com
Netgrocer.com
www.amazon.com (search for Sugar in the Raw)

**SWEETLEAF STEVIA**
Netgrocer.com
www.amazon.com (search for SweetLeaf Stevia)

**TREASURE CAVE REDUCED-FAT BLUE CHEESE**
Netgrocer.com

**VICTORIA ALL NATURAL MARINARA SAUCE**
www.newyorkflavors.com
www.amazon.com
(search for Victoria All Natural Marinara Sauce)

**WALDEN FARMS CALORIE-FREE PANCAKE SYRUP**
www.waldenfarms.com
www.amazon.com (Search for Walden Farms Calorie-Free Pancake Syrup)

**WALDEN FARMS SUGAR-FREE CHOCOLATE SYRUP**
www.waldenfarms.com
Netgrocer.com
www.amazon.com (Search for Walden Farms Sugar Free Chocolate Syrup)

**WELLSHIRE FARMS REDUCED-FAT CHORIZO SAUSAGE**
www.wellshirefarms.com
(Search for chorizo; you have to buy 18 pounds.)

**WHEAT ORZO**
www.amazon.com (search for wheat orzo)
www.delallo.com

**WHOLE WHEAT BAKED PITA CHIPS**
www.amazon.com
(search for Athenos Whole Wheat Baked Pita Chips)

**WHOLE WHEAT PASTRY FLOUR**
www.amazon.com
(search for whole wheat pastry flour)

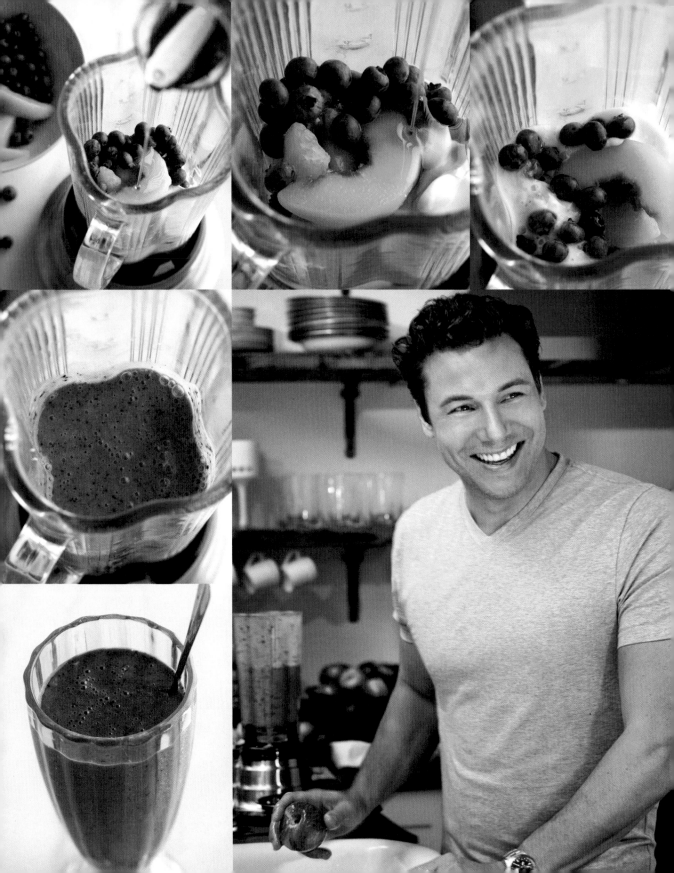

# INDEX

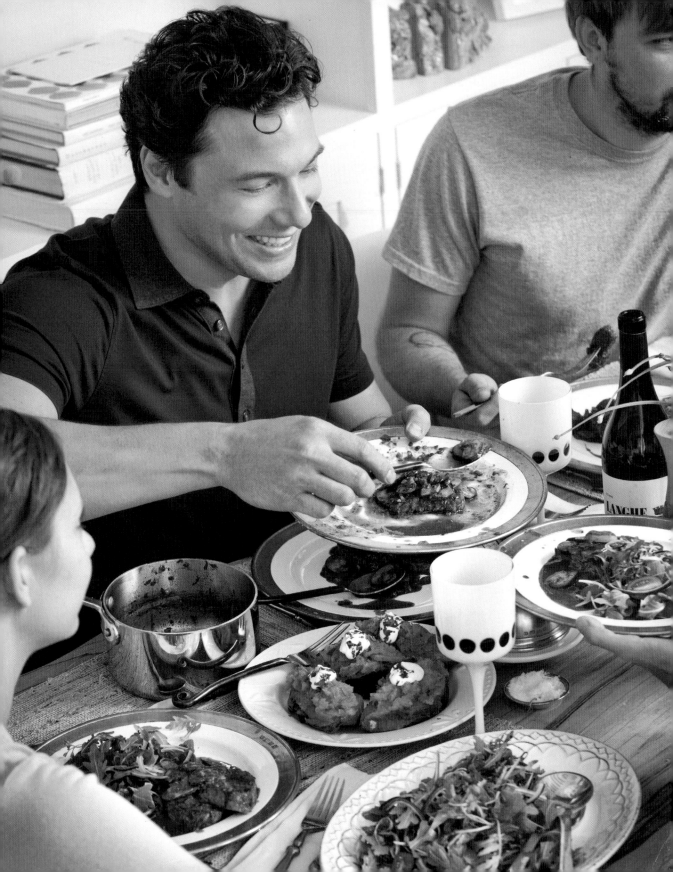

# About the Author

Celebrated chef Rocco DiSpirito is the author of six highly acclaimed cook books, including the #1 *New York Times* bestseller *Now Eat This!*, in which he transformed America's favorite comfort foods into low-fat, low-calorie dishes, that are still packed with flavor.

Rocco first gained widespread acclaim after opening his multi-starred New York City restaurant Union Pacific. He was the first chef to grace the cover of *Gourmet* magazine as "America's Most Exciting Young Chef," and was voted America's Best New Chef, by *Food & Wine* magazine. In her three-star review, the venerable *New York Times* restaurant critic Ruth Reichl said: "I have yet to taste anything on Mr. DiSpirito's menu that is not wonderful. I was moaning as I ate." Additionally, Rocco's culinary skills have earned him several significant awards, including the cherished James Beard Award for his first cookbook, *Flavor*.

Rocco is a native New Yorker who learned his early culinary skills in his Italian mother's kitchen and is a cum laude graduate of both the prestigious Culinary Institute of America, and Boston University. Over the last twenty-five years, working in the United States and abroad, Rocco developed his unique sense of flavor, which is distinguished by his unmatched combinations of ingredients that leave those who try his creations "breathless," according to the Zagat restaurant guide.

In addition to his classical chef training, Rocco starred in the Food Network series *Melting Pot*, the NBC hit reality series *The Restaurant*, and the A&E series *Rocco Gets Real*. He is a regular on the Food Network's *The Best Thing I Ever Ate*, and his latest TV show, *Rocco's Dinner Party*, debuts in spring 2011 on Bravo. He is a frequent guest on the *Rachael Ray* show, *Good Morning America*, and *The Dr. Oz Show*. Rocco has also appeared on *The Tonight Show with Jay Leno*, *The Oprah Winfrey Show*, *Late Night with David Letterman*, *Live! with Regis and Kelly*, *The View*, the *Today* show, *The Ellen DeGeneres Show*, *Jimmy Kimmel Live!*, and *Chelsea Lately*; competed on ABC's *Dancing with the Stars*; and was the guest chef on NBC's *The Biggest Loser* for multiple seasons.

Rocco has been featured in hundreds of national magazine articles and is a current member of the *Fitness* magazine advisory board as well as a regular contributor to *Runner's World*. In 2003 he was named the "Sexiest Chef Alive" by *People* magazine.

An avid triathlete and an advocate of healthy living, Rocco, is a spokesperson for Feeding America, Food Bank for New York City, and Dr. Oz's Healthcorps. Rocco believes healthy and delicious are no longer mutually exclusive. You can contact Rocco at www.roccodispirito.com and twitter.com/roccodispirito.